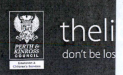

THE PRIMAL BLUE- PRINT

MARK SISSON

1 3 5 7 9 10 8 6 4 2

This edition published in 2012 by Vermilion, an imprint of Ebury Publishing
A Random House Group company

First published in USA by Primal Nutrition in 2009

The Random House Group Limited Reg. No. 954009

Addresses for companies within the Random House Group can be found at
www.randomhouse.co.uk

The Random House Group Limited supports The Forest Stewardship Council
(FSC®), the leading international forest certification organisation. Our books
carrying the FSC label are printed on FSC® certified paper. FSC is the only forest
certification scheme endorsed by the leading environmental organisations,
including Greenpeace. Our paper procurement policy can be found at
www.randomhouse.co.uk/environment

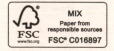

MIX
Paper from
responsible sources
FSC® C016897

Printed and bound by CPI Group (UK) Ltd, Croydon, CR0 4YY

ISBN 9780091947835

To buy books by your favourite authors and register for offers visit www.
randomhouse.co.uk

ACKNOWLEDGEMENTS

My editor, Brad Kearns, made a tremendous contribution in the preparation of this manuscript. His extensive writing experience and insights on health and fitness were invaluable to the creation of the final product.

Aaron Fox, my ace general manager and webmaster at MarksDailyApple.com, was a brilliant strategist, researcher and project manager for *The Primal Blueprint*. MarksDailyApple.com staffers, Bradford Hodgson and Reagan Smith, offered excellent insights to help improve the text and provided extensive research and fact-checking support. Catherine Fisse's unique and often devil's-advocate viewpoint helped me present a clear and focused message. The outstanding copy-editing skills of Laura R. Gabler helped get this book to the finish line triumphantly. Devyn Sisson made Dad look good with her cover photography. Don Derenthal designed the Grok and Korg figures. The provocative insights and opinions of numerous authors and bloggers have inspired me; among them are Loren Cordain (author of *The Paleo Diet*), Jared Diamond (author of *Guns, Germs and Steel*), Dr Michael and Dr Mary Dan Eades (authors of *Protein Power*), Gary Taubes (author of *Good Calories, Bad Calories*), and bloggers Art DeVany at arthurdevany.com, Peter at *Hyperlipid,* and Stephan at *Whole Health Source.*

For an expanded list of my favourite books and websites, and a comprehensive index of books, newspaper and magazine articles, research papers, and Internet links that were used in the research and preparation of this text, please visit MarksDailyApple.com.

Olympic triathlon Gold and Silver Medallist Simon Whitfield has shown that the power of living primally can indeed apply to high-level endurance athletics. Dr Walter Kearns' consultations helped me present the medical and scientific material in an organised, factually accurate, and easy to understand manner. My wife Carrie and children Devyn and Kyle keep me grounded and balanced when my primal obsessions threaten to take over my days and nights! I owe you guys a vacation – and this time I'm coming along too!

CONTENTS

WELCOME FROM MARK

> '*The doctor of the future will give no medicine, but instead will interest his patients in the care of the human frame, in diet, and in the cause and prevention of disease.*'
> THOMAS EDISON

When I began the journey to produce this book nearly five years ago, it felt like David versus Goliath redux. Yes, I had readers of my MarksDailyApple.com blog egging me on to produce a Primal manifesto attacking conventional wisdom (a recurring term throughout the book, akin to a yellow highway hazard sign), and had a few fitness books under my belt from years past, but this endeavour was doing battle against the mighty opponent of the status quo, conventional wisdom … not to mention the staid publishing industry. More than a few doors were shut in my face and phones politely hung up as I breathlessly wrapped up my pitch. 'Mark, you're not a doctor. You have no credibility.' 'Clever idea, but you need a celebrity attached or it won't go anywhere.' 'Ditching grains? Eating more fat? Making workouts slower, or shorter? This stuff will never fly with today's reader.'

After literally pounding the pavement for two days making the publisher/agent rounds in New York City, I collapsed in a heap in my hotel room. My feet ached from wearing real shoes for hours (ah, the side-effects of a mostly Vibram Five Fingers lifestyle …), but I had a big smile on my face. I was ready for battle. If the mainstream channels wouldn't bow down to receive the exciting new Primal Blueprint, I would be distinctly honoured to become my own author, agent and publisher!

Now, I wouldn't call myself the gloating type, but I think the Primal community as a whole can gloat like crazy these days. The movement has grown from a wacky, extreme grassroots scene to mainstream acceptance. The hardcover version of this book, published by an unknown outfit out of Malibu, CA (can ya' get any further away from the publishing epicentre of Park Ave?), sold through six printings (over 130,000 copies), climbed the charts to hit number 2 overall best-seller on amazon.com in March of 2010, and occupied the number-one spot on Amazon's Exercise & Fitness, and Diet & Weight Loss lists, on and off, for nearly a year. Many of my friends in the primal/paleo/ancestral health community have also published popular books in the last couple of years. The influence of conventional wisdom on our collective psyche has never been more tenuous, as people are sick of being sick, fat, tired and stressed. The time has come to ditch once and for all the methodology dispensed by the decades-long succession of gimmicky best-selling diet books and return to our genetic roots as hunter-gatherers.

This work represents the culmination of my primal philosophy, which has taken shape over the past 20 years through extensive research and life experience. I'm not a scientist or doctor; I'm an athlete, a coach and a student on a lifelong quest for exceptional health, happiness and peak performance. I have an insatiable curiosity about what we need to do to achieve such goals and a growing mistrust of the answers that have been heaped upon us by the traditional pillars of health 'wisdom' (Big Pharma, Big Agra, the AMA, the FDA and other government agencies), the health and fitness profiteers glorified by Madison Avenue, and even the know-it-all multilevel marketer next door.

The Primal Blueprint is my effort to distil the information I've studied from the world's leading evolutionary biologists, paleontologists, geneticists, anthropologists, physicians, nutritionists, food scientists, exercise physiologists, coaches, trainers and scientific researchers into a concise list of behaviour laws that have moulded this perfect human genetic recipe and hence assured our survival over the millennia. While the book you are holding is a product of the new millennium, the behaviour laws are as old as the dawn of mankind; they merely re-inform us about the fundamentals of health that seem to have been forgotten, or misinterpreted, in the modern world.

The content in this book comes to you unfiltered by pretence or decorum. I am not beholden to any employer, government agency, professional licensing board or sponsor or to any other higher power that might result in the filtering of my message. I don't have any agenda – except, I suppose, to sell you a book and change your life! I simply don't trust many of the major elements of 'conventional wisdom' that we have blindly accepted as gospel for decades.

In my case, the mistrust has been well earned over the past 35 years of trying to do 'the right thing' (another recurring theme) by diligently following conventional wisdom. For several years of my youth, I ran in excess of 100 miles a week with a single-minded focus towards competing in the 1980 US Olympic Marathon Trials. At my peak, I was considered by many around me to be a picture of health: 6 per cent body fat, a resting heart rate of 38 beats per minute, and a marathon time of two hours, eighteen minutes that had placed me fifth in the US National Marathon Championships.

While I reached some notable heights during my endurance career, I also experienced some devastating lows. Soon after my best marathon performance, the monumental physical stress of my training regime and the state-of-the-art 'high-energy' diet that fuelled it resulted in a succession of serious overuse injuries, illnesses and burnout. While I looked like a picture of health, I was really an example of overstress and inflammation.

I was the fittest person my friends knew, yet I suffered from recurring bouts of fatigue, osteoarthritis in both of my feet, severe tendonitis in my hip joints, stress-related gastrointestinal maladies, and six or more upper respiratory tract infections each year. Most people have travelled a less extreme path than I, yet nearly all of us have experienced similar results by following the conventional wisdom of our time: weight-loss efforts doomed to a 96 per cent long-term failure rate, workout programmes leading to fatigue and increased appetites for sugar, and medications that exacerbate the underlying cause of pain while barely alleviating symptoms (not to mention the unpleasant side effects). So if you have followed this path up until now, I applaud your efforts and desires to do the right thing, and I deeply empathise with your frustration in trying to succeed amidst a whirlwind of conflicting and confusing advice.

My goal with *The Primal Blueprint* is to expose large sections of the lucrative health and fitness industry as ethically and scientifically bankrupt; to peel back the many layers of marketing blather, folk wisdom and manipulative dogma and replace it with 10 simple Primal Blueprint behaviour laws modelled on the evolutionary success of our ancestors.

Pause and reflect on the following simple statement for a moment, for it is the most powerful and compelling rationale for living according to the Primal Blueprint: Human beings have prevailed, despite incalculable odds, by adapting to the selective pressures in their environment over thousands of generations. Our primal ancestors were lean, strong, smart and productive, which enabled them to survive, reproduce, rule over more physically imposing members of the animal kingdom and exploit virtually every corner of the earth. This is no mean feat, yet conventional wisdom has essentially dismissed the legacy of our ancestors in favour of quick fixes.

Today, at the age of 58, I feel healthier, fitter, happier and more productive than ever. I am no longer a marathon or triathlon champion (nor do I want to be), but I maintain a weight of 165 pounds (75kg) with 8 per cent body fat. I eat as much delicious food as I want, I am not beholden to regular mealtimes or even regular meals, I exercise just three to four hours per week (instead of the 20 to 30 I put in back in the day) and I almost never get sick. My personal clients (ranging from world-champion triathletes to ordinary citizens just trying to lose a few – or a lot of – pounds), as well as tens of thousands of readers at MarksDailyApple.com, report similar life-altering benefits from following the Primal Blueprint.

Now it's your turn.

YOUR WAY OR THE HIGHWAY

Throughout the following chapters I hope to show you the immense personal power you have to determine your own health and fitness destiny, and to give you the tools you need to reprogramme your genes, reshape your physique and enjoy a long, healthy, energetic and productive life. The Primal Blueprint principles are wonderfully simple, practical and inexpensive, and they require minimal, if any, sacrifice or deprivation. Unlike many of the gimmicky diet and exercise books that have graced the best-seller shelves in recent decades, the Primal Blueprint is intuitive and easy to follow – not just for the first 21 days or the first four months, but for the rest of your life.

I have a deep understanding and empathy for the real-world concerns that we all share, such as lack of time, budget issues, motivational challenges, dysfunctional social circumstances, eating disorders, ingrained bad habits and other powerful influences that can sabotage the picture-perfect diet plan served up by the celebrity of the moment. On numerous occasions I've felt the disappointment of taking a plunge, heart and soul, into a new diet or athletic training regime only to fall well short of the ambitious goals I had set. Adding insult to injury, I often discovered later that I'd been given bad advice – by slick advertising or a less-than-knowledgeable coach, peer or professional expert. Few things in life are more frustrating!

The Primal Blueprint should not make you feel trepidation; this is not a regimented programme where I shove my ideas down your throat and cajole you to go against your own common sense or pleasure-seeking human nature. My experience with the MarksDaily Apple.com community has taught me the value of the collaborative approach to health and well-being. Whenever I think I might raise an interesting theory or discussion point that could be considered contrary to conventional wisdom, I put it to the thousands of readers of my blog, who can all contribute freely to the discussion. Many of these readers are forward-thinking doctors, scientists, researchers or coaches whose valuable input and suggestions I could not have otherwise easily solicited.

This interplay often forces me to substantiate – or at times even restructure – my position. It also always requires me to adapt my message so that it resonates with real people and their real-life experiences. So, you can see that the philosophical positions and practical guidelines that shape the message of this book have been heavily battle-tested, scrutinised, refined and finally approved by thousands of 'Primal' enthusiasts (as well as sceptics).

> *'The Primal Blueprint is the centrepiece of a vibrant community of people connected by the Internet and committed to living their lives to the fullest potential, challenging the status quo, and not being afraid to try something old.'*

The Primal Blueprint is more than just a book. It's the centrepiece of a vibrant community of people who are connected by the Internet and who are committed to living their lives to the fullest potential, challenging the status quo, and trying something *old*. I encourage you to participate at MarksDailyApple.com; share your experiences with the programme and connect with an audience that can relate to you in a way that goes beyond what a book or even a paid trainer can offer. Every day, *The Primal Blueprint* features an easy-to-read, hard-hitting, but light-hearted commentary on all manner of healthy lifestyle topics, including delicious recipes, workout tips and videos, evaluation of the latest research, and an extensive library of bite-sized inspiration and reminders to keep you eating, exercising and living to your potential.

In this book I will provide you with a basic framework of diet, exercise and lifestyle guidelines that you must observe to be successful. However, how you make the pieces fit comfortably into your own life is best left to you. I strongly support you making allowances for, adjustments to, and occasional deviations from the Primal Blueprint based on your particular real-life concerns and constraints. After all, our ancestors had to constantly adjust to their unpredictable environment and have given us the tools to do the same. That's the primal part; the blueprint in the title connects us to the familiar analogy of construction plans that provide the foundation for action but are often altered during the actual construction project. A programme that allows you to go with the flow and frees you to listen more deeply to your own intuitive knowledge – which is far more expert than any outside resource.

The fact that you are in control will give you the most powerful source of motivation you can imagine – instant and ongoing direct feedback that the Primal Blueprint is working. No more exercising until exhaustion or obsessing about the arduous restrictions common to popular weight-loss programmes; the Primal Blueprint is a way of life that is attainable for everyone. It's time to pursue your own unique peak-performance goals and enjoy your life to the absolute maximum, carrying on a tradition that humans have pursued for tens of thousands of years. Thank you for agreeing to take this journey with me. Now, let's have some fun and get primal!

Mark Sisson
Malibu, CA
December 2011

PRIMAL BLUEPRINT PAPERBACK – ADDITIONS

This streamlined edition of the 2009 hardcover *Primal Blueprint* contains numerous updates and enhancements to the text, reflecting the evolving Primal movement in 2012. Many of the revisions have been inspired by reader feedback and Internet forum commentary. Areas that were confusing to more than a few have been reworded or explained differently. Areas where I might have made points a few more times than necessary have been edited to keep the story flowing!

After extensive consultation with experts and my own research, I've clarified and/or elaborated upon some of my dietary positions. For example, the importance of balancing your dietary ratio of omega 6:omega 3 fatty acids warrants more selectivity on nuts and seeds than I communicated in the 2009 hardcover. Hence, in this book you'll see macadamia nuts earning special distinction above other nuts and seeds due to their favourable fatty acid profile. The year-round availability of highly cultivated, overly-sweetened fruit warrants more selectivity and moderation to be truly Primal-aligned, particularly if you want to reduce excess body fat. I've tried to assert these and other important points stronger than ever in this book. Finally, at the end of the book you will find extensive bonus material as follows:

- **Common Stumbling Blocks:** Derived from thousands of MarksDailyApple.com forum posts, we provide quick tips to help overcome the most common challenges to transitioning to a Primal lifestyle.
- **'Hacks'** for each of the 10 Primal Blueprint lifestyle laws to promote quick results in body composition, fitness, athletic performance and daily energy levels and to reduce disease risk factors and reliance on medication.

- **Workout suggestions:** Detailed descriptions of the Primal Essential Movements; dynamic outdoor strength workouts that integrate the Primal Blueprint strength-training principles and various options for all ability levels to conduct safe, fun all-out sprint sessions.

- **A few words about diet and dieting:** I attempt to eliminate confusion about contrasting dietary advice by examining how the basic assumptions, and entire paradigm, of Primal eating differs from that of the Standard American Diet, causing differing conclusions to be reached. I clarify some misconceptions about vegetarianism, low-fat eating and programmes that promote an amazing rate of weight loss.

- **Internet appendix:** MarksDailyApple.com has extensive supporting material, including text references, suggested reading (blogs, magazine articles and books), resources for shopping and information and wide-ranging Q&A about all aspects of the Primal Blueprint.

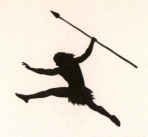

INTRODUCTION

WHAT IS GOING ON HERE?

PRIMAL BLUEPRINT VS. CONVENTIONAL WISDOM

In the Primal Blueprint (PB), we reframe these major elements of Conventional Wisdom (CW). Consider these alternatives with an open mind; we will discuss each in detail throughout the text.

Grains – wheat, rice, corn, cereal, bread, pasta, etc.

CW: "Staff of Life" – foundation of healthy diet. 6-11 daily servings recommended by US Government and numerous other experts. Main energy source for brain and working muscles. Whole grains provide extra nutrition and fiber.

PB: "Worst mistake in the history of the human race" (UCLA evolutionary biologist Jared Diamond). Drives excess insulin production, fat storage, and heart disease. Allergenic, immune-suppressing, nutritional value inferior to plants and animals. Whole grains possibly worse due to "anti-nutrients" that compromise immune and digestive function and promote systemic inflation

Saturated Animal Fat

CW: "Eating fat makes you fat." Heart disease risk factor. Replace saturated fats (meat, dairy) with polyunsaturated vegetable oils.

PB: Major dietary calorie source (from animal foods). No direct correlation with heart disease risk. Drove human evolution/advancement of brain function for two million years. Promotes efficient fat metabolism, weight control and stable energy levels.

Cholesterol

CW: Strictly limit intake. Elevated levels = elevated heart disease risk. Take statin drugs and eliminate animal foods (especially eggs) if total is 200 or over or family history of heart disease.

PB: Essential metabolic nutrient, no direct correlation with heart disease risk. Only dangerous when oxidation and inflammation occur (from poor diet and exercise habits). Statins have considerable side effects and minimal, if any, direct benefit.

Eggs

CW: Minimize consumption due to high cholesterol content of yolk.

PB: No correlation between egg intake and blood cholesterol levels. Yolk among the planet's most nutritious foods.

Fiber

CW: Important dietary goal, derive mostly from grains. Improves gastrointestinal function, lowers cholesterol, speeds elimination, helps control weight by minimizing caloric intake.

PB: Incidental fiber from vegetables and fruit is optimum. Grain-based diet causes excess fiber - inhibiting nutrient absorption, and hampering gastrointestinal function and elimination.

Meal Habits

CW: Three squares (or six small meals) daily to "keep flame burning". Skipped meals = slowed metabolism, lower energy levels, muscle breakdown, sugar cravings, and future binging risk.

PB: No need for regular meals when insulin production is moderated and you reprogram your genes to become a fat burning beast. Intermittent Fasting becomes effective weight management tool.

Strength Training

CW: Focus on form and deliberate work/return rhythm. Lift to "failure" in sequence through numerous stations (takes about an hour for a complete workout). Isolate body parts to get desired size, toning and "cuts".

PB: Emphasize explosive movements over deliberate pace. Conduct full body, functional exercises to develop broad athletic competency and an excellent strength-to-weight ratio. Finish workouts in 30 minutes or less.

Cardio Workouts

CW: "60 minutes of moderate-to-vigorous intensity on most days of the week" (US Government recommendation). A consistent schedule of vigorous workouts helps control weight by burning tons of calories.

PB: US Government recommendation results in "Chronic Cardio", leading to overstress, fatigue, burnout, injury, accelerated aging, and increased disease risk. Calories burned during chronic workouts simply increase appetite (particularly for sugar) – ineffective for weight loss. Slow down for better health and peak performance!

Weight Loss

CW: High-complex carb/low-fat diet, regimented meals, portion control and Chronic Cardio exercise. It's all about "calories in/calories out"... and lucky genes!

PB: High-fat/moderate protein/low-carb diet; intuitive, sporadic meals; and a strategic blend of Primal workouts. Don't worry about portion control, regimented meals, fanatical workouts or even family genetic predispositions. Eat Primal foods, ditch SAD foods, and reprogram your genes to enjoy effortless lifelong weight control.

Play

CW: Ah, brings back fond memories of childhood. But who has time these days?

PB: Integral component of overall health and balanced lifestyle. Outdoor, active, unstructured fun is appropriate for all ages. Scientifically proven to increase work productivity and help manage stress of hectic daily life.

Sun Exposure

CW: Avoid the sun to prevent skin cancer! Lather up with SPF 20, 30, 40, 50 – all you got!

PB: Get plenty of sun to avoid skin cancer! Vitamin D synthesis promotes healthy cellular function and prevents all forms of cancer, including melanoma. Expose large skin surface areas enough to maintain slight tan, but of course avoid burning with clothing, shade, and sunscreen.

Footwear

CW: Sturdy, cushioned shoes minimize injury, improve comfort. Custom orthotics can provide additional support and protection.

PB: Get primal - go barefoot (or minimalist)! Perpetual use of "big" shoes increases impact trauma, weakens foot muscles, and increases pain and injury rates throughout lower extremities.

Prescription Drugs

CW: Relieve pain, speed healing, prevent/cure disease, and address genetic frailties. Everyday use can enhance quality of life (Viagra, etc.).

PB: Mask/exacerbate underlying causes, compromise homeostasis and thus health, and produce disastrous side effects. Simple lifestyle changes can replace vast majority of pills. Wonderful in case of emergency!

Goals

CW: Set specific, measurable goals to stay motivated and focused. "Consistency is key". Missed workouts = guilt, weight gain, and lost fitness.

PB: De-emphasize specific, results-oriented goals (potential to discourage – a la weight loss failure or "post-marathon blues"). Stay motivated by focusing on fun, and release attachment to outcome. Consistency = overstress. Vary routine to minimize stress and improve adaptive response by genes. Missed workouts drive recovery, improvement and freshness.

> *'Americans will always do the right thing – after they've*
> *exhausted all the alternatives.'*
> WINSTON CHURCHILL

I'm going to ask you to forget almost everything you thought you knew about diet, exercise and health. There is a distressing amount of *flawed* conventional wisdom that confuses, misleads, manipulates and complicates even the most devoted efforts to do the right thing: eat healthily, exercise effectively, control weight and avoid today's incredibly common health conditions, such as obesity, arthritis, indigestion, insomnia, diabetes, heart disease and cancer.

In *The Primal Blueprint* I will reveal why eating a low-fat diet rich in whole grains such as bread, rice, pasta and cereal can easily make you fat and malnourished, and why millions of joggers and gym-goers who put in the time and effort to lose weight routinely compromise their health and accelerate the ageing process as a direct result of their devotion to fitness. I'll also explain why cholesterol level and saturated fat intake are *not* the major risk factors for heart disease that we have been led to believe, and why a relatively high-fat diet in fact promotes health and longevity. I'll show you that weight loss does not have to involve the suffering, sacrifice and deprivation we've been conditioned to accept but instead is a matter of eating the right foods (plants and animals), avoiding the wrong foods (processed fats and carbohydrates – including grains – and trans- and partially hydrogenated fats) and exercising strategically, for far fewer hours than you might assume, to reach your desired fitness level.

All the answers are found in a set of 10, simple, logical, Primal Blueprint diet, exercise and lifestyle behaviours. Modelling your 21st-century life on that of our primal hunter-gatherer ancestors will help you greatly reduce or eliminate almost all of the disease risk factors that you may falsely blame on genes you inherited from your parents.

Unfortunately, too many of us narrowly define genes as largely unalterable inherited traits – height, body type, eye colour, physical or intellectual abilities and 'family history' health conditions and diseases. While some genes are indeed responsible for traits that are largely unaffected by lifestyle, many more play a bigger role in your health than you might realise. As later chapters will explain, your genes – guided by what you eat, how you move, and even how you think – are the traffic cops that direct the functioning of every single cell in your body, every moment of every day.

Whatever you throw at them, your genes are going to respond in an effort to promote survival and, beyond that, homeostasis (the balanced and synchronistic functioning of all systems in the body). After all, this is the essence of human evolution.

However, be forewarned that when you are sitting on the couch late at night chowing down Cheetos and Dr Pepper, your body will still valiantly pursue homeostasis (releasing insulin and stress hormones into the bloodstream), *regardless of whether or not it benefits your long-term health*. I am merely presenting the steps you can take to reprogramme your genes to trigger *desirable gene expression* and achieve 'effortless weight loss, vibrant health and boundless energy' – if these happen to be of interest to you!

> 'Instead of falling victim to your genetic vulnerabilities, you can control how your genes express themselves in constantly rebuilding, repairing and renewing your cells.'

The idea that we can reprogramme our genes through lifestyle behaviour is the central premise of *The Primal Blueprint*. It represents a clear departure from today's fatalistic conventional wisdom, which suggests that our genes, for better or worse, determine our destiny and that we have little say in the matter – unless prescription drugs or the Human Genome Project discoveries can come to the rescue. True, you might have a genetic tendency towards accumulating excess body fat or a family history of type 2 diabetes, but you'll be more likely to see these traits expressed when you make poor lifestyle choices and send the wrong signals to your genes. Instead of falling victim to your genetic vulnerabilities, you can control how your genes express themselves in constantly rebuilding, repairing and renewing your cells. Briefly, here are the most critical, life-altering elements of *The Primal Blueprint*:

- **Become a Fat-Burning Beast** by removing processed carbohydrates from your diet to minimise your body's insulin production. This means eliminating not only sugars and sweets but also grain products including wheat, rice, pasta, cereal and corn. A diet that emphasises meat, fish, poultry, eggs, nuts, seeds and colourful natural carbohydrates, such as vegetables and fruits, is the primary way to improve your general health, control your weight and minimise your risk of heart disease, cancer, diabetes, arthritis and other diet-influenced medical conditions. If you are carrying excess body fat, it will disappear virtually effortlessly when you focus on eating the delicious, filling, nutritious foods that have nourished humans throughout the course of evolution for two million years. Seriously, it's as simple as choosing the right foods to moderate insulin production. You will not have to struggle or suffer to shed excess body fat.

- **Optimise your exercise programme** by engaging in a genetically desirable blend of frequent, low-intensity movement (walking, hiking, easy cardio), regular brief, intense strength-training sessions and occasional all-out sprints that help improve body composition and delay the ageing process. This strategy is far superior to the conventional wisdom approach of following a consistent schedule of frequent medium-to-difficult-intensity sustained workouts, such as jogging, running or cycling, cardio machines, or group classes. That workout plan – which I refer to derisively as 'Chronic Cardio' – places excessive and prolonged physical stress on your body, leading to fatigue, injuries, compromised immune function and burnout. Sometimes, less really is more.

- **Manage stress levels** with plenty of sleep, play, sunlight, fresh air and creative outlets and by avoiding the trauma that often arises from making stupid mistakes. Rebel against the tremendous cultural momentum that is growing in which sedentary lifestyles, excessive digital stimulation and insufficient rest are becoming a major part of everyday life. Honour your primal genes by slowing down and simplifying your life. Your ancestors worked hard to survive, but their regular respites from stress gave them the peace of mind and body that is so highly coveted today.

IS DYING OF OLD AGE GETTING OLD, OR WHAT?

As you will soon discover, our genes were not only designed through evolution to keep us healthy, but they desperately *want and expect* us to be healthy. Today, with the hectic pace of the high-tech modern world, we struggle with the idea of how to do the right thing by our genes. The ensuing failure creates a level of frustration and confusion that causes many of us, whether overtly or deep down inside, simply to give up. Experience teaches us how difficult it is, if not impossible, to be lean, fit, energetic and healthy when following conventional wisdom, so instead we succumb to the forces of consumerism designed to placate our pain with silly shortcuts, comforts, conveniences and indulgences. Consequently, the popular 'Hey man, life is short!' rationalisation becomes a self-fulfilling prophecy.

The consequences of eating processed foods, exercising excessively (or, conversely, being inactive) and making poor lifestyle decisions, work in concert against your genetic mandate for health. At the very least, you can experience excess body fat storage, subpar fitness, aching joints, gastrointestinal problems, frequent minor illnesses, sugar cravings, energy-level swings and recurring fatigue. This sounds bad enough as it is, but continuing to misdirect your genes with the wrong choices over years and decades will likely result in obesity, diabetes, heart disease, cancer and/or the vast majority of degenerative conditions requiring a doctor's care or medication in later life. A huge percentage of all visits to the doctor today are a direct consequence of lifestyle choices that are misaligned with the environmental and survival conditions that shaped our primal genetic make-up.

These consequences are painfully obvious to almost everyone, and our collective interest in doing the right thing has in recent years fuelled a booming fitness industry, incredible advancements in medicine, much greater awareness of healthy foods and lifestyle choices, significant declines in smoking and sharp increases in restaurants offering salad bars and smoothies. Ironically, though, the collective health of the USA – and other Western countries that have adopted our fast-paced culture – is worse than ever. A study released in 2008 by Johns Hopkins University, Maryland, suggests that by the year 2030, 86 per cent of all adults in the United States will be overweight or obese (up from the current estimate of 65 per cent); what's more, a National Institutes of Health conference report stated that 'our trends predict that *all* Americans will be obese by 2230!'

We reluctantly accept as fact that the normal human life span consists of growing up to reach a physical peak in our early 20s, followed by an inevitable steady decline caused by the ageing process. Under this faulty assumption, we allow ourselves to gain an average of one and a half pounds (two-thirds of a kilo) of fat per year, starting at age 25 and continuing until we are around 55[1] (we also lose half a pound of muscle per year, resulting in adding a pound a year in the wrong places as we age). Our last decade or two (until we reach the average life span of about 78 years)[2] is commonly characterised by inactivity, insufficient muscle mass and excess body fat, assorted medical conditions and a host of prescription drugs which are required to alleviate the pain and symptoms of chronic disease.

Twenty-seven per cent of us will die from cardiovascular disease, and another 23 per cent will die from cancer.[3] I know that 100 per cent of us will die from something, but personally I'd prefer to actualise a motto I crafted in honour of our hunter-gatherer ancestors: 'Live Long, Drop Dead!' Yes, many primal humans succumbed to primitive hazards (death by predator, or infection from a deep cut) before they hit today's voting age, but many of those who avoided misfortune could live six or seven decades in exceptional health and fitness. In almost all cases, primal humans were healthy and strong for their entire lives, until they met their sudden demise. There was simply no such thing as today's abysmal decline into old age. After all, the clan couldn't support any excess baggage in their daily battle for survival.

While 21st-century longevity statistics are vastly superior to any other time in human history, these increases are mostly due to science, not healthier lifestyle behaviours. Furthermore, modern longevity is often undesirably inflated by things that keep us alive but do not improve quality of life: hospital machinery, pharmaceuticals and the ability to reel in the years, doing little more than putting spoon to mouth and thumb to remote control.

Of the two and a half trillion dollars America spends annually on health care, the Center for Disease Control and Prevention (CDC) estimates that 70 per cent of that is spent on lifestyle-related chronic diseases, such as obesity, diabetes and heart disease. A surprising number of people accept this, believing that some of us are just fortunate to have 'good genes' and the rest must cross their fingers against bad luck.

Of course, millions of modern citizens contributing to these woeful statistics are completely disconnected from what's required to be healthy, and it might be hard for you even to relate to this segment of humanity that hasn't a clue or a care about this stuff. However, even the most health conscious among us often struggle. Despite a sincere commitment to do the right thing according to conventional wisdom, we have collectively failed to lose those last 5, 10 or 50 pounds of weight. Injuries, fatigue and burnout plague all exercisers, from the weekend warriors to the professionals. We have been programmed by the healthcare establishment to turn to prescription drugs to treat symptoms of distress in a reflex action, even though most conditions are minor and easily corrected by simple dietary and lifestyle changes. In the process, we interfere with normal gene-driven metabolic processes and thwart our innate ability to heal naturally – paving the way to one day join the masses on the wrong side of the stats.

'70 per cent of today's health care expenditures are for lifestyle-relate chronic diseases, such as obesity, diabetes and heart disease.'

The story is sad, but the good news is that, for the most part, your destiny is in your hands. By the time you complete this book, you will understand the big picture and all the necessary details of how to eat, exercise and live in order to reprogramme many of your genes for lifelong good health. In the process, you will take control of your own body and your own life. This is really the only sensible way to counter the tremendous momentum that pushes us away from health, balance and well-being in our hectic modern world.

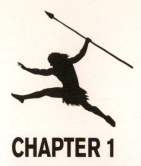

CHAPTER 1

THE TEN PRIMAL BLUEPRINT LAWS

('COMMANDMENTS' WAS ALREADY TAKEN)

'Nothing in biology makes sense except in the light of evolution.'
THEODOSIUS DOBZHANSKY

IN THIS CHAPTER

I introduce the 're:evolutionary' premise that we should model our diet, exercise and lifestyle behaviours after our primal ancestors from 10,000 years ago, adapting them strategically to the realities of high-tech modern life. The inexorable technological progress of civilisation has diverted us from the dietary habits and active, stress-balanced lifestyles that allowed primal humans to prevail under the harsh, competitive circumstances of evolution. However, we are genetically identical (in virtually all respects relevant to human health) to our hunter-gatherer ancestors, owing to the fact that evolution ground to a halt when the major selection pressures of starvation and predator danger (eat or get eaten!) were eliminated.

Genes are more than just the largely unalterable inherited traits with which we typically associate the term. They are the 'traffic cops' that direct the function of all the cells in your body, at all times. Your genes don't have to be your destiny; you can 'reprogramme' them with healthy lifestyle behaviours and thereby make even strong genetic predispositions to disease, excess body fat and other adverse health conditions irrelevant.

The 10 Primal Blueprint laws are:

1. Eat lots of plants and animals
2. Avoid poisonous things
3. Move frequently at a slow pace
4. Lift heavy things
5. Sprint once in a while
6. Get adequate sleep
7. Play
8. Get adequate sunlight
9. Avoid stupid mistakes
10. Use your brain.

The quote by Dobzhansky that begins this chapter was also the title of a famous 1973 essay in which the noted evolutionary biologist and devout Russian Orthodox Christian acknowledged that, whether or not you believed in the existence of a higher power, you could not begin to understand even the simplest concepts in biology unless you understood how evolution had worked to shape and differentiate the genes of every single one of the several million species on the planet.

Within the past hundred years, tens of thousands of anthropologists, evolutionary biologists, paleontologists, epigeneticists and other scientists have worked diligently to piece together a fairly detailed interpretation of the environmental and behavioural factors that have directly influenced our development as a species since our creation. As a result, we now have a very good picture of the conditions under which we emerged as *Homo sapiens*.

Some seven million years ago, hominids (our pre-human ancestors) split from apes and branched out into various new species. Then, about two million years ago, the humanlike species *Homo erectus* began to take charge of the food chain with their large brains, upright stature, skilled use of tools and fire and organised hunter-gatherer societies.

Over time, *Homo erectus* branched into various species and subspecies (*Homo neanderthaensis*, *Homo habilis*, *Homo sapiens* and others). Most researchers believe that the modern *Homo sapiens* species evolved in Africa between 200,000 and 100,000 years ago, prevailing over all other *Homo erectus* subspecies. Then, about 60,000 years ago, a small number of modern humans left Africa and began their great migration across the planet.

Recent archaeological findings strongly support this 'out of Africa'[1] theory: that the entire human population of the planet, amazingly, can trace its origins to a small pool of intrepid *Homo sapiens* in Africa. There were only an estimated 2,000 to 5,000 African humans at that time, and some scientists believe that only about 150 people crossed the Red Sea to begin the migration. Talk about six degrees of separation!

'ARE WE NOT MEN? WE ARE DEVO!'
(DEVO ALBUM COVER, 1978)

I hope you are sitting down to absorb one of the most critical – and quite possibly mind-blowing – tenets of *The Primal Blueprint*:

> *'Our primal ancestors were likely stronger and healthier than we are today.'*

'How can this be?' you ask. Well, it's all about survival of the fittest. The human body is the miraculous result of millions of years of painstaking design by evolution. Through natural selection, involving countless small genetic mutations and adaptations in response to a hostile environment, our ancestors were able to prevail over unimaginably difficult conditions and opponents and populate all corners of the earth.

Many anthropologists suggest that the human species reached its evolutionary pinnacle (in terms of average muscularity, bone density and brain size) about 10,000 years ago. After that, we started to take it easy and get soft. Our physical decline was a natural consequence of a couple of things: first, we had already spent thousands of generations leveraging our increasingly proficient brain function to manipulate and tame the natural environment (with tools, weapons, fire and shelter) to our advantage. The second factor was perhaps the most significant lifestyle change in the history of humanity: the gradual advent of agriculture. When humans began to domesticate and harvest wheat, rice, corn and other crops as well as livestock (this happened independently around the globe, becoming prominent about 7,000 years ago in modern-day Egypt; North America was one of the last areas to implement agriculture, about 4,500 years ago)[2], the ability to store food, divide and specialise labour and live in close civilised quarters eliminated the main selection pressures that had driven human evolution for two million years – the threats of starvation and predator danger.

When humans no longer faced these constant selection pressures, evolution essentially ground to a halt in conjunction with the flourishing of civilisation. Consequently, many researchers assert that today we are genetically identical to our primal ancestors at least relating to behaviours that promote human health. Some challenge this assertion by pointing to examples of recent genetic variations, such as higher lactose tolerance rates among those of herding ancestry. (I clarify confusion about this topic in the Primal Blueprint Q&A supplement at MarksDailyApple.com). For now, let's stay focused on the big picture: discovering the most important evolution-tested lifestyle behaviours that promote optimal gene expression – which have not changed in 10,000 years.

This idea that human DNA – the genetic 'recipe' for building a healthy, lean, thriving human that resides in each of our 60 trillion cells – is almost exactly the same today as it was 10,000 years ago has been most notably promoted by the work of Dr Boyd Eaton, chief anthropologist at Emory University in Atlanta and author of *The Paleolithic Prescription*, and the late James V. Neel, founder of the University of Michigan's Department of Genetics, and supported by hundreds of other leading anthropologists, evolutionary biologists, and genetic researchers.

While our primal ancestors made the most of their genes (remember, they had no choice; the alternative was to starve or become some other creature's dinner!), we have fallen far short. The development of agriculture and civilisation caused humans to become smaller (including our brain size) and sicker (originally due to contagious diseases and other repercussions of civilisation but lately more because of our vastly inferior diet, exercise and lifestyle behaviours).

'The development of agriculture and civilisation caused humans to become smaller and sicker, leading to a dramatic decline in life expectancy.'

Human life expectancy 10,000 years ago was about 33 years. While not too impressive by 21st-century standards, primal man actually lived longer than his civilised successors all the way into the early

20th century! Average life expectancy reached a low of 18 during the Bronze Age (3300–1200 BC, Ancient Egypt, etc.), rose only slightly to between 20–30 through Classical Greek (500–300 BC) times, the Roman Empire (0–AD500) and the Middle Ages (700–1500), and was still only between 30 and 40 as late as the early 20th century. Around that time, medical advancements (antibiotics, hospital and community sanitation, decreased infant mortality rates, etc.) helped life expectancy statistics skyrocket.

Fossil records show that primal humans who could steer clear of fatal misfortune could routinely live six or seven decades in excellent health and fitness and had a 'maximum observed life span' of an astonishing 94 years! [3] Among present-day hunter-gatherers (e.g., Ache, Hadza, Hiwi and !Kung – groups that have almost no modern conveniences or medical care), it is not uncommon to see strong, healthy people living well into their 80s. More than a quarter of the Ache people of Paraguay make it to 70. Moreover, 73 per cent of Ache adults die from accidents and only 17 per cent from illness. Think about the extraordinary implications of hunter-gatherer longevity: with no medications or medical care of any kind, a massive lifelong struggle for food, clothing and shelter completely devoid of any modern comforts, primal humans (and modern humans living primally) can still live to what even we softies consider old age.

Of course, the civilisation-driven decline in life expectancy didn't matter in a pure evolutionary context. As long as civilised humans made it to reproductive age and had children, they could pass their genes along to the next generation without penalty. While progressing beyond survival of the fittest conditions is definitely a good thing, the sober reality is that today's technological age is enjoyed by the fattest, laziest humans in the history of humanity. Hence, the Ultimate Human award goes to *Grok*, my nickname for the prototypical pre-agricultural human being. Grok[4] is the central character of both this book and my blog. He's a lean, smart, healthy character whom you will grow to love.

'The human species reached its evolutionary pinnacle about 10,000 years ago. After that, we started to take it easy and get soft....Hence, the Ultimate Human award goes to **Grok,** *my nickname for the prototypical pre-agricultural human being.'*

Unlike Grok, who ruled the planet with little more than a spear and a thatched hut in his portfolio, even the most impoverished humans of the last several thousand years, extending up to the present day's Third-World inhabitants, have not really 'competed' genetically. The presence of the most rudimentary modern influences, such as grain consumption, food storage, permanent shelters and basic weapons to thwart potential predators, all suppress the true Darwinian survival of the fittest playing field that allowed Grok to thrive.

Sure, being a maths whiz or a natural athlete may significantly influence your path through life and give you a competitive edge in pursuits to which you are inclined, but these genetic attributes no longer provide a survival advantage in the evolutionary sense. Tour de France legend Lance Armstrong has a genetically superior cardiovascular system, but he could have easily cruised through life as a candy-chomping, video-gaming fat kid and still have reproduced successfully due to lack of selection pressure for human endurance in the modern world.

In fact, considering all the comforts and medical advancements of modern life, we could easily argue that we currently exist in a state of *devolution*. For the most part, this is great (many of us have suffered illnesses or traumas over the course of our lives that would have killed us a century ago, let alone 1,000 or 10,000 years ago). However, we must be vigilant not to let the advantages of modern life compromise our health (e.g., heading to the pharmacy instead of the gym to combat back pain).

The challenge is in applying the Primal Blueprint laws to modern life. How do we use the lessons and benefits of natural selection against the pressures of a complex modern society bent on promoting consumerism and quick fixes over the pursuit of health? How do we reprogramme our ancient genes to recapture excellent health? We simply have to ask ourselves: 'What would Grok do?'

> *'Genes don't know – or care – whether these environmental signals promote or compromise your health; they simply react to each stimulus in an effort to promote your immediate survival.'*

YOU HAVE TO FIT YOUR GENES TO FIT INTO YOUR JEANS

In order to begin to understand the concept of reprogramming your genes, it will help to understand what they actually are and how they work. Each of your 50 or 60 trillion cells contains a nucleus with a complete set of DNA instructions divided into handy subsets called genes. There are approximately 20,000 different genes located on the long strands of DNA in each cell. These DNA strands are further organised into the 23 pairs of chromosomes with which we are familiar. In any given cell, only a small fraction of the total number of genes is actively involved in carrying out the main 'business' of that particular type of cell. Depending on environmental signals, genes trigger the manufacture of certain specific proteins and enzymes to perform the various tasks required of them. For example, the beta cells in your pancreas manufacture insulin but they don't grow bigger when you lift weights; liver cells can synthesise nutrients, but they don't grow new bone tissue – and yet each cell has the entire 'recipe' for a human residing on the DNA.

The most important thing to understand here is that most genes are not self-determining. They do not turn on or off by themselves; they respond to signals they receive from their immediate environment. You have the power to turn on or turn off certain genes that have a profound influence on your health. You may not be able to reprogramme your eyes from blue to brown, but you can certainly avoid getting a pot belly, even if your dad, grandpa and brothers all exhibit a strong disposition in their familial genes for such an attribute.

Genes actively control cell function all the time, so the overall health and survival of your body are primarily dependent on which genes get turned on or off in response to their immediate environment. Genes don't know – or care – whether these environmental signals promote or compromise your long-term health; they simply react to each stimulus in an effort to sustain your short-term survival, just as they have been designed to do by evolution, having been moulded by the precise behaviours of our ancestors.

Sprint or lift weights and the biochemical 'by-products' from that specific activity turn on certain genes that repair and strengthen the exercised muscle. Do too much exercise and other genes will promote excessive production of catabolic hormones, leading to prolonged inflammation and hindered recovery. An allergic reaction represents your body's (misdirected) genetic response to a perceived airborne or ingested threat. An autoimmune disease is often a genetic overreaction of that same system caused by unfamiliar foods (see Chapter 5). Similarly, type 2 diabetes typically develops after prolonged periods when your genes are trying to protect you from the dangers of eating too many carbohydrates.

In a profound example of our genes' ability to switch on and off, researchers studying the link between smoking and lung cancer have discovered that tobacco smoking causes *hypermethylation* (a complete or partial deactivation) of a single gene known as MTHFR. Turning off MTHFR triggers an opposite effect – *hypomethylation* (systemic dysfunction) – in many other genes, setting the stage for further cancer development.

The idea that the environment influences whether genes are turned on or off is not a new one; in 1942 the geneticist and evolutionary biologist C. H. Waddington first coined the term *epigenetics* to describe how genes might interact with their surroundings to create a unique individual. Today, the study of epigenetics is one of the fastest-growing subdisciplines of genetics. Moreover, the burgeoning field of *nutrigenomics* has identified hundreds of ways in which nutrients (foods or supplements) impact on gene expression. You may be familiar with the direct influence folic acid has on reducing neural tube birth defects, which is why all women who are pregnant or are trying to conceive are advised to take folic acid supplements. This is but one small example of the powerful influence diet can have on reprogramming genes.

An Australian study suggested that human genes are adversely affected by sugar ingestion for two weeks (genetic controls designed to protect the body against diabetes and heart disease are switched off as an acute reaction to eating sugar) and that prolonged poor eating can cause genetic damage that can potentially be passed through bloodlines! On an even grander scale, research shows that certain cells within the body, called mesenchymal stem cells, can become bone cells, fat cells, muscle cells, or even cancer cells in adults, depending upon the environmental signals they receive.

Clearly, your lifestyle behaviours can either destroy or support many aspects of your health and can often be far more relevant than inherited predispositions to allergies, diabetes, or even more serious conditions. Not to make light of the serious genetically influenced health challenges that many face over their lifetimes, I would argue that we are *all* predisposed to heart disease, cancer, arthritis and today's other leading lifestyle-related health problems if we programme our genes with the wrong diet and lifestyle behaviours – and even thoughts.

Obviously, you cannot encourage your kids to grow to seven feet tall simply by feeding them healthy foods and making sure they get plenty of sleep; we all have profound limitations when it comes to how our genes can express our unique individual potential. For confirmation, just take a look at the physical marvels in the Olympic 100-metre race. These athletes, some of the most physically gifted on the planet, might be one in a million genetically, but they are still an example of *optimal gene expression*. The choices they have made – the foods they've eaten, how they've trained, even how they've thought – have all helped them make the most of their natural-born talents to rise to the top in very competitive arenas. This is all you ought to be concerned with – making the most of your own genetic recipe to enjoy a long life of excellent health and peak performance through the 10 Primal Blueprint laws.

The following chapters will explore the rationale, benefits and practical suggestions for living according to the 10 simple Primal Blueprint laws. These laws represent the specific behaviours that led directly (shaped by two million years of evolution) to the genetic recipe for a healthy, lean, fit, happy human being. Almost nothing has changed in this recipe since pre-agricultural times – except the endless new ways in which we modern humans discover to mismanage our genes and compromise our health.

By understanding how these behavioural laws shaped our genome, we can reprogramme our genes to express themselves in a direction of health. And when I say simple laws, I really mean it. If you read just this chapter and never opened the book again, you'd have all the information you need to live a long, healthy, disease-free life.

Here then is a brief description of the laws of living 10,000 years ago and a quick primer on how to adapt them to your 21st-century lifestyle.

> 'Play by the rules, but be ferocious.'
> PHIL KNIGHT, FOUNDER OF NIKE, INC.

PRIMAL BLUEPRINT LAW NUMBER 1: EAT LOTS OF PLANTS AND ANIMALS

Plants and animals encompass everything our ancestors ate (from a huge list of individual foods) in order to obtain the protein, fats, carbohydrates, vitamins, minerals, antioxidants, phenols, fibre, water and other nutrients necessary to sustain life, increase brain size, improve physical fitness and support immune function. Ironically, the primal human diet differs greatly from what conventional wisdom recommends. Because the various diet camps passionately argue conflicting positions to a confused public, it's essential to reflect on how profoundly important and logically sound it is to model our diets on those of our ancestors, whose bodies evolved to survive, reproduce and thrive on these foods. Talk about a lengthy and severely scrutinised (as in, 'life or death') study protocol!

For one, primal humans across the globe ate widely varied diets due to environmental circumstances, such as climate, geography, seasons and activity level. There is no single regimented diet of narrowly defined foods that trumps all. Once you ascribe to the broad guidelines of the Primal Blueprint (eat plants and animals, avoid modern foods foreign to our genes), personal preference will be the driving force behind your food choices each day.

Also notable about our ancestors' diet is that they ate sporadically – mostly due to the lack of consistently available food (not a big issue in the developed world these days, eh?). Consequently, we became well adapted to store caloric energy (in the form of body fat, along with a little bit of muscle and liver glycogen) and burn it when dietary calories were scarce. You may be disturbed at the idea of possessing the genetic trait to store extra food calories efficiently as fat; however, by simply eating the right kinds of foods you can use this bank account 'savings and withdrawal' mechanism to your advantage – maintaining ideal levels of body fat while stabilising those of your daily appetite and energy. *Hint:* it's mostly about moderating the wildly excessive insulin production resulting from the Standard American Diet (SAD).

Today, similar principles apply for healthy eating. Focus on quality sources of animal protein (local, pasture-raised or organic sources of meat, poultry, fish and eggs), an assortment of colourful vegetables and fresh fruits, and healthy sources of fat (animal fats, avocados, butter, coconut products, nuts and seeds, olives and olive oil). You also need to realise that a significant amount of conventional wisdom about healthy eating is simply marketing fodder which grossly distorts the fundamental truth that humans thrive on natural plant and animal foods, or relies on gimmicks to support the dogma of flawed, manipulated 'research'. For example, eating at particular times (three square or six small meals a day), combining or rotating specific food types at meals, structuring your meals according to pre-programmed phases or stages, eating foods supposedly aligned with your blood type, striving for specific macro-nutrient ratios, or keeping score of your portions and weekly treat allowances, are all gimmicks that have no credibility in the context of evolutionary biology.

Furthermore, regimented programmes are virtually impossible to enjoy and stick to over the long term, because they run counter to human nature. We humans thrive on eating a variety of natural foods that satisfy and nourish us, in times, amounts and variations that fluctuate according to personal preference, environmental circumstances, activity levels, stress levels and many other factors. I suggest you enjoy eating as one of the pleasures of life and reject most of everything you've ever heard about that dictates when and how much you should eat. Instead, eat when you are hungry and finish eating when you feel satisfied. Realise that Primal foods are intrinsically the most delicious, because they satisfy your cravings and distinct tastes, stabilise mood and energy levels, and promote health and well-being.

PRIMAL BLUEPRINT LAW NUMBER 2: AVOID POISONOUS THINGS

The ability of humans to exploit almost every corner of the earth was partly predicated on consuming vastly different types of plant and animal life. Primal humans developed a keen sense of smell and taste, along with liver, kidney and stomach function, to adapt to new food sources and to avoid succumbing to poisonous plants that they encountered routinely when foraging and settling new areas. For example, the reason we have a sweet tooth today is probably an evolved response to an almost universal truth in the plant world that anything that tastes sweet is safe to eat.

While we have little risk of ingesting poisonous plants unless we're on a woodland walkabout today, the number of toxic agents in our food supply is worse than ever. By *toxic* I mean man-made products that are foreign to your genes and disturb the normal, healthy function of your body when ingested. The big offenders, including sugars and fizzy drinks, chemically altered fats and heavily processed, packaged, fried and preserved foods, are obvious. It's not a stretch to directly compare the poisonous berries of Grok's day with much of the stuff shelved at eye level in your local supermarket.

What are less accepted, and therefore more insidious, as a dietary 'poison' are processed grain foods (wheat, rice, corn, pasta, cereal and derivative products, such as bread, crisps, crackers, muffins, pancakes, tortillas, waffles, etc.); cooking grains such as barley, millet, rye and amaranth; and – to a slightly lesser extent – legumes (beans, lentils, peanuts, peas and soy products). These staple ingredients of diets across the globe are generally inappropriate for human consumption for the simple reason that our digestive systems (and our genes) have not had ample time to adapt to both the unfamiliar protein structure of grains and the excessive carbohydrate load of all forms of cultivated grains and legumes. Essentially, the advent of grains and civilisation has eliminated the main thing that's made humans healthy: selection pressure to reach reproductive age – and to care for ourselves, and others, beyond!

Ingesting grains (yep, even whole grains, as we'll discuss in detail in Chapter 5), legumes and other processed carbohydrates causes blood glucose levels to spike (both simple and complex carbohydrates get converted into glucose – at differing rates – once they enter the body; we'll use the accurate term *blood glucose* to convey what many call *blood sugar*). This spike is a shock to our primal genes, which are accustomed to natural, slower-burning foods. Your pancreas compensates for this excess of glucose in the bloodstream (a condition that is toxic and can quickly become life-threatening, as experienced by diabetics) by secreting excessive levels of insulin. While insulin is an important hormone that delivers nutrients to muscle, liver and fat cells for storage, excessive insulin released in the bloodstream causes glucose to be removed so rapidly and effectively that it can result in a 'sugar crash'. This occurs in the form of mental and physical lethargy and (because the brain relies heavily on glucose to fuel it) a strong craving for quick replacement energy in the form of more high-carbohydrate food. This leads to a vicious cycle of another ill-advised meal, another excessive insulin response and another corresponding blood glucose decline.

Because insulin's job is to transport nutrients out of the bloodstream and into the muscle, liver and fat cell storage depots, its excessive presence in the bloodstream inhibits the release of stored body fat for use as energy. Insulin's counter-regulatory hormone, glucagon, accesses carbohydrates, protein and fat from your body's storage depots (muscle, liver, fat cells) and delivers them into the bloodstream for use as energy. When insulin is high, glucagon is usually low. You don't have energy in your bloodstream, so your brain says, 'Eat now! And make it something sweet so we can burn it immediately!'

The mobilisation of stored body fat has been humans' preferred energy source (and weight-control device) for a couple of million years, and now you've just bypassed that whole process. It's as simple as this: you cannot reduce body fat on a diet that stimulates high levels of insulin production. Full stop.

Beyond the weight-loss frustrations, overstressing your insulin response system over years and decades can lead directly to devastating general system failure in the form of type 2 diabetes, obesity, cardiovascular disease (thanks to vascular inflammation, peripheral oxidative damage and other insulin-related troubles which we will learn more about later) and diet-related cancers. Chapter 5 will explain in detail that even whole grains (brown rice, whole wheat bread, etc.) are not particularly healthy, because they still trigger excessive insulin production, contain anti-nutrients that promote inflammation and hamper digestion and immune function, and (even though they have more nutritional value than refined 'white' grain products) displace the far more nutritious plants and animals from being the caloric emphasis of your diet.

> '*The mobilisation of stored body fat has been our preferred energy source (and weight-control device) for a couple of million years. It's as simple as this: you cannot reduce body fat on a diet that stimulates high levels of insulin production.*'

PRIMAL BLUEPRINT LAW NUMBER 3: MOVE FREQUENTLY AT A SLOW PACE

Grok spent several hours each day moving about at what today's exercise physiologists might describe as a very low-level aerobic pace. He hunted, gathered, foraged, wandered, scouted, migrated, climbed and crawled. This low-level activity prompted his genes to build a stronger capillary (blood vessel) network to provide oxygen and fuel to each muscle cell and readily convert stored fat into energy (fat is the main fuel used for low-level aerobic activity). His daily movement also helped develop strong bones, joints and connective tissue. What Grok did not do was deplete his energy and muscle glycogen supply with regularly scheduled sustained efforts of moderate-to-difficult intensity. This counter-intuitive behaviour could have left him vulnerable to a predator, starvation or some other misfortune. You may have heard the recently popularised sentiment that humans were 'born to run'? More accurately, we were born to walk extensively and run (long distances or sprint) once in a while – after or away from something when life depended on it.

Today most of us either are too sedentary or conduct workouts that are too stressful and misaligned with our primal genetic requirements for optimum health. The exercise gospel for decades has been to pursue a consistent routine of aerobic exercise (jogging, cycling, cardio machines, group classes, or any other sustained effort), supposedly leading to more energy, better health and weight control. However, too many lengthy workouts at elevated heart rates (above 75 per cent of maximum) can put you at risk of exhaustion, burnout, injury and illness. The high-carbohydrate diet required to perform these workouts day in and day out only adds to the problem. At the extreme – such as with the overtrained marathon runner or ironman triathlete – a commitment to fitness can actually accelerate the ageing process and elevate risk of heart disease.

Over-exercising is a common scenario when you consider how our active population has such strong focus, dedication and will-power to push through signs of fatigue. Our bodies are simply not adapted to benefit from chronic aerobic exercise at intense or even mildly uncomfortable heart rates, nor to slog through exhausting circuits of resistance machines several days a week. The mild to severe difficulty of these Chronic Cardio or strength workouts overtaxes the stress response (commonly referred to as the fight-or-flight response) in your body. Here, your pituitary gland tells your adrenal glands to release cortisol into your bloodstream (cortisol is a powerful stress hormone that is critical to a variety of physical functions and energy production). The spike of cortisol in the bloodstream from a stressful event increases respiration, heart rate, blood circulation and mental focus and even converts muscle tissue into glucose for quick energy. This is a great example of how we abuse a system that was genetically designed to respond to emergencies, such as Grok facing a predator.

Even today, the fight-or-flight response is highly desirable and effective in the face of true danger or peak performance stimulus, such as an Olympic sprinter crouching in the starting blocks or an emergency worker summoning superhuman strength for a rescue effort. Unfortunately, when the stress response is triggered repeatedly (by the constant hectic pace of modern life coupled with workouts that are too long, too difficult or too frequent), your adrenal glands can so overproduce cortisol that they eventually become fatigued and release less-than-normal levels of cortisol and other hormones critical to many aspects of health. Thyroid hormones and testos-terone also decrease from prolonged stress, resulting in a decline in energy levels, loss of lean muscle tissue, a suppressed immune system and the general condition best described as burnout.

What our genes truly crave is frequent movement at a slow, comfortable pace: walking, hiking, easy cycling, or other light aerobic activities with a heart rate range of 55 per cent to no more than 75 per cent of maximum. These efforts are far less taxing than the typical huffing and puffing, struggling and suffering exertion level that we've been conditioned to think leads to fitness. So find ways every day to move more often, such as walking (even across the car park instead of cruising for a close space; take the stairs instead of the lift – it all adds up over a lifetime!), hiking, swimming, easy cycling or anything else that moderately elevates heart rate. Strive to accumulate two to five hours per week of low-level exercise. More is better as long as you have the time and can resist the temptation to 'go hard'. If possible, make an effort to go barefoot frequently to develop natural balance, flexibility and lower extremity strength.

PRIMAL BLUEPRINT LAW NUMBER 4: LIFT HEAVY THINGS

Grok's life demanded frequent bursts of intense physical effort – returning gathered items (firewood, shelter supplies, tool material and animal carcasses) to camp, climbing rocks and trees to scout and forage, and arranging boulders and logs to build shelter. The biochemical signals triggered by these brief but intense muscle contractions prompted improvements and adaptations in muscle tone, size and power.

Today, following a strength-training programme featuring natural, total-body movements (squatting, push-ups, pullups, etc.) helps you develop and maintain lean muscle mass, increases metabolism to maintain low levels of body fat, increases bone density, prevents injuries and enables you to enjoy balanced hormone and blood glucose levels. An approach of short-duration, high-intensity workouts – conducted fairly regularly but without excessive regimentation (always aligned with your energy levels) – will produce superior results to a routine of going to the gym too often for workouts that last too long. The latter is a recipe for fatigue and undesirable gene expression. You can enjoy extraordinary benefits doing as little as two focused, intense, 25-minute sessions per week, with minimal risk of overtraining or mental burnout.

PRIMAL BLUEPRINT LAW NUMBER 5: SPRINT ONCE IN A WHILE

In a primal world where danger lurked around every corner, Grok's ability to run was a strong indicator of whether he would live long enough to pass those superior genes down to the next generation. Whether he was dashing off to avoid a charging herd of mastodons or running down small game for dinner, Grok's sprints triggered gene expression within fast-twitch muscle that allowed him to go a little faster the next time.

Today, occasional maximum-effort sprints help increase energy levels, improve athletic performance and minimise the effects of ageing by promoting the release of testosterone and human growth hormone (these are beneficial for women as well as men). Once every 7–10 days, when energy and motivation levels are high, choose a simple, brief sprint workout and go all out! Novices can choose low-impact options (stationary bike) and work up to actual running sprints.

PRIMAL BLUEPRINT LAW NUMBER 6: GET ADEQUATE SLEEP

Our ancestors' activity and sleep patterns were shaped by sunrise and sunset. Days started early (they actually caught the worm … and ate it!), and after the sun went down, it was safer to huddle together and rest. Furthermore, hunter-gatherers required plenty of downtime to repair and rejuvenate from their active lifestyles. Sleep researchers believe evolution wired us for *bi-phasic* sleep patterns: a major night-time chunk (likely interrupted in primal times by security or family issues) along with a mid-day siesta, well timed to correspond with a natural circadian rhythm dip that we all experience in the afternoon hours.

Today, with life exponentially more hectic and stressful than at any time in human history, adequate sleep and restoration are widely neglected. Primarily to blame is excess artificial light and digital stimulation after dark, along with ingestible toxins (e.g. sugar, alcohol and prescription and over-the-counter medications) and, of course, the ubiquitous alarm clock. It's critical to minimise your exposure to artificial light after dark, create calm, relaxing transitions into sleep time and then obtain sufficient hours of sleep such that you wake up naturally (no alarm, except on occasional special circumstances) refreshed and energised.

Adequate sleep helps the immune system function optimally and promotes the release of the key hormones that enhance brain and endocrine function, and plays a major role in regulating appetite and metabolising fat optimally. Go to sleep at the same time each night after a calm, deliberate wind down – no television, heavy exercise, big meals or other high stimulation before bed. Your sleep requirements will vary according to lifestyle circumstances (early airplane flights, etc.), but establishing a solid foundation of excellent habits is essential. Don't be afraid to take naps when your afternoon energy levels lull. The world will not miss you while you grab a few winks, and you will refresh the optimum balance of brain chemicals to increase productivity when you get back at it. Even a 20-minute siesta can provide awesome benefits when you are deficient in sleep.

PRIMAL BLUEPRINT LAW NUMBER 7: PLAY

Our ancestors spent hours every day involved in various forms of social interaction not related to their core 'careers' of securing food and shelter and caring for their young. Studies of modern hunter-gatherers, such as the !Kung Bushmen of the Kalahari Desert in Africa, reveal that they generally work far fewer hours and have more leisure time than the average 40-hour-plus modern worker. Anthropologist Marshall Sahlins's popular theory of the 'original affluent society' argues that hunter-gatherers are able to achieve affluence (indeed a more literal definition than the consumerism-tainted one that we are familiar with) by desiring little and thereby meeting those desires in normal daily life.

Once the day's catch was complete, or the roots, shoots, nuts and berries had been gathered, it was time for Grok to play. Youngsters would chase each other around and wrestle, vying for a place higher up in the tribe's social strata. Primal humans might also have practised spear- or rock-throwing for accuracy, chased small animals just for sport, or spent time hanging out and grooming each other. The net effect of their play was to support family and intergenerational bonding, unwind from frequent life-threatening stress and also keep their bodies primed for the physical challenges of daily life.

Today *play* is a four-letter word. We still pick blackberries in our spare time, but now a BlackBerry is on a website and comes with various calling plan options and messaging features. The unrelenting stimulation of modern life, combined with the consumerism mentality of the free market economy, makes play more important than ever, yet more difficult to schedule. Take some time every day to unplug from the office or daily chores and have some unstructured fun. If you have children, you can model that play is a lifetime endeavour and you can learn a few things from them while you're at it! Besides being fun and socially redeeming, play offers biochemical benefits in the form of endorphins released into the bloodstream, while also providing a healthy cognitive balance to the excessive mental strain and endless stimulation thrust upon us in the digital age.

PRIMAL BLUEPRINT LAW NUMBER 8: GET ADEQUATE SUNLIGHT

Cavemen (and women) didn't spend their days inside caves, they were outdoors pursuing their various survival tasks and leisure endeavours. Regular sun exposure allowed Grok to manufacture plenty of vitamin D, which is critical to healthy cell function. Adequate vitamin D is nearly impossible to obtain from diet alone, and we must manufacture this hormone internally through the exposure of large skin surface areas to sufficient amounts of sunlight over the long term (vitamin D can be stored up in summer and dispensed during the winter months).

Today getting plenty of sunlight – and hence vitamin D – is nowhere near a given, what with our penchant for spending much of our time in confined spaces, such as cars, offices and homes – and screening obsessively when we do venture out into the big, bad sun. Experts believe a variety of serious health problems result from this relatively abrupt change in human lifestyle (sound familiar from our advent of agriculture discussion?). Besides the critical vitamin D requirement, sunlight also has a powerful mood-elevating effect, which can enhance productivity at work and comfort with interpersonal relations.

Getting regular sunlight implies that you are spending time outdoors, appreciating the open space and breathing fresh air. The net effect of taking time to enjoy these positive environmental surroundings (perhaps during your daily moderate exercise sessions!) is an excellent stress-balancer to being in confined spaces with artificial light and stale air. Your cells become truly energised on a biochemical level when you obtain regular doses of sunlight, fresh air and open space. While burning is certainly not healthy, maintaining a slight tan over much of the year indicates that you have adequate vitamin D exposure.

PRIMAL BLUEPRINT LAW NUMBER 9: AVOID STUPID MISTAKES

Our ancestors required a keen sense of observation and self-preservation to avoid danger. They were always scanning, smelling and listening to their surroundings, ever aware of potential trouble from saber-toothed tigers, falling rocks, poisonous snakes or even a twisted ankle from a careless step. Hypervigilance and risk management were premium skills honed to perfection every day. Even minor mistakes could prove disastrous, such as scraping a knee on a rock and dying from an ensuing infection gone unchecked.

Today, vicious tigers are not a life-threatening safety concern (except at the San Francisco Zoo in 2007, but I digress …), but we humans carelessly (can you say, 'multitasking'?) find ways to invite pain and suffering of a different nature into our lives. Buckle your seat belt, don't drink, text or talk while driving, and be prepared and hypervigilant when you go backpacking in the wilderness, descend a steep hill on your 15-pound racing bike, or use a blowtorch, chain saw, or tile cutter. Devote a little more attention and energy to risk management in your daily choices so you can enjoy a long, happy life and pass your own superior genes to the next generation.

PRIMAL BLUEPRINT LAW NUMBER 10: USE YOUR BRAIN

One of the most important things that separate humans from all other animals is intellectual ability. The rapid increase in the size of our brains over just a few thousand generations was the combined result of optimum dietary choices (including consuming high levels of healthy fat and protein – see Law Number 1) and a continued reliance on complex thought – working the brain just like a muscle. The best proof of this is the fact that hunter-gatherers all around the world developed language, tools and superior hunting methods independently.

While you might argue that we use our minds a lot to navigate and make money in today's world, the reality is that many of us are stuck in unfulfilling or rote jobs or are otherwise disconnected from continued intellectual challenge and stimulation. Numerous studies of general intelligence qualities identify curiosity as one of the most profound markers of intelligence. Opportunities for intellectual stimulation are everywhere in daily life. Commit to some personal challenges, such as learning a new language, playing a musical instrument, or taking an evening college class. Research indicates that the risk of devastating mental conditions including depression, dementia and Alzheimer's can be reduced by keeping your brain active as well as your body.

THAT'S IT

Aside from – ahem – the reproductive act, I challenge you to name any other significant behaviour that shaped our genes and today plays a critical role in our health and well-being.

Could it really be this simple? Could the prevention of and cure for obesity, diabetes, heart disease, physical decline, most cancers and the general overstressed existence of the modern human be contained in our genes? While you may be able to find detractors to extract bits and pieces of this blueprint and offer up a critical view, the premise is absolutely unassailable: our genes are suited for a hunter-gatherer existence, because that is how we *Homo sapiens* have evolved and spent the great majority of our time on earth.

The same genes that turn against you to develop heart disease, diabetes, atherosclerosis, high blood pressure, high cholesterol, arthritis and most other degenerative diseases can also be reprogrammed to unlock a leaner, fitter, more energetic body, a substantial slowing of the ageing process and a reduced risk of illness, injury and burnout. The secret is to do the right thing: follow lifestyle habits that promote desirable gene expression and avoid those that promote negative outcomes.

That statement alone – to do the right thing – is no revelation. The revelation here is how easy, natural and fun the lifestyle behaviours are that will help you build your ideal body. Now you can enjoy natural, delicious, nutrient-dense foods that promote good health and effortless weight management by moderating insulin production. Now you have permission to back off from uncomfortable workouts and regimented schedules and instead enjoy an active lifestyle with

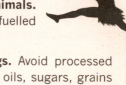

LEARN THEM, KNOW THEM, LIVE THEM!

Law Number 1: Eat Lots of Plants and Animals. Enjoy the natural, satisfying foods that fuelled two million years of human evolution.

Law Number 2: Avoid Poisonous Things. Avoid processed foods (trans- and partially hydrogenated oils, sugars, grains – even whole grains – and legumes) that are foreign to our genes and make us fat and sick.

Law Number 3: Move Frequently at a Slow Pace. Enhance fat metabolism and avoid burnout by keeping active but taking it easy.

Law Number 4: Lift Heavy Things. Brief, intense sessions of functional, full-body movements support muscle development and delay ageing.

Law Number 5: Sprint Once in a While. Occasional all-out sprints trigger optimal gene expression and beneficial hormone flow.

Law Number 6: Get Adequate Sleep. Avoid excessive artificial light and digital stimulation after dark to align your natural circadian rhythm with the sun and enjoy optimal immune, brain and endocrine function.

Law Number 7: Play. Balance the stresses of modern life with some unstructured, physical fun! Both brief breaks and grand outings are essential to mental and physical well-being.

Law Number 8: Get Adequate Sunlight. Don't fear the sun; adequate sun exposure helps synthesise vitamin D to ensure healthy cell function.

Law Number 9: Avoid Stupid Mistakes. Cultivate hyper-vigilance and risk management to avoid those mistakes that bring 'avoidable suffering' to modern humans.

Law Number 10: Use Your Brain. Engage in creative and stimulating activities to nurture your mental health and overall well-being.

regular low-intensity aerobic movement punctuated by occasional brief and very intense efforts. You can even hang out in the sun and take a nap in the name of health!

You will notice the benefits of the Primal Blueprint lifestyle laws in a matter of days, not weeks or months. Your genes are active all the time, either helping you build, regenerate and maintain homeostasis or unintentionally tearing you down. It's all based on the environmental signals you provide them through your food, exercise and lifestyle choices.

> '[My] greatest error has been not allowing sufficient weight to the direct action of the environments, ie, food, climate, etc., independently of natural selection [upon evolution].'
> CHARLES DARWIN

CHAPTER SUMMARY

- **Grok:** The survival of the fittest drove two million years of evolution to create the ultimate human being – 10,000 years ago! Grok is the nickname for our primal human lifestyle role model, who was bigger, stronger and, in many respects, healthier than us. Soon after Grok's time, the advent of agriculture across the globe eliminated the main selection pressure on humans: starvation. Civilisation effectively resulted in a slowing of our evolution and we have gone soft as a consequence. However, because our DNA is virtually identical to Grok's, we can adapt his evolutionary-based lifestyle behaviours into our 21st-century lives in order to pursue optimum health. The overall functioning of your body is primarily dependent on how your genes respond to signals in their immediate environment. *The Primal Blueprint* is an instruction manual consisting of 10 simple behaviour laws that direct our genes to build a healthy, energetic, happy, lean, strong, bright, productive modern human.

- **Diet:** Eat plants and animals and avoid processed foods (sugar products, grains, legumes and manufactured foods with chemically altered fats). Grains, while a global food staple long believed to be healthy, should be avoided because they stimulate an excessive release of insulin and are far less nutritious than vegetables, fruit, nuts, seeds and animal foods. A diet emphasising grains (and legumes, to a lesser extent) inhibits fat metabolism, precludes us from eating more nutritious plant and animal foods, and also paves the way for serious disease.

- **Exercise:** Move frequently at a slow pace (walking, jogging, hiking – avoiding excessive medium-to-high intensity cardio), lift heavy things (regular strength-training sessions that are brief and intense), and conduct occasional all-out, short-duration sprints to stimulate growth hormone release, build muscle, reduce fat and delay the ageing process.

- **Lifestyle:** Get adequate sleep (it restores muscles and rejuvenates the brain), find time in your busy schedule for unstructured play (which relieves stress and improves emotional and mental well-being on a chemical level), get plenty of sunlight (to stimulate the production of important vitamin D and help balance the negative effects of spending excessive time confined indoors), avoid making stupid mistakes by practising hypervigilance and risk management for today's hazards, and use your brain for creative pursuits that balance the often repetitive or intellectually rote elements of your existence.

- **Blueprint for Success:** The Primal Blueprint laws are simple and intuitive, unlike many elements of conventional wisdom that suggest you have to struggle and suffer to attain your fitness and weight-loss goals. You will notice the benefits of Primal Blueprint living immediately – more even energy, better immune function, more enjoyable eating and exercising – as your genes direct your cells to function optimally at every moment.

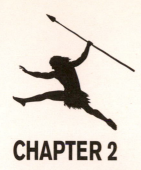

CHAPTER 2

GROK AND KORG

FROM INDIGENOUS TO DIGITAL: ONE GIANT STEP (BACKWARDS) FOR MANKIND

IN THIS CHAPTER

We will examine the contrasting daily lives of Grok and his primal family with their modern-day antithesis, the Korg family. No, not to see who can travel 20 miles quicker (the Korgs' SUV beats Grok's bare feet with a few hours to spare … although the story might be different if it were a race on foot!), but to examine the benefits of adapting primal behaviours to the modern world and the damage caused by living in conflict with our genetic predisposition to be fit, healthy and happy.

The extremely unhealthy saga of the Korgs might seem embellished, but it's actually a statistically accurate indicator of many lifestyle trends today: hectic schedules compromising quality family time; an emphasis on quick-cook processed foods in place of natural, home-prepared foods; prescription drugs used in place of making a lifestyle change; digital entertainment replacing physical activity; and overly stressful exercise programmes that cause even the most devoted to fail their weight loss and fitness goals.

While the story is distressing, the good news is that with some simple, enjoyable lifestyle modifications the momentum can turn immediately in the direction of better health (including freedom from dependence on prescription medications), higher energy, successful long-term weight loss and a more enjoyable life for you and your family.

> *'A man's health can be judged by which he takes two at a time – pills or stairs.'*
> JOAN WELSH

As we contrast a day in the life of our primal and modern families, we must refrain from the common knee-jerk rationalisations about the superiority of today's technological world. While infant mortality rates and death from tiger attacks are way down (notwithstanding that 2007 taunting incident at the San Francisco Zoo), it is sobering (pardon the pun) to consider that motor vehicle accidents heavily influenced by alcohol use are the leading cause of death for youths aged between 15 to 24, followed by suicide and homicide. While no one is arguing that we should disavow our worldly possessions and go back in time to live in mud huts and wield spears, even so, we must take a hard look at our lifestyles and absorb some powerful lessons offered by the legacy of our ancestors.

LIVIN' LARGE 10,000 YEARS AGO

Your impression of primal life might be negatively coloured by sensationalised portrayals of pre-civilisation humans as filthy, grunting savages dwelling in caves or by the harrowing vision of man potentially meeting his doom in the jaws of a beast or by the fangs of a snake. Unpleasant camping experiences (you know – too many mosquitoes, strange night noises, or no hot showers) might add to a dark vision of what it might have been like to live in hunter-gatherer times. Indeed, life was rough in many ways – much time and energy was devoted to getting food and other basic essentials that we take for granted. However, in many other ways – including the most simple and fundamental areas necessary for a healthy, happy life – Grok actually had it pretty good.

Ten thousand years ago, in a time period coinciding with the ending of the last major Ice Age, the continent of North America was populated with small bands of hunter-gatherer tribes. Many theorise that this migration (probably driven by the tracking of big game herds) originated in Russia and moved very slowly eastwards over dozens of generations across the Bering Land Bridge (which became submerged about 10,000 years ago) and then south into Canada and the United States. These tribes typically numbered 10 to 30 people and were comprised of nuclear or extended families. While the average human life expectancy was about 33 in Grok's time,[1] if Grok had been able to avoid misfortune by accident, predator or illness, his life expectancy would have increased dramatically. Shortly after Grok's time, the advent of agriculture drastically changed the nature of human life on earth and caused numerous markers of human health to steadily decline. Matt Ridley, author of *The Agile Gene*, reports that the average brain size in 50,000 BC was 1,567cc for males and 1,468cc for females. Strange as it may seem, average brain sizes today are 1,248cc for males and 1,210 for females, with the onset of the shrinkage closely related to the advent of agriculture.

GROK'S WALK

Grok and his longtime mate have two children: a 12-year-old boy and a one-year-old girl. Two other children didn't make it past infancy, a traumatic yet unavoidable part of life that the couple likely mourned deeply but from which they quickly moved on. Grok and his small band of 20 relatives live in what is now known as the great Central Valley of California. It's a cool, moist climate supporting vast pine forests, owing to the lower mean temperatures of the era (the mean earth temperatures have continued to rise over the last 10,000 years).

The gathering of berries and other fruit, leafy greens, primitive roots, shoots and other vegetation, nuts and seeds provide the bulk of Grok's food supply. Grok probably enjoys fish from nearby rivers and hunts a variety of small mammals, such as beaver, rabbit, squirrel and mole. He might score occasional big game (mammoth, mastodon, bison, bear, lion, saber-toothed tiger, wolf, deer and moose), but these animals are nearing the end of their era. He also enjoys the rich nutrition offered by various juicy, high-protein insects (remember, I said we'll strive to model *most* of Grok's lifestyle behaviours …).

Naturally, we'll start our day with Grok's family at sunrise. They awaken easily to the sound of birds chirping and begin their morning routine amidst the ageless singsong babble of a one-year-old. First things first – time to put together the morning meal. Grok's mate provides the baby with the most nutritious food ever known to human kind: breastmilk. The baby will begin to eat solid food within a few months but will continue to rely heavily on breastmilk for three years. This not only will provide nutrition for physical growth but will give her immune system a head start in dealing with potential health issues that her mother has already overcome.

Grok's son will also enjoy a power breakfast. Because it's now late summer, special treats abound in the form of fat grub worms and local berries in their narrow ripening window. The current bounty is a far cry from the severe reduction in their caloric intake the previous winter, caused by unusually heavy rains. Fortunately, Grok and his family had been able to tap into their genetic ability to efficiently mobilise their stored body fat and make up for the caloric deficits in their diet. The family had also adapted to their winter circumstances by sleeping more and reducing their daily activity level.

The son gladly handles the chore of picking a basket of berries and quickly returns to camp. After breakfast, they turn their attention to preparing items for their daily endeavours: tidying up woven storage receptacles, sharpening rudimentary weapons such as spears and packing food rations (mostly nuts and seeds) for their planned journey. Today they are going for a long walk, heading east towards the Sierra foothills to gather more berries and perhaps score some small game. Everyone is eager – even though the temperature will be warm and the walk will be longer than their typical daily wanderings – because they will get to enjoy a cool dip in a river at the midpoint of their journey.

After a nutritious breakfast, the family heads out, mother carrying the baby and the pre-teen keeping busy harassing squirrels with rocks. Arriving at the river, they feast on more berries and a few freshwater clams, sip clean water, and blissfully bathe, splash and jump off rocks into the crystal clear and brisk river. Grok's occasional brief exposure to cold water offers more than fun.[2] He doesn't know it, but this activity is considered a 'natural' healer that helps boost immune function and antioxidant defence, decreases inflammation and pain, and increases blood flow and lymphatic function – something which is particularly therapeutic for tired muscles.

After his splash, Grok lounges on a sunbaked rock. His eyes gradually begin to shut, and he nods off for a power nap. As soon as his eyes fully close, positive hormonal changes occur in Grok's body.[3] Humans have adapted to obtain great benefits from even brief naps; one reason for this is that the need for continued vigilance at nighttime against predators or other dangers made uninterrupted sleep difficult. Another is because the relaxed pace of primal life lends itself to afternoon shut-eye opportunities. Grok quickly drifts into the deepest, most restorative 'delta' sleep cycle. Stress hormone levels are moderated and his brain chemicals are rebalanced, allowing him to wake up 20 minutes later refreshed and relaxed. The daughter takes the opportunity to doze off for far longer, even as she is hoisted up into her carrying sling as the family heads off.

Clad in skirts made of plant fibres and animal skin, the family moves effortlessly in bare feet over undulating terrain and makeshift animal trails. The ground is covered with rock and plant debris, including sharp burrs discarded by native plants, but they deftly cruise along for hours without so much as cramp or a stubbed toe. Even at 12 years old, Grok's son has already developed excellent cardiovascular endurance, muscle strength and balance. And because a physically challenging life is routine to him, he probably doesn't moan or complain about the length of the journey or the boredom factor ('Are we there yet?'). After all, no video games await for him back at home .... The parents pause on numerous occasions to teach their son about native plant life, point out animal markings, and dispense other environmental lessons that will serve him well and keep him safe and well fed as he grows to assume ever more challenging and valuable hunter-gatherer responsibilities.

> *'Typical of humans 10,000 years ago, Grok and his family are of similar height and weight (but with more muscle and less body fat) to a modern family.'*

Typical of humans 10,000 years ago, Grok and his family are of similar height and weight (but with more muscle and less body fat) to a modern family. Grok sports a single-digit body fat percentage and the well-balanced physique of today's Olympic decathlete. Pardon the expression, but Grok's mate, by today's standards, would probably qualify as a 'hottie'. Her active lifestyle gives her the striking attributes of a ballerina, a gymnast and an ironman triathlete rolled into one enviable primal physique.

While Grok initially had planned to return to their permanent settlement that same evening, he chats briefly with his mate to discuss a spontaneous change of plans – to rest for the day and camp out. Because expectations and complexities are so minimal in Grok's life, the family easily goes with the flow of significant decisions like these without a second thought – this despite being unprepared for an overnight stay. It simply means a couple of hours' additional work to gather up materials and construct a temporary shelter, build a fire and get some dinner. No worry – they are safe together and accepting of every circumstance nature brings them.

Grok and his son head out for a quick hunt. We'd be surprised at how primitive their weapons are, but the duo are able to use their extraordinary intelligence and instinct about the natural world to quickly procure a couple of rabbits for dinner. Walking back to camp, their celebratory banter is rudely interrupted by the appearance of a brown bear, drawn by the smell of the carcasses and wishing to make an unfair trade of human lives for dead rabbits. A surge of fight-or-flight hormones floods the bloodstreams of Grok and his son. Grok immediately delivers a stream of detailed instructions to his son (back up slowly, maintain eye contact, etc.). His son nods calmly, stifling his instinct to scream or run in the interest of survival. Grok, seemingly fearless in the face of this menacing creature, calmly lays the rabbits down on the ground and carefully joins his son in deliberate retreat. The bear issues a couple of loud roars just to be sure everyone knows who's boss, gathers his 'kill' and moseys along. For good measure, Grok and his son take off on a dead sprint for 60 seconds, until they are safely out of the predator's sight.

Twenty minutes later, the fight-or-flight chemicals have worn off, the father-and son debriefing is complete and Grok arrives back at camp with empty hands and, most likely, a smile and shrug of the shoulders. This gesture epitomises the requisite disposition for the uncertainty of primal life. It's a coping mechanism we have hardwired into our genes: 'Don't worry, be happy.'

Meanwhile, Grok's mate has discovered some leafy green vegetation that they can eat raw or cook briefly over the campfire with a few wild potatoes. A computer analysis of the nutrient content of the food they consume, even without the rabbits, over the course of a typical month (a sufficient time period to account for the feast-or-famine realities of primal life and our graceful genetic ability to deal with it effectively) would reveal optimum levels of carbo-hydrates, protein, fat, vitamins, minerals, fibre, antioxidants and other elements they need to sustain a lifetime of exceptional fitness and vibrant health. Similarly, if we were to draw Grok's blood for laboratory analysis, this primitive human would likely come up a big winner by today's health standards: he would be free of disease markers such as high C-reactive protein levels (indicative of unde-sirable systemic inflammation); he would possess ideal levels of cholesterol, triglycerides, blood glucose and insulin; and he would be free of common modern-day nutrient deficiencies.

After dinner, the family lingers around the campfire for perhaps an hour or two, relaxing, telling stories and winding down the day as the sun sets. This routine of quality family time in the evening is likely more than today's average working parents spend with their children in an entire week (families average 19 minutes together per day of time free from television and other distractions).[4] As the sun sets, Grok and his family are ready for a good night's sleep.

> *'Don't bother about being modern. Unfortunately it is the one thing that, whatever you do, you cannot avoid.'*
> SALVADOR DALÍ

THE AMERICAN DREAM – UNPLUGGED (OR SHOULD WE SAY, 'PLUGGED IN?')

Our modern family, the Korgs (Korg is Grok spelled backwards – fitting when you consider the Korgs' dramatic departure from Grok's simple, healthy lifestyle), live where Grok did in California's Central Valley, in what is now known as Stockton.

Stockton is a medium-sized, middle-income community located

on the Sacramento River delta, only an hour's drive from the metropolitan San Francisco Bay Area, which has a population of some seven million. The Korgs – and thousands of other families like them in bedroom communities outside the Bay Area proper – believe they have the best of both worlds: an 'easy' commute to the Bay Area and its salaries, combined with affordable housing (Stockton's median home price is several hundred thousand dollars less than most comparable homes in the Bay Area), less congestion, and good recreational, educational and cultural opportunities. Ken Korg's two hours a day in the car seems like a routine cost of living the American Dream.[5]

AN ALARMING MORNING

Waking up naturally with the sun? Not the Korgs. Ken's wife, Kelly, is up and out of the house when it's still dark, heading to the gym for a 6am Spinning class. It's a struggle for her to get onto the bike for that class three days a week, but Kelly knows that her only chance to get a workout – or, for that matter, to enjoy some personal time – is before the family stirs and the responsibilities pile up. Besides, Kelly has struggled all her life with her body weight and would dearly love to drop the 20 or more pounds suggested by her physician to get her body mass index (BMI) into the healthy range.

When the alarm clock emits its digital chirping bird signal (very similar to Grok's; you can also choose breaking waves or wind chimes!) in the darkness of 5.15am, an immediate stress reaction initiates throughout Kelly's body. Even the benign digital birds jolt her abruptly out of a restful sleep cycle and stimulate a mini fight-or-flight response by spiking her cortisol levels. Rising in the dark further disrupts her circadian rhythm (since a variety of hormones and brain chemicals are sensitive to light and dark cycles), resulting in a stressful start to Kelly's day – ironic in that her early-morning workout is part of her sincere commitment to becoming more healthy.

The rest of the Korg family avoids Mum's cortisol spike, but due to a host of other factors, they have their own issues waking up. Ken is already awake when his alarm sounds at 7am, but his mind and body are in no hurry to get up and out of bed. Part of his situation is psychological – he is not terribly excited at the prospect of an hour on the roads, but other factors in his body's slug imitation are the medications he's taking and the previous night's late dessert – a generous slice of cheesecake made with 60g of processed carbohydrates, partially hydrogenated vegetable oil and assorted unpronounceable chemical preservatives.

Ken's cheesecake spiked his blood glucose just as he was attempting to fall asleep, interfering with the release of melatonin that naturally triggers sleepiness. Instead of spending the first hour in bed drifting into ever deeper cycles of sleep, Ken was fidgeting and twitchy because of the excess blood glucose in his system. Besides the glucose coursing through his veins, Ken's brain waves were jacked up from spending the final 90 minutes of his evening watching television. Even though he was exhausted and thus attempting to wind down after a long day, the fast-moving, flickering images on the screen (often violent or otherwise arousing) caused irregular stimulation to Ken's retina. This type of stimulus is transferred directly to the brain via the optic nerve and disturbs the normal function of the hypothalamus, the control centre for many vital body functions, including the initiation of proper sleep patterns.[6]

Alas, Ken is one of more than 30 million Americans to hold a prescription for sleep medication,[7] which he reaches for on occasions like these. The quick-acting sleep medication, combined with the eventual heavy insulin release to counter the cheesecake, has Ken dead to the world within 20 minutes of taking the pill. Seven hours later, the effects of his Ambien pill are still pronounced; he feels sluggish and groggy instead of naturally refreshed and energised.

Nevertheless, it's time to get the Korg clan moving, so Ken drags himself out of bed and heads over to the bedrooms of his 14-year-old son and six-year-old daughter. Rousing them is no easy task. Kenny Korg is experiencing his greatest need for sleep since infancy, and, like most modern teenagers, he isn't getting enough.[8] Kenny is also affected by a couple of other common adolescent conditions: drowsiness during the day and a delayed circadian phase, which has him naturally wanting to stay up later and wake up later.

Kenny would feel fantastic with a regular afternoon power nap, but of course napping isn't cool, so he usually fights his body's need by ingesting a caffeine-laced energy drink or soda. He effortlessly stays up late playing computer games or cruising MySpace and texting his friends. Because he often doesn't power down until 11pm or sometimes midnight, the 7am alarm comes far too early for him to feel rested and energised.

Young Miss Cindy Korg has her own troubles waking up. The mind-numbing effects of the cherry-flavoured antihistamine/decongestant/cough suppressant/analgesic over-the-counter medication her mum gave her the previous evening are still lingering after a fitful sleep. She wakes up groggy, with blocked sinuses, but must rally to get to school on time. Cindy's third upper respiratory tract infection this year was chalked up to 'the bug that's going around'; however, bugs are always going around; it was really her suppressed immune system –weakened by the ever-present processed carbohydrates and sugars in her diet – that prevented her from easily containing the virus after the first contact.

Kelly, always wanting to do the right thing as a mother, unknowingly prolonged Cindy's ordeal by giving her a common cold 'remedy' that was intended to ease her suffering but in fact interfered with her daughter's natural defences. Pounding the cough syrup every four hours for a few days more than likely doubled the time required for complete recovery by quelling the mild fever that was her primary defence against the virus, blocking the production of mucus intended to drain the virus into the stomach (where it can easily be killed by stomach acid), drying out the sinuses so she could breathe easier (but causing them to swell to the point that she can't breathe out of her nose at all this morning), and suppressing a productive cough that might have kept her up at night but would have allowed her lungs to expel the virus-laden mucus. These 'symptoms' were actually Cindy's potent gene-based natural defences – all thwarted by modern medicine.

Cindy's tendency to get sick more often than other kids her age is partly due to immune-suppressing dietary factors but also may be strongly associated with Kelly's choice to stop breastfeeding her after only three months. Tired of waking up every few hours at night or having to interrupt her work day to pump breast milk, and having been sold on the benefits of infant formulas by TV and magazine ads, Kelly made the switch at least a year earlier than many progressive pediatricians would have recommended. Simply by the mother coming into contact with the baby's skin and picking up any pathogens on the body, the mother's immune system manufactures the antibodies and immune cells required to resist infections. She then passes those antibodies and lymphocytes ('natural killer' white blood cells) to the baby through breast milk. For that reason, many cultures breastfeed for two or three years. At any rate, Cindy finally summons the strength to get dressed and head downstairs.

Kelly bursts through the door as the family is shuffling around trying to get ready for the day. She's chipper and energised from her 50-minute class, which elevated her heart rate to 85 per cent of maximum or higher for most of that time period. The intensity of the effort has released a flood of stress hormones into her bloodstream, so she's on a 'runner's high' (due to the effects of natural painkilling endorphins) as she greets her family. Kelly quickly sticks three waffles into the toaster. Trying to shop healthy, she always chooses wholegrain waffles for her family. (I'll detail on page 190 in Chapter 5 – 'The Holes in the Whole Grain Story' – why whole grains can even be considered *less healthy* than refined.)

Kelly dutifully cracks open a can of meal-replacement drink. Main ingredients: skimmed milk powder, sugar, fructose and cocoa, along with plenty of chemicals, synthetic vitamins and vegetable oils – not much nutrition but plenty of simple carbohydrates (38g) to raise blood glucose temporarily and stimulate an insulin surge. The 'good' news is that it contains only 240 calories. A minute later, the Korgs' power breakfast is ready: orange juice and wholegrain waffles with some DNA-disturbing margarine and 'low sugar' maple syrup (made with artificial sweeteners[9] and woefully far removed from the sweet nectar that flows out of a hole drilled in a Vermont maple tree). Kelly's second shake at lunch will result in a total of only 480 calories consumed since seven o'clock the previous evening – a period of 17 hours. While our bodies are adept at supplying adequate energy through intermittent food consumption (such was the reality of daily life for Grok), Kelly's high-intensity dawn workout coupled with the energy demands of her busy day make it not a good time to skimp on healthy food. As a consequence, her body's genetically programmed mechanisms (the same used by Grok in wintertime or when facing starvation) will attempt to slow down her metabolic rate to conserve fat stores and send a powerful signal to the appetite centre in her brain to consume excessive carbohydrate calories (to quickly replace lost muscle glycogen and protect against this perceived starvation).

Unlike Grok, Kelly's calorie-restriction efforts will not result in the burning of stored body fat, because the frequent insulin spikes after her high-carbohydrate shakes, eating binges and even 'healthy' American meals can inhibit fat burning and, in fact, (with high-insulin eating habits followed over time) produce metabolic changes that make it increasingly difficult to mobilise stored fat for energy. This condition is obviously affecting Kelly – such an active, disciplined person failing so miserably to reduce body fat. The net effect of Kelly's punishing (elite athletes spend a substantially lower percentage of total exercise time at elevated heart rates than Kelly) 10 early-morning workouts and devoted calorie restriction is a reduction in muscle mass (which further lowers her metabolic rate and certainly doesn't improve her body image), an increase in body fat (due to the binge eating and slowed metabolic rate), and recurring fatigue, mood swings and frustration.

The sting of failure is intensified every time Kelly sees her peppy neighbour Wendy, who has dropped eight pounds in two weeks since following her new multi-level marketing-driven cleansing diet. Upon further examination of these remarkable results, however, it's evident that the eight pounds consist almost entirely of water and muscle tissue. Wendy's severe calorie-restriction programme kicks into gear a fight-or-flight response mechanism known as gluconeogenesis (gluco is Latin for 'sugar', neo for 'new', genesis for 'make'), where her muscle tissue is converted into glucose to supply her energy needs. The depleted state of her muscles results in significant water loss, considering that every gram of stored glycogen binds with four grams of water in the body. The eight pounds will return in a matter of days when exhaustion causes a return to normal, or supernormal, calorie intake.

'THAT PROBLEM'... AMONG OTHERS

Ken hates these first few minutes after Kelly gets home from her morning workout, because her energy level makes such a stark contrast to the slow-moving household. On the flip side, Kelly is famous for shutting down around 8.30pm, after the stress hormone buzz wears off and insulin floods her system following dinner. With Ken's contrasting late-evening pattern, time for couple intimacy is virtually non-existent. Furthermore, Ken has recently been experiencing 'that problem' but is hesitant to share his concerns with anyone, let alone make an appointment with a physician to receive a prescription for Viagra. After all, Ken is still in his forties and thinks Viagra is for old guys. Ken would be surprised to learn that about a third of all erectile prescriptions are dispensed to men under 50 and that use by men under aged 45 tripled between 1998 and 2002.

Biochemically, Ken has several issues that contribute to his poor performance. The sustained high levels of cortisol in his bloodstream from his stressful lifestyle factors, such as inadequate sleep and job stress, suppress testosterone production which leads to diminished energy levels, weakened immune function, and, of course, reduced sex drive. His higher-than-optimum body fat levels and excessive insulin production from his high-carbohydrate diet and insufficient exercise also contribute to low testosterone, poor blood circulation and other common-but-curable impotency factors.

Oh, and I almost forgot to mention Ken's Lipitor (the world's best-selling drug, having made nearly $13 billion in sales in 2005), a statin medication he takes for 'high' cholesterol that can cause muscle and liver problems, deplete CoQ10 (coenzyme Q10; a natural anti-oxidant and cofactor that is critical to cellular energy metabolism) and, yes, inhibit sexual performance.

Ken only recently (and reluctantly, to his credit) started on Lipitor, at the behest of his doctor, who was concerned about his total cholesterol count of 205. This is not in the high-risk range by any means, but is high enough for the doctor to want to bring it down a little, which the statins manage to do quickly. Unfortunately, statins also produce serious side effects,[11] mainly by blocking the production and flow of CoQ10 into cell mitochondria. This disturbance of mitochondria hampers the body's ability to generate normal amounts of energy (hence the common statin-user complaint, 'I feel tired and weak'), as well as fight free radicals and moderate inflammation. Furthermore, statins do not affect triglyceride (blood fat) levels or LDL (the so-called bad cholesterol) particle size (bigger is worse), nor do they decrease risk of death in any women, in men over 65, or in men under 65 who have not had a heart attack.

Kelly, in turn, struggles with her self-esteem and body image, leading to reduced desire for intimacy. Furthermore, her stressful exercise regime and poor nutritional habits interfere with healthy female hormone balance and contribute to the reduction of her sex drive.

Ken fills his commuter mug with coffee, hustles Cindy (with her cold medication hangover) into the car, and they depart. The first stop is four-tenths of a mile away at her school.[12] It's four minutes until the tardy bell, and the front entrance is mobbed with a conga line of cars waiting to reach the drop-off zone. By the time Ken's car reaches its destination, Cindy is in a panic, as she will once again chase the tardy bell. Fear of a tardy slip may not be on par with a surprise visit from a bear, but the same fight-or-flight response occurs in Cindy as it did in Grok. The parting is anything but warm and comforting – a few choice words from Cindy and a quick admonishment in return from Ken: 'Fine, maybe I'll just make you walk next time!' An excellent idea, considering the short trip from home to classroom by auto has taken six minutes, whereas even a leisurely walk (say, the pace that Grok and his family maintained for several hours, while trading off carrying a small child) from home to classroom would not have taken much longer.

Ken extracts his sedan from the campus swarm and soon begins his navigation of main roads and motorways. As he drives up and over the small mountain range that marks the geographic boundary of the Bay Area, Ken spends his hour of 'solitude' listening to talk radio – bouncing back and forth between sports and news talk – and taking several phone calls from friends or co-workers in the office. This constant and distracted stimulation to a brain still experiencing the effects of Ambien leads to mental fatigue before he even sets foot in the office. What's more, at the 40-minute mark of Ken's journey, he is suffering from heartburn and bloating (from his regular consumption of fried and fatty foods, dairy products, alcohol, sugars and desserts, sodas and other carbonated beverages and substantial caloric intake before bed) as well as his typical recurring back pain (an affliction he shares with 60 to 80 per cent of the general population).

Ken reaches into his briefcase and whips out his pill container, extracting a purple pill and a white capsule. The 'healing purple pill' is Nexium (the third best-selling drug in the world with $5.7 billion in sales in 2005), which is used to treat the increasingly common condition known as gastroesophageal reflux disease (GERD) and its main symptom of heartburn. Nexium, classified as a proton pump inhibitor, blocks the production of hydrochloric acid in the stomach. This provides immediate relief for Ken's pain but seriously inhibits the digestive process, which relies on hydrochloric acid and other powerful acids to break down and assimilate nutrients from food.

Next is the white capsule Celebrex, a popular nonsteroidal anti-inflammatory (NSAID) prescription medication that reduces levels of hormone-like substances called prostaglandins which are part of a natural inflammation response occurring in Ken's body. He takes it to alleviate the back pain that accompanies the inflammation. He will pop another Celebrex this evening, as per the recommendation of his physician, who also suggested at his last visit that he schedule an appointment at a physical therapy clinic to obtain a customised back and core strengthening exercise routine. He's been meaning to do that but hasn't yet found the time.[13] Instead, Ken grabs some exercise here and there when the stars align and gaps open up in his schedule. Owing to his athletic youth, his competitive appetite is bigger than his physical condition. His forays into adult pickup basketball at the health club usually produce more tweaks and pulls than inspiration and motivation to pursue a regular, balanced total-body fitness programme.

If Ken proceeds with the typical behaviour pattern, he will use these prescription NSAIDs for years and neglect sufficient regular exercise. Down the road, owing to Ken's long-term use of such a powerful systemic anti-inflammatory medication, the drug's impact will diminish (at which point his doctor will probably put him on something stronger) and his body's natural ability to control all types of inflammation will have been steadily decimated. This will set the tone for a variety of serious health conditions to take root, including (owing to his poor diet and lifestyle habits) many cancers and heart disease. Yep, that's right, studies suggest a significant increased risk of heart attack when taking NSAIDs. Vioxx was a very popular NSAID taken by 80 million people worldwide from 1999 until 2004, when it was taken off the market due to concerns about side effects that increased heart attack risk. Celebrex sales skyrocketed as a result, until research suggested that it too posed similar risks. Celebrex sales then dropped sharply but later steadily resumed to exceed $2 billion in 2006.

> *'The idea on the medical horizon is that chronic inflammation is a root cause of degenerative disease. It is time for medical schools to improve nutrition education. If physicians are trained to use "food as medicine" they may not need to rely on drugs and their distressing side-effects to treat the inflammatory process.'*
> DR ANDREW WEIL

SPREADSHEETS AND CHOW MEIN

After an hour and eight minutes of driving from the school, Ken arrives at his office. He works as an accountant for a software company. The hours are regular (unlike many of his co-workers, who are selling or developing software and routinely working 10- to 12-hour days), and he makes a third more than he could in the same position in Stockton. Aside from the set hours and compensation benefits, the working conditions are challenging. Executives and division sales managers constantly enroll the accounting team in their hyperdrive, desperate mentality. They have a penchant for requesting ridiculously fancy presentations at short notice, or strolling into Ken's office and literally breathing down his neck to obsessively review sales figures in the days counting down to quarterly close.

The perk of being able to leave promptly at 6pm each evening is muted by the feeling of complete mental exhaustion that overcomes Ken as soon as he opens his car door in the car park. In his previous position (closer to home and for significantly less pay), Ken would take a leisurely lunch hour to eat a sandwich in the park or even join a co-worker for a light workout at the gym. He'd return to work refreshed and then proceed at a sensible pace through the afternoon hours, pausing often to share a laugh with his colleagues. Lately, he has stayed at his desk to eat lunch, which is typically procured via a 40-second drive to a busy nearby intersection which offers numerous quick food options.

Ken, inspired by Kelly's commitment, is also making a concerted effort to 'do the right thing' and eat more healthily. He eschews the burger bars for a Chinese buffet, which sounds healthier but is actually just as bad. He returns to the office armed with chow mein noodles and sweet-and-sour chicken, trying not to spill the mostly simple carbohydrate meal onto his spreadsheets. Laughter in the hallways has been replaced by the discernible buzz of anxiety, the unspoken fear that heads will begin to roll if Ken's spreadsheets don't impress stockholders and executives. In contrast to the few brief moments of Grok's life-or-death encounter with a bear, Ken's workplace is essentially a daily nine-hour grind of unrelenting moderate stress. Ken and the rest of us would still choose the spreadsheets over being held to ransom by a bear, but the impact of prolonged chronic stress is far more destructive to human health (and misaligned with our genes) than a pattern of brief intermittent stresses coupled with adequate downtime and a relaxed lifestyle.

The post-lunch, insulin-driven sugar crash hits Ken hard, so he scarfs down one of the PowerBars Kelly had thrown into his brief-case (PowerBar Energize Tangy Tropical has 42g of carbohydrates – 25 of them sugar) and heads to the break room for his daily after-noon coffee. Ken consumes two cups and one to two diet sodas each day, a total of about 250 milligrams of caffeine.[14] While this is not quite enough to classify him as an addict (actually, that's about the daily average for Americans), it is definitely another substance, along with the several prescription and over-the-counter meds, that he is dependent upon to make it through his day.

LOVE, MONEY AND INSULIN

Even while making a comfortable income by any reasonable defini-tion, the Korgs are experiencing financial stresses that are familiar to many.[15] After deductions for taxes and, of course, the enticing employee stock purchase programme (where 5 per cent of his gross income is fed back to the monster), a third of his annual net goes to mortgage and related tax and insurance costs. Other healthy chunks go to car payments and insurance, food shopping and dining out, medical expenses not covered by Ken's skimpy company policy, and the occasional whopper, such as two grand for a major surgery at the vet, two grand for Kenny Korg's class field trip to Washington, D.C., 800 bucks for Kelly's last-minute bereavement trip to the East Coast for a family friend's funeral, yet more for a weight-loss 'starter kit' that gung-ho neighbour Wendy basically forced upon them (a 28 per cent discount when buying an entire case!), and so on.

Kelly contributes to the family's bottom line by running her own stimulating but stressful business as a freelance graphic designer. The flexible hours are great, although the healthy boundary between work and personal life often gets blurred. One favourite ritual is picking up her daughter from school every day and taking her out for a treat – carrying on a fond family tradition she and her sisters enjoyed with their mother. As Eric Shlosser details in *Fast Food Nation*, Kelly is cooperating with the food industry's institutional-ised exploitation of American families that allows parents to replace quality time (particularly the nearly extinct family home mealtime, and the guilty conscience that goes with being too busy) with instant gratification – and therefore love – for their children.

The treat time coincides with Kelly's daily affliction of the afternoon blues, owing to her pre-dawn wake-up call, the caloric depletion brought about by her crash diet, and the work/parent/personal health and fitness juggling act that is her life. The colourful, peppy, healthy lifestyle messaging inside the local juice bar franchise helps Kelly rationalise about her impending insulin flash flood. She confidently orders a 24-oz Strawberry Surf Rider for herself and a 16-oz Mango-a-go-go for her daughter. Cindy excitedly suggests adding a couple of baked goods from the child's-eye-level display case to the tab. Ever vigilant, Kelly scans the choices to pick the healthiest and settles on a couple of reduced-fat blueberry-lemon loaves, 'part of a complete breakfast – complement with a smoothie or freshly squeezed orange juice,' says the menu. Each loaf offers 290 calories, 73 per cent of which come from processed carbohydrates (lead ingredients: sugar and flour) with virtually zero nutritional value and a guaranteed strong insulin response. Cindy finishes only half her loaf, but Kelly makes sure it doesn't go to waste.

The discipline of Kelly consuming fewer than 500 calories in the previous 19 hours is no match for a depleted brain and body. While the 24-oz Strawberry Surf Rider will provide Kelly with some much-deserved antioxidants and other healthy nutrients from the frozen fruit, 87 per cent of its 490 calories come from sugar. Along with one and a half blueberry-lemon loaves, Kelly has ingested 925 calories (make that an even thousand, counting a few long pulls on her daughter's straw to try the Mango-a-gogo), including 187g of refined carbohydrates (that's more than the Primal Blueprint's recommended range of 100 to 150g for an entire day!). Her sugar/insulin roller-coaster will again hamper her fat-burning efforts for hours after this onslaught and lead to fatigue and sugar cravings come dinnertime.

Young Cindy Korg's drink and half loaf send more than 100g of sugar into her little body, stressing her insulin system – and her immune system – yet again. The previous day, at a classmate's birthday party, she had consumed typical party fare of two slices of thin-crust cheese pizza (460 calories), a small slice of chocolate cake (235) with a small scoop of vanilla ice cream (150), some box juices with high-fructose corn syrup (she opened three over the course of the party and drank only half of the fluid [a typical ratio, as any parent who's hosted a birthday party can confirm] = 130 calories), and several assorted bite-sized sweets from the take-home party bag (150 calories). Her total calories in the three-hour period came to 1,125, more than half in the form of simple sugar. That's enough to stimulate a significant insulin response in a 300-pound man, let alone a 55-pound child.

Naturally (owing to family genes, her parents rationalise), young Cindy is already significantly overweight. Fortunately (from a psychological perspective only), unlike in past generations, her plump physique is shared by many of her classmates.[16] While this certainly protects her self-esteem, it makes it difficult to change the popular chartered course of this young ship, sailing towards peril and doom. Studies suggest that overweight kids are highly likely to become overweight adults and consequently suffer from serious health problems and life-threatening diseases.

> 'Studies suggest that overweight kids are highly likely to become overweight adults and consequently suffer from serious health problems and life-threatening diseases.'

KENNY'S WORLD

We haven't heard much about the Korgs' teenage son, Kenny, which is appropriate because he is already emotionally disconnected from his busy family and pulled by the powerful force of peer influence in directions that create conflict with stable family life. In his early years, Kenny was naturally active and spent hours outside running and playing. Unfortunately, each passing pre-teen year saw more sedentary technological distractions commandeering his time and innocent play in the garden being exchanged for competitive organised sports.[17]

While Kenny has some innate athletic ability, he lacks the naturally healthy aggression and competitiveness that allow young athletes to move to the front of the pack. Lacking time to connect with his son, Ken makes the common mistake of overpressurising his son's athletic experience with misplaced emotion and 'encouragement' that feels to his son like results expectations and criticism. By the time Kenny becomes a teen, he is finished with organised sports and deep into a new cultural phenomenon called MMORPG (massive multiplayer online role-playing games),[18] such as *World of Warcraft* and *Runescape*, where a player creates a digital persona and interacts with many others in a virtual world, often immersed for eight or ten hours at a time. At school, he maintains grades that are decent yet below his potential, but he is incurring increasing reports of misbehaviour in class. During a telephone conversation with the school counsellor, the topic of attention deficit hyperactivity disorder (ADHD) is broached as a potential reason for Kenny's misbehaviour.

Kenny's feelings of alienation are exacerbated at the dinner table that evening, when Ken peppers him with the exact same questions heard at breakfast about his son's decision to skip the basketball tryouts. The teen is naturally offended, unaware that one of the most common side effects of Ambien is short-term memory loss and that Ken truly has no recollection of the conversation from 12 hours before (and some eight hours after popping the Ambien).

The exchange escalates into a blowout which covers various pent-up resentments. Ken decides to make an appointment for his son to visit a psychiatrist. After two sessions, the psychiatrist diagnoses Kenny with ADHD and promptly prescribes the amphetamine Adderall[19] – despite growing controversy surrounding its overprescription to children who lack serious symptoms and a true clinical diagnosis, the potential link to serious cardiovascular side effects, and the high incidence of abuse among teenagers using the stimulant recreationally. (An estimated seven million American children take stimulants prescribed for attention disorders, a 500 per cent increase since 1991.) It's more likely that emotional factors, lack of sufficient vigorous exercise and poor dietary habits (sugar binges, regular caffeine intake and lack of healthy fats) are to blame for Kenny's adverse classroom behaviour, but unfortunately, Kenny now has another hurdle on the path to getting his mind and body back into balance for the challenging school years ahead: the powerful effects of stimulant medication on his growing body.

When critiquing the particulars of kids and their exercise, sleep, dietary habits and school high jinks, you might default to thinking, 'What's the big deal?' Kenny and millions of his peers will continue their mildly objectionable ways, but they'll get through high school just fine (provided they heed Primal Blueprint Law Number 9, Avoid Stupid Mistakes). They'll go off to college and pull all-nighters fuelled by pizza, Red Bull and Top Ramen, then they'll unwind after exam pressure with lots of alcohol, more pizza and maybe a few cupcakes at the college bash. I don't think previous generations can claim they are unfamiliar with this routine.

It's true, young people are incredibly resilient, in case you've forgotten. With metabolism accelerated and the endocrine system flooding the bloodstream with peak levels of key growth and reproductive hormones, the raw (indeed, primal) energy of youth can often override any potential insulin-driven fatigue from a Red Bull buzz wearing off. We can all attest to the difference between being at our physical peak and being beyond it. At 55, I'm proud to be able to (more or less) hang out with my teenage son, Kyle, when we play Ultimate Frisbee (the official name of the game is simply Ultimate, given that Frisbee is a brand name and you can use any type of disc to play) till we drop. Then, while I'm sunk deep into the couch/ottoman licking my wounds and icing my strains, he'll grab an apple and his skateboard (and his helmet of course ... remember Law Number 9) and bust out of the door to the next activity!

However, if we consider the concept that our genes – even young genes – are predisposed to all kinds of problems if we give them the wrong environment (and, hence, the wrong signals), we can conclude that it's just a matter of time until the fountain of youth runs dry. Remember in college those boys with six-pack abs drinking small kegs every weekend? A decade later, you can find most of them with pony keg guts drinking six-packs every weekend. As a parent or an influential figure in a child's life (or perhaps an evolved young person reading *The Primal Blueprint*!), you can assert the importance of having a foundation of healthy lifestyle habits and a deep respect and understanding for how to get the best out of your body. This will pave the way for a future different from today's extremely disturbing one in which many experts predict a shorter life expectancy for children than for their parents – for the first time since … (Anybody? Bueller? Anybody?) … the advent of agriculture 10,000 years ago.[20]

'WE HAVE MET THE ENEMY, AND HE IS US'

This classic quote uttered by Walt Kelly's popular comic strip character, Pogo, captures the Korgs' plight perfectly: their well-intentioned efforts to do the right thing seem continuously sabotaged by cultural norms and misguided conventional wisdom. We are conditioned by the powerful forces of consumerism to pursue flawed solutions to our problems and ailments. The prescription drugs downed by Ken (and now Kenny, too), Kelly's overly stressful exercise routine and overly restrictive diet, the massive amount of unhealthy food ingested by the family on a daily basis, and the lack of simple, quality family time, might be disturbing to read about, but are all absolutely the norm today.

If you felt the Korgs' tale was an appalling, melodramatic and unrealistic example of a modern family, you have lifestyle reference points that are significantly more healthy and balanced than those of the average American family. The references to the Korgs' daily routine, prescription drug use, weight-loss battles, eating and exercise habits, childhood obesity, teenage behaviour challenges and digital media use are provided in detail in the 'Grok Chapter References' appendix.

As they say, your kids grow up – and you grow old – before you know it. A lack of awareness, lack of knowledge and sometimes, sadly, a defiant, ignorant stance of disrespecting the essentials of health and well-being (including our genetic programming) tragically degrade the precious time families have together. This loss plays out every day and touches virtually every family in the modern world. It's time to stand up and take control of your health and well-being, to honour your genes by living according to *The Primal Blueprint* and, finally, to reject many tenets of conventional wisdom that are flawed and hazardous to your health. In this book, we will do just that, further building momentum and crushing obstacles in our path as we march towards the ultimate expression of our human potential.

HOW GROK PROBABLY SPENT HIS DAY

Hunting or gathering food **5 hours**

Sleep, nap, rest, relax **10 hours**

Habitat-, shelter-, basic human needs-related chores **3 hours**

Leisure time consisting of play and family or group socialising **6 hours**

Estimates derived from studies of the modern hunter-gatherer culture of the !Kung Bushmen in Africa.

HOW KEN KORG SPENDS HIS DAY

Workplace **9 hours**

Commute **2 hours**

Sleep **6.7 hours**

Television, computer, digital entertainment **4 hours 21**

Grooming, household chores, free time **2.3 hours**

(components: leisure/educational reading: 24 minutes; meaningful conversation with child: 3.5 minutes)

Estimates derived from TV Free America in Washington, D.C., American Time Use Survey Summary (U.S. Department of Labor, Washington, D.C.), A.C. Neilsen Company, and Kaiser Family Foundation.

CHAPTER SUMMARY

- **Grok's Lifestyle:** Grok faced unimaginable hardships in primal life, but in many ways he enjoyed superior health to that of modern humans. While rates of infant mortality and death by predator or accident were far higher than today, if Grok were able to avoid such tragedy, he could enjoy robust health and supreme physical fitness into his 60s or 70s. Grok's hunter-gatherer existence involved a diet of natural plants and animals, hours of low-level aerobic exercise every day, and occasional short bursts of maximum effort. Primal existence was simpler and slower paced, with life-or-death stressful events coming infrequently and lasting only briefly. This type of existence is more aligned with our genetic make-up than the unrelenting stress of modern life.

- **Korg's Lifestyle:** Our modern suburban family, the Korgs, have diverged dramatically from the lifestyle basics modelled by Grok that are essential for good health. Long commutes, packed schedules and excessive digital entertainment compromise family camaraderie. Financial pressures, insufficient sleep and downtime, extensive use of prescription drugs, poor dietary habits and exhausting exercise programmes lead to an excessively stressful modern existence and consequent health problems.

   The Korgs' diet features excessive processed foods and insufficient nutritious foods. In particular, they eat too many simple carbohydrates and grains that lead to excess insulin production. These dietary mistakes lead to assorted health problems, particularly undesirable body composition, beginning in childhood and continuing for a lifetime. Kelly Korg's well-meaning devotion to exercise and careful dieting does not lead to fat loss, because the workouts are too stressful and she regularly has excessive insulin in her bloodstream (from consuming too many carbohydrates), which inhibits fat burning. Ken's lack of exercise, poor eating habits, work-related pressures and reliance on prescription drugs to counter lifestyle errors make him tired and stressed and put him on the path to the eventual onset of serious disease. The

Korg children are victimised by the disastrous cultural trends of today's youth, such as insufficient activity, excessive digital media use, high-insulin diets and overpressurised athletic and academic experiences that lead to alienation and rebellion.

- **Your Family:** It's critical to depart from these harmful cultural trends and create a different reality for you and your family. Modifying dietary habits to Primal Blueprint recommendations and placing limits on technology and jam-packed schedules in favour of relaxing family interaction will help reverse the appalling family dynamics characterised by the Korgs' story.

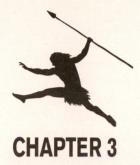

CHAPTER 3

PRIMAL BLUEPRINT EATING PHILOSOPHY

'DO THESE GENES MAKE ME LOOK FAT?'

'I bought a talking refrigerator that said "Oink" every time I opened the door. It made me hungry for pork chops.'
MARIE MOTT

IN THIS CHAPTER

Here I will present the philosophy, rationale and benefits of Primal Blueprint eating, emphasising the importance of moderating insulin production by limiting intake of processed carbohydrates – not only sugars but all cultivated grains (yep, even wholegrains). This simple dietary modification – perhaps the single most critical take-away action item from the Primal Blueprint – will allow you to avoid the immediate unpleasant physical effects of high-carbohydrate eating, succeed with long-term weight-loss goals, and prevent most common lifestyle-related health problems and diseases.

I will also reveal to you why the conventional wisdom story about cholesterol as a direct heart disease risk factor is deeply flawed. The true culprits that trigger the development of atherosclerosis are oxidation and inflammation, created largely by the Standard American Diet of excess carbohydrates and chemically altered fats. There are dietary steps you can take to virtually eliminate your risk of heart disease, including regulating your omega 6:omega 3 (O6:O3) balance to prevent systemic inflammation and virtually eliminate your risk of heart disease .

In the next few pages I will outline how each macronutrient (protein, carbohydrate, fat and the 'fourth fuel' of ketones) affects your eating strategy, energy levels and overall health, and the Primal Blueprint Carbohydrate Curve on page 107 will reveal how carbohydrate intake impacts on your health and weight management success. The concept of 'eating well' means more than just making healthy food choices; it means eating sensibly and intuitively, in a relaxed environment conducive to maximum appreciation of food and avoiding regimented, restrictive diets that lead to negativity, guilt and rebellion. To help you on your way, included here are tips on how to succeed in converting to Primal Blueprint eating without causing the stress or disappointment that is so common with unrealistic diet programmes.

> *'Obesity is really widespread.'*
> JOSEPH O. KERN II

Primal Blueprint eating offers many health benefits, which served Grok and his ancestors well for over two million years. The most important goal of eating like Grok is to minimise the wildly excessive insulin production caused by the Standard American Diet. Making this simple change will allow you to lose unwanted fat, maintain an ideal body composition for the rest of your life and eliminate the major disease risk factors that will kill more than half of all Americans. Here are some other major benefits of the Primal Blueprint eating style:

- **Fat-burning Beast!** When you reduce your consumption of grains, sugars and other simple carbohydrates in favour of plants and animals, your levels of insulin and glucagon will be in an ideal balance, enabling you to utilise fatty acids (from both food intake and stored fat) as your preferred fuel source. This helps regulate daily energy levels, even if you skip meals. In contrast, excess insulin production from a sugar-burner diet requires that you eat every few hours to bump up blood glucose levels that have crashed.

- **Effortless Weight Management:** Plants and animals are much more nutritionally dense than processed carbohydrate foods, which comprise a large percentage of calories in the typical modern diet. Eat like Grok and you'll meet your nutritional needs with fewer calories, and dramatically boost your antioxidant intake. Second, the protein and fat you will be eating have been shown by food scientists to provide deeper and longer-lasting satisfaction levels (what they call *satiety*) than you get from a high-carbohydrate diet. Finally, when you consume fewer carbohydrates and, as a result, produce less insulin, your hunger and cravings (caused by insulin removing glucose from the bloodstream after high-carbohydrate meals or snacks) will subside, and you'll intuitively moderate your caloric intake.

- **Enhanced Cellular Function:** The high-quality fat found in Primal Blueprint foods provide optimal structural components for cell membranes and encourage your body to convert stored fat efficiently into energy. This includes the well-known omega-3s, monounsaturated fats such as avocados, macadamia nuts and olive oil, and even the saturated animal fat that conventional wisdom has warned us to avoid.

- **Lean Muscle Development and Maintenance:** The high-quality protein found in Primal Blueprint foods will help you build or maintain lean muscle mass, achieve ideal bone density and control your body's day-to-day repair and renewal requirements. When you moderate insulin production, exercise sensibly and eat adequate amounts of protein, you become more *insulin sensitive*. This means the receptor sites in your muscle cells can assimilate amino acids and glucose efficiently, which is the key to muscle building and recovery.

- **Reduced Disease Risk Factors:** Ditching grains, sugars, other simple carbohydrates and processed foods, especially 'bad fats' (trans and partially hydrogenated), will reduce your production of hormone-like messengers that instruct genes to make harmful pro-inflammatory protein agents. These agents increase your risk for arthritis, diabetes, cancer, heart disease and many other inflammation-related health problems.

A SEPARATE SHELF FOR THE BLUEPRINT

You may be familiar with the decades-old best-selling Atkins diet programme, named after Dr Robert Atkins, the original proponent of 'low-carb' dieting. Over the years, numerous other programmes (e.g., *South Beach Diet* and the *Zone*) have battled for shelf space supremacy. Diet best-sellers have varied from mostly credible to completely ridiculous. Followers of Atkins, South Beach, and other low-carbohydrate diets will indeed lose fat by strictly limiting carbohydrates and thus insulin production; however, an obsessive 'ultra-low-carb' strategy can be unhealthy over an extended time period because it limits your intake of some of the most nutritional foods known to humans – vegetables and fruits.

While the Primal Blueprint also advocates eliminating the extremely harmful processed carbohydrates and sugars from your diet, vegetables and fruits are a central component of the Primal Blueprint eating strategy. Vegetables and fruits (which consist mainly of carbohydrates) are nutrient-dense yet calorically sparse, so that even generous portions of these foods will usually prompt minimal insulin production. I should really say 'seasonal fruits' and add a caveat that some moderation of fruit intake is warranted today. If you wish to reduce excess body fat, be advised that fructose (the carbohydrate form found in fruit) is more easily converted to fat in the liver than other carbohydrate sources such as simple sugar. This is particularly true if you are not exercising much and your glycogen stores are routinely full. Furthermore, we have only recently enjoyed year-round access to heavily cultivated modern fruits that are sweeter than the wild stuff Grok encountered during narrow ripening seasons. Bottoms up on the locally grown berries in the summer time, but ease off on that daily bowl of mangoes and pineapples as you strive to transform into a fat-burning beast.

One of the online Primal Blueprint appendices at MarksDaily Apple.com compares and contrasts the Primal Blueprint with popular diets such as *Atkins,* Low Fat (e.g., Ornish, MacDougall, Pritikin), Metabolic and Blood Typing, paleo-themed diets, South Beach, vegetarian and the Zone. Of all these mentioned, the paleo eating approach is the most similar to the Primal Blueprint. However, I refrain from even calling the Primal Blueprint a 'diet', due to its comprehensive nature. The Primal Blueprint is a lifestyle – with some important but extremely flexible eating guidelines. I prefer to apply the eating laws in conjunction with the other eight Primal Blueprint lifestyle laws for best results.

80 PER CENT OF YOUR BODY COMPOSITION IS DETERMINED BY HOW YOU EAT

The Primal Blueprint eating philosophy might seem a little unusual at first for those trying to do the right thing by conventional wisdom. After all, here's a plan that suggests that most fats are not bad at all. In fact, pundits might describe the Primal Blueprint as a high-fat, moderate protein, fairly low-carbohydrate diet – particularly in comparison to the exceedingly high-carbohydrate diet that has been recommended for years by the USDA Food Pyramid and Food Plate Visuals, American Heart Association and American Medical Association.

We now know that these outdated and unwarranted suggestions to eat 300 or more grams of carbohydrates each day has contributed greatly to the destruction of human health. It's not unusual for an average American now to consume 500 or 600 grams of insulin-generating, fat-storing carbohydrates daily. Keep in mind that Grok and his clan probably worked hard to gather an average daily intake of only 80 to 100 grams of carbohydrates, most of which was contained inside slow-burning fibrous wild plants. By averaging between 100 and 150 grams daily (certain extremely active folks may adjust this upwards, which I'll discuss later) of vegetable- or fruit-sourced carbohydrates, and incidental carbohydrates from nuts, seeds and moderation foods such as high-fat dairy and dark chocolate, you can achieve optimally low levels of insulin, enjoy stable energy levels and easily reduce excess body fat and keep it off. If you want to accelerate your fat loss for a period of time, lowering your average carbohydrate intake to 50 to 100 grams or less per day will allow you to easily drop an average of one to two pounds (a half to one kilogram) of body fat per week. (We will discuss this strategy in Chapter 8.) And you can do all this while eating until you're satisfied – no suffering!

Sitting down again? Here's another zinger that will blow your mind and set you straight about what the secret to weight loss and long-term body composition success really is…

> 'Eighty per cent of your ability to reduce excess body fat
> is determined by how you eat, with the other 20 per cent
> is dependent on proper exercise, other healthy lifestyle
> habits and genetic factors.'

It's as simple as this: if you have excess body fat, it's directly reflective of the amount of insulin you produce from your diet combined with your familial genetic predisposition to store fat. In plain-speak: if you eat like crap and have bad (genetic) luck, you'll get fat and sick and you'll probably die early. On the other hand, bad diet and good luck (having the 'skinny gene') might allow you to avoid a plump figure but also might result in a physique that I call 'skinny fat' – having minimal subcutaneous fat, minimal lean body mass and poor muscle definition but with dangerous amounts of visceral fat surrounding the organs.

Furthermore, skinny fat folks can and do get heart disease, hypo-glycemia, arthritis, sarcopenia (loss of muscle mass), chronic fatigue, compromised immune function, exhausted stress-management mechanism and a host of other adverse health consequences heavily attributed to diet. A slender type 2 diabetic can experience an even greater risk for serious disease, because he or she is less able to acti-vate the so-called thrifty genes that efficiently store excess dietary glucose in fat cells and as a result that glucose floats around in the bloodstream causing intense cellular damage. While the outward visibility and overall impact severity of poor lifestyle habits vary widely due to luck of the draw, we all share an evolutionary genetic predisposition to suffer chronic disease when we eat foods that are misaligned with our genes.

On the positive side, if you eat right, you can look your absolute best even if you have bad genetic luck. Your ability to reduce excess body fat and maintain desirable body composition is directly related to your ability to moderate insulin production with healthy dietary habits and, to a lesser extent, your willingness to follow a sensi-ble exercise programme that combines extensive low-level cardio: frequent brief, intense strength-training sessions and occasional all-out sprints. Even if you have struggled with excess body fat for your entire life, you can quickly and dramatically alter your destiny by following the simple laws of the Primal Blueprint.

I'm not talking about achieving 'success' with a short-term crash programme; the Primal Blueprint is based on eating as much as you want, whenever you want, from a long list of delicious foods – and simply avoiding eating from a different list. When I say you will notice results quickly and dramatically, I'm referring primarily to the immediate increase and stabilisation of energy levels, less hunger and mood swings related to 'bonking' (running low on blood glucose), improved immune function and a reduction in the symptoms of allergies, arthritis and other inflammatory conditions exacerbated by the anti-nutrients in a grain-based diet.

Regarding weight loss, we must recognise that our minds are so messed up on this topic that it's hard to even have a sensible conversation about it. The stories of losing massive amounts of weight in a short time are so commonplace that we seem to expect nothing less when we pursue weight-loss goals. First, the Primal Blueprint is really about improving body composition, instead of just losing weight. This means a reduction in body fat percentage and an increase or maintenance of muscle or lean body mass.

Clearly, gaining muscle and losing fat produces more impressive appearance changes than someone who drops 20 quick pounds on a crash diet that depletes muscle mass and water. Lean body mass (muscle, skeleton and all the rest of you that is not fat) is also directly correlated with 'organ reserve' – the highly desirable ability of all your vital organs to function optimally beyond basal level (e.g., when your heart rate elevates during exercise). We'll discuss this critical longevity component further in Chapter 6.

When you trigger your genes to stop storing body fat and start burning it, as well as to build or maintain muscle mass, you can sensibly and realistically lose a pound or two of body fat per week. You can even do this with minimal exercise, but the fat loss (and the gaining, sculpting or toning of lean muscle) will be accelerated significantly when you choose the right exercise regime. Mostly, your success depends on how diligent you are in keeping dietary insulin levels low, thereby allowing your body to obtain more of your caloric needs from your stored body fat .

Not a day goes by without a friend, client or MarksDailyApple. com commenter relating to me how he or she notices improvements within days of switching to the Primal Blueprint eating style. As I will explain in this chapter, you have the chance to alter your biochemistry at each meal – to stimulate a fat-burning metabolism and maintain consistent energy levels, or to do the opposite with poor food (and exercise) choices. The momentum you build with good choices will make it easier to discard old habits, while you gain instant gratification from satisfying meals and stable energy levels, as well as positive long-term health and metabolic consequences.

INSULIN – THE MASTER HORMONE

The insulin story is perhaps the most health-critical concept in this book, so I want you to fully understand it on both a practical and a biochemical level. Like so many things in life, a moderate amount of insulin is good and a lot can be bad – very bad. By now you understand insulin's role as a storage hormone and that eating more carbohydrates results in more insulin production. Insulin delivers nutrients to all cells, but for our purposes, we'll focus on insulin's role delivering nutrients to liver, muscle and fat cells. When the system works as designed by evolution, cell receptors use insulin as a key to unlock pores within the membrane of each cell. With the cell door open, nutrients can then be stored inside the cell. It's an elegant way for cells to gather the nutrients they need and also to eliminate excess glucose from the bloodstream (remember, excess glucose is highly toxic) and store it as fuel for a later date.

Unfortunately, when you produce too much insulin over a period of time, as happens when a modern diet is high in processed carbohydrates, several things go wrong. First, muscle and liver cells just aren't able to store a whole lot of glycogen (the stored form of glucose), so it's easy to exceed storage capacity. The average person can only store a total of about 400 grams (less than one pound) of glycogen in liver and muscle tissue (even a highly trained athlete can only store perhaps 600 total grams). When your liver and muscles become filled with glycogen, any glucose remaining in the blood-stream that isn't used in 'real time' by your brain or muscles (such as during an intense workout) gets converted into triglycerides in the liver and sent to fat cells for storage.

When blood insulin levels are high, those same fat cells store not only the excess glucose but the fat you ate at your last meal.

Moreover, high insulin signals the fat cells to hold on to the fat and not release it for energy. If the pattern of high-insulin-generating meals continues, fat cells swell up and you gain weight. Eventually, especially among people who don't exercise much, muscle and liver cells start to become *insulin resistant* – their receptors become desensitised to insulin's nutrient storage signals (the afore-mentioned insulin key doesn't unlock the cell membrane to allow nutrients in). Inactive people generally have plenty of muscle and liver glycogen stored at all times; because they are unpractised at burning energy and are inefficient at restocking energy from dietary nutrients, insulin takes ingested carbohydrates and fats on an express train, passing right through the liver to their ultimate destination in fat cells.

Continuing this process can lead to obesity and other Meta-bolic Syndrome symptoms (a combination of medical disorders). Eventually, even fat cells become resistant to further storage because we only have a fixed amount of fat cells. At that point, the body's last line of defence against glucose (the complete gorging of a finite number of fat cells) has maxed out. Consequently, all hell breaks loose in terms of blood glucose toxicity and insulin damage – leading to even greater risk for diabetes, heart attack, blindness, the need for limb amputation and other disasters.

Unless you are exercising incessantly to burn stored glycogen and fat, the more insulin your pancreas produces, the more resistant your muscle and liver cells can become. This happens because the genes responsible for these receptor sites turn themselves off or 'down-regulate' in response to – and as a defence against – the exces-sive insulin in your bloodstream. This is all part of the body's quest for balance and your genetic response to environmental signals.

This doesn't mean your daily Power Bar is going to lead to limb amputation any time soon, but as you gain further understanding of the insulin story, it becomes clear how the shocking statistic of the average American gaining one and a half pounds (two-thirds of a kilo) of fat a year for 30 years is achieved. Conversely, when insulin levels are moderated (as happens with low carbohydrate eating and/or frequent exercise), your liver and muscle cell receptor sites become *insulin sensitive* – more effective at absorbing ingested nutrients transported by insulin. Furthermore, moderated insulin levels signal genes to make more receptor sites.

An insulin-resistant liver exacerbates the situation. The 'No Vacancy' sign hanging on the liver (glucose is turned away due to insulin resistance) tricks some cells in your liver into believing they are starved of glucose. In response to the liver's storage cells refusing to accept glucose, your genes signal other specalised liver cells to commence gluconeogenesis and dump more glucose into the bloodstream, despite the fact that there's already plenty there (talk about a communication breakdown!). Of course, your resistant muscle cells are deaf to insulin signalling as well, so the new, extra glucose your liver just made is also diverted to the eager fat cells – unless they too are over-gorged with fat. Here is a quick summary of some of the unpleasant consequences of becoming insulin resistant:

- **Fat cells can't release their stored energy into the bloodstream**, where the fatty acids could be used as fuel, because insulin keeps the fat locked inside.
- **Fat cells get bigger** (and fatter), so you gain weight.
- **More glucose stays in your bloodstream longer**, causing damaging AGEs (advanced glycation end products). AGEs are chemical reactions that occur when blood-borne glucose molecules bind randomly with important proteins, rendering them useless. This can result in increased inflammation and risk of heart disease, as well as the circulation problems and neuropathies (nervous system disorders) that characterise type 2 diabetes.
- **Pancreatic beta cells**, continually sensing high levels of sugar in the bloodstream, keep working harder and harder to pump out more and more insulin. Eventually, the beta cells can become exhausted and stop working entirely – similar to the plight of insulin-dependent type 1 diabetics. All of this happens as a result of eating too many carbohydrates for too long and/or not exercising enough to maintain insulin sensitivity.

But wait, there's more! As bad as all that glucose remaining in the bloodstream is, chronically high levels of insulin are almost worse. Excessive insulin is very pro-inflammatory and can wreak havoc throughout the body. Scientists know that within any species, those that produce the least amount of insulin over a lifetime generally live the longest and remain healthiest.

Excessive insulin is also now believed to be a central catalyst in the development of atherosclerosis. Insulin promotes platelet adhesiveness (sticky platelets clot more readily) and the conversion of macrophages (a type of white blood cell) into foam cells, which are the cells that fill with cholesterol and accumulate in arterial walls. Eventually, a cholesterol and fat-filled 'tumour' blocks circulation in the artery, a situation further aggravated by increased platelet adhesiveness and thickness of the blood. In addition, insulin reduces blood levels of nitric oxide (a compound that relaxes the endothelium, the lining of your arteries), causing your artery walls to become more rigid. This drives up blood pressure and increases the sheer force of blood against the arterial wall, further exacerbating the atherosclerotic condition. (I will explain the chain of events causing atherosclerosis, and what you can do to prevent it, in more detail in the cholesterol section on page 3.)

Once you understand the process, it's instructive to take a step back and realise how important exercise is to creating insulin sensitivity (along with low-insulin eating, of course). If you frequently empty your liver and muscle cells of glycogen with brief, intense workouts (you burn a little bit of glucose during the long, slow stuff, too), you become adept at not only burning calories but replenishing nutrients. Insulin will transport nutrients into your liver and muscle instead of just having them go straight to fat. If you are sedentary and eat a moderate or high-carbohydrate diet, there is no selection pressure (to borrow an apropos term from our evolution discussions) to be insulin sensitive. My foolproof prevention plan – or, dare I say, cure – for those with type 2 diabetes, obesity and heart disease, no matter how overwhelming their genetic predisposition is to these conditions, is to exercise according to the Primal Blueprint laws and to moderate dietary insulin production.

It's interesting to note that levels of growth hormone and other important health-enhancing hormones are also adversely affected by insulin resistance. The pituitary gland makes the growth hormone, which is then sent to the liver to signal the production of insulin-like growth factors (IGFs). Many of our cells have surface receptors for IGFs. Because of its similar structure, insulin binds to IGF receptors and prevents growth hormone-stimulated IGFs doing their job. Excessive insulin also interferes with thyroid function. The thyroid gland produces a hormone called T4, which is converted in the liver to T3, the primary hormone that controls energy metabolism. When your liver becomes insulin resistant, conversion of T4 to T3 declines drastically. This leads to a decrease in metabolic rate, increased fat storage and diminished energy levels and brain function.

High insulin levels over long periods of time also hamper sex hormone synthesis, causing levels of testosterone, DHEA and other sex hormones to decline steeply as we age. Hormone levels naturally decline over time, but this flagship premise of the multibillion-dollar anti-ageing industry is very likely exacerbated by insulin resistance as opposed to the mere passing of the seasons. Remember, if Grok was lucky, he could enjoy dramatically better health and physical fitness into his 70s than most of today's baby boomers. Sex hormones are supposed to be transported through the bloodstream by globulin (a blood protein) to act upon target organs and tissues. When excessive insulin is present, these hormones can stay bound to globulin instead of getting dropped off at the target cells (e.g., the adrenal glands, sex organs and brain) and doing their thing. Even an expensive anti-ageing hormone regime cannot override this undesirable condition caused by excessive insulin.

Clearly, the ideal strategy is to use only the insulin you need to re-stock muscle and liver glycogen stores, to rebuild muscle and other tissue with amino acids and, finally, to transport fatty acids for a variety of essential metabolic functions (including energy storage). By maintaining an optimal balance between insulin and glucagon, you become like an ATM machine, always open for deposits and withdrawals based on your daily energy needs. Clearly, insulin is absolutely essential to life; it's just that chronic overproduction of insulin (also known as hyperinsulinemia) turns a good thing into a bad thing. It's as simple as this: when you eat the Primal Blueprint-style foods that fit your genes, you'll be able to fit into your jeans!

BUT A LITTLE BIT WON'T HURT, RIGHT?

If these clinical details about the long-term damage from a high insulin-producing diet are not sufficient to get you to change your breakfast order today, consider the short-term unpleasant effects of high-carbohydrate, insulin-producing meals and snacks (on otherwise healthy, non-diabetic folks).

Ingesting a high-carbohydrate food or meal (sugary foods and beverages, desserts, processed grains, etc.) generates an immediate increase in blood glucose levels, which has the short-term effect of elevating your mood, energy level and alertness. In a matter of minutes, however, your pancreas secretes a requisite amount of insulin to quickly remove glucose from the bloodstream before it becomes toxic. Depending on the type and amount of carbohydrates you consumed and your degree of insulin sensitivity, this insulin rush can eventually cause your blood glucose levels to decline so much that your glucose-dependent brain soon becomes low on fuel. As a result, you may soon feel sluggish, foggy and cranky and have trouble focusing. While this explains the familiar post-lunch afternoon blues, extensive data also suggest a strong link between attention deficit/hyperactivity disorder (ADHD) and processed carbohydrate consumption/insulin production.

The ingestion of lots of carbohydrates, followed by the secretion of lots of insulin, which causes low blood glucose levels, is perceived as a stressful event by the hypothalamic-pituitary-adrenal (HPA) axis. This homeostasis-monitoring part of your endocrine system triggers the fight-or-flight response, causing your adrenal glands to release epinephrine (commonly called 'adrenaline') and cortisol into your bloodstream. Cortisol breaks down precious muscle tissue into amino acids, some of which are sent to the liver and converted into glucose through gluconeogenesis. The ensuing blood glucose rush gives you the boost your brain thinks you need – commonly at the expense of your muscle tissue! Depending on your individual sensitivity to glucose and insulin, the stress response to this seesaw process may make you feel jittery, edgy and hyper, and you may have a racing heartbeat.

Others may not experience any stress hormone buzz, likely because years of abusing this delicate life-or-death energy boosting mechanism (high-carbohydrate eating, excessive artificial light/insufficient sleep and high-stress lifestyle) have exhausted their adrenal glands and pancreas. Instead, they'll just feel like taking a nap after high-carbohydrate meals. Consequently, your roller-coaster ride will consist of a brief glucose high after meals, followed by sugar cravings (to repeat the cycle) and/or a desire for a nap once insulin starts going to work. However the particulars of your daily energy level and appetite fluctuations play out, all roads in this saga lead to burnout and elevated risk of disease and dysfunction mentioned in the previous section.

Besides the unsettling energy swings and added stress, sugar also seriously hampers immune function as soon as it's ingested. We know that excessive and/or prolonged production of cortisol is a potent immune suppressor (the fight-or-flight mechanism diverts resources to provide an immediate energy boost). Research also shows that sugar itself can impair the function of immunity-related phagocytes (immune system cells that remove bacteria or viruses from the bloodstream) for at least five hours after ingestion.

This impairment happens through a process known as competitive inhibition, when excess glucose prevents the all-important antioxidant vitamin C from being transported inside certain immune cells. Because both molecules use the same mechanism and entry point to gain access to the inside of the immune cells, the presence of excessive glucose can overwhelm the transporter site and block vitamin C from entering. With your guard down, oxidative stress on your body increases as free radicals are allowed to run wild. Furthermore, your blood thickens as a response to these immune stressors, which is why heart attacks (in people predisposed to them) tend to occur after a meal.

Note that the chain of events described here happens routinely in a normal, healthy person who overdoes carbohydrate or sugar intake. Experiencing these high-low, high-low cycles from sugar ingestion is no fun, but it does mean you still have some sensitivity to the negative effects of sugar ingestion and insulin production. If you *don't* experience significant noticeable symptoms from eating lots of carbohydrates (particularly sugar), you are likely well on your way, or have already developed, the extremely problematic condition of insulin resistance. The analogy of a smoker feeling minimal to no immediate ill effects from his or her habit applies here. I'd argue that a vast majority of the population is somewhere on this continuum, far outside of the healthy ideal of a diet that moderates carbohydrate intake and insulin production in line with our genetic requirements for health. Naturally, grain or sugar products will jack up blood glucose levels quickly and produce a greater insulin response than consuming a similar amount of calories from vegetables and fruits, or combining a few carbohydrates with slower-burning protein or fat calories.

While it's obviously preferable to mute the immediate insulin spike, your diet's total insulin production is the most important element to consider. If you are routinely eating 150 to 300g (or more) of carbohydrates per day, you will likely gain weight insidiously (unless you exercise like crazy) and still increase your risk of developing other associated health problems, including the 'oxidation and inflammation' syndrome that is the major culprit behind heart disease. (I will discuss this in the next section.)

CHOLESTEROL – THE WHOLE STORY

The debate over the theory known as the lipid hypothesis of heart disease has raged for years. The pharmaceutical industries and government and medical experts have done a great job of vilifying cholesterol and saturated fats as the major causes of atherosclerosis and heart disease via the well-accepted lipid hypothesis of heart disease. You know their story by now: your arteries are like pipes and cholesterol is the fatty, sticky gunk that clogs them up if you eat too many high-cholesterol animal products (meat, eggs) or saturated fats in general. According to conventional wisdom, you should eat a low-fat, low-cholesterol, high complex-carbohydrate diet. If your diet or genetic 'bad luck' results in a total cholesterol level of over 200, you simply take cholesterol-lowering statin medicines to safely reduce your risk.

In recent years, many elements of conventional wisdom about cholesterol have been called into question. While there is significant dispute and uncertainty on the issue among respected experts, there is compelling evidence that freely dispensing powerful statin medications to reduce all forms of cholesterol offers only minimal protection from heart disease and stroke. Furthermore, it's almost universally agreed that lifestyle modifications (such as losing weight, reducing intake of processed carbohydrates and fats, consuming omega 3 oils, exercising and managing stress levels) can do a much better job than statins in eliminating the major heart disease risk factors.

Because I highly respect the valiant battle medical professionals are fighting with today's heart disease pandemic (after all, they often have little or nothing to do with patients until they show up in the waiting room with clogged pipes), I'd like to assert here that this is not a 'Mark versus your doctor' battle of the egos. Rather, I believe this is an unbiased interpretation of cutting-edge data that extends beyond the narrow and dated 'eating fat drives cholesterol drives heart disease' story that most of us are familiar with, including physicians. Remember, physicians don't *necessarily* have any specialised knowledge about the link between diet and heart disease from their medical training. Or if they do, it might be very outdated information. Like your plumber, their expertise is in dealing with already-clogged pipes.

> 'Using total cholesterol level – or even your LDL cholesterol value – is irrelevant in the absence of further context, such as Metabolic Syndrome and other accomplices to heart disease.'
> FRAMINGHAM HEART STUDY

The following discussion will give you a deeper understanding of exactly what causes heart disease (*hint*: it's oxidation and inflammation, driven primarily by poor food choices, excessive insulin production and all forms of stress in excess, including overexercising) and help you do a better job of minimising heart disease risk than just following the party line of 'Don't eat cholesterol – and take drugs if your numbers are high.'

Among the most notable research refuting the cholesterol story is the highly respected Framingham Heart Study. The study (which I reference often at MarksDailyApple.com) has followed the dietary habits of 15,000 participants (residents of Framingham, Massachusetts) over three generations. It is widely regarded as the longest (it began in 1948 and is still going strong!), most comprehensive study of health and illness factors on a population assessment in medical history. It has led to the publication of more than 1,200 research articles in leading journals. Study director Dr William Castelli summarised the issue unequivocally when he said, 'Serum cholesterol is not a strong risk factor for coronary heart disease.' Among the study's highlights are these:

- **There is no correlation** between dietary cholesterol and blood cholesterol levels.
- **Framingham residents who ate the most** cholesterol, saturated fat and total calories actually **weighed the least** and were the most physically active.

Luckily for us, over the past decade hundreds of bright, clear-thinking researchers have re-examined this data, conducted new research and written extensively on how and why the conventional wisdom lipid hypothesis of heart disease is deeply flawed. (Google the term *cholesterol sceptics* and you'll discover an organised group called the International Network of Cholesterol Skeptics, populated by dozens of leading MDs and PhDs in the field from across the globe.) Their research now shows that atherosclerosis is caused mainly by the excessive oxidation (and the ensuing inflammation) of a certain type of cholesterol that constitutes a small fraction of the mostly good stuff flowing through your bloodstream.

Ironically, in many cases, it appears that this oxidation might be made worse by consuming the very cholesterol-free polyunsaturated fats in vegetable and grain oils that the medical establishment led us to believe were healthier than animal fats! Furthermore, the drugs to lower cholesterol have done little or nothing to improve the health of most of the people taking them, while the side effects and expense have been devastating to millions more.

THE LOWDOWN ON LIPOPROTEINS

Cholesterol is a little waxy lipid (fat) molecule that happens to be one of the most important substances in the human body. Every cell membrane has cholesterol as a critical structural and functional component. Brain cells need cholesterol to make synapses (connections) with other brain cells. Cholesterol is the precursor molecule for important hormones such as testosterone, estrogen, DHEA, cortisol and pregnenolone. Cholesterol is needed for making the bile acids that allow us to digest and absorb fats. Cholesterol interacts with sunlight to convert the all-important vitamin D. The bottom line is that you can't live without cholesterol, which is why your liver actually makes up to 1,400 milligrams a day, regardless of how much food-borne cholesterol you consume – or how much you avoid it like the plague – in your diet.

Because cholesterol is fat-soluble (it does not dissolve in water – think balsamic vinegar staying intact in a dish of olive oil) but must travel to and from cells in the watery environment of the bloodstream, it needs to be carried by special spherical particles called lipoproteins (the name means 'part protein and part lipid'). There are several varieties of lipoproteins with different transporting functions – chylomicrons, LDLs, IDLs, HDLs and VLDLs (as well as subfractions of those) – but the three we are concerned with here are VLDLs, LDLs and HDLs (very low-density, low-density and high-density lipoproteins, respectively). Each of these lipoproteins carries a certain percentage of cholesterol, triglycerides and other minor fats. Your blood test values for triglycerides and HDL, LDL and VLDL cholesterol represent the combined total in your bloodstream of what all the lipoproteins are transporting.

VLDLs, the largest of these cholesterol complexes, are manufactured in the liver in the presence of high levels of triglycerides. Hence, VLDLs comprise 80 per cent triglyceride and a little cholesterol. After leaving their birthplace in the liver, these lipoproteins deliver their cargo to fat and muscle cells for energy. Once these VLDLs have deposited their triglyceride load inside a fat or muscle cell, their size decreases substantially and they convert into either large, fluffy LDLs or small, dense LDLs – in both cases bearing mostly cholesterol and a little bit of remaining triglyceride. Large fluffy or 'buoyant' LDLs are generally harmless, even at relatively high levels (this has a strong genetic component), as they go about their assigned task of delivering cholesterol to the cells that need it.

The real trouble starts when triglycerides are unusually high in the bloodstream causing your body to convert VLDL into small, dense LDL. This condition can occur routinely when you eat a high-carbohydrate diet (even if it's a low-fat diet), because excessive insulin production drives the conversion of ingested carbohydrate into fat (triglycerides). Obviously, the condition can also occur when you eat a moderate-carbohydrate, high-fat diet, because insulin will see to it that both excess carbohydrates and fat get circulated in the bloodstream and stored in fat cells.

Dr Dean Ornish and other proponents of low-fat eating will tell you that reducing fat intake quickly reduces cholesterol and triglyceride levels. This is absolutely true, as confirmed by numerous best-selling books as well as newspaper and magazine feature stories touting quick and dramatic results (lowered cholesterol and triglyceride levels) from fat-restrictive diets. But the reason why this happens is this: your liver makes cholesterol as a raw material for the bile salts that help you digest fat, so if you aren't eating much fat, your genes will be given the signal to down-regulate cholesterol production.

However, low-fat eating requires you to consume excessive carbohydrates, by default, to obtain your daily energy requirements. This leads to excessive insulin production and, as you recall, kick-starts the cycle that eventually leads to heart disease. Any way you slice it, consuming too many carbohydrates leads to high triglycerides (not to mention the other risk factors detailed in the sidebar 'How to Sneeze at Heart Disease').

> 'Low-fat eating requires you to consume excessive carbs, by default, to obtain your daily energy requirements.'

With high triglycerides in your blood, VLDL production skyrockets to handle the extra load and these particles can be altered into the small, dense LDLs that have been shown to be a major factor in atherosclerosis and heart disease. Being small and dense, these LDLs (why can't all medical nomenclature be this easy?) can become stuck in the spaces between the cells lining the artery and then become oxidised. This oxidative damage causes inflammation and begins a process of destruction that I will explain shortly. Research has shown that people with Metabolic Syndrome and/or type 2 diabetes all have elevated levels of both triglycerides and these small, dense LDL particles. Of course, these same people also have substantially increased risks for heart disease and stroke.

The remaining cholesterol complex with which you might be familiar is the high-density lipoprotein (HDL), which takes cholesterol back to the liver for recycling. HDLs also clean up any damaged or oxidised cholesterol that might cause problems later – including removing the small, dense LDL particles and oxidised cholesterol that have become stuck in the artery wall. These tiny but powerful HDL cholesterol complexes are often called the 'good cholesterol' or 'nature's garbage trucks'. Scientists generally agree that the more HDL you have, the lower your risk for heart disease. As you might have imagined, people with Metabolic Syndrome and/or type 2 diabetes also typically have low levels of beneficial HDL. Exercise is one of the cheapest, easiest and most effective ways to raise HDL. Consuming saturated fat is another!

MURDER MYSTERY DINNER – OXIDATION AND SMALL, DENSE LDL ARE GUILTY!

As mentioned earlier, because lipoproteins have a lipid surface, they are subject to oxidation. Like oils left open in your kitchen, they can go rancid when they come in contact with oxygen. When this happens they – and the cholesterol inside – can become damaged. Of course, oxidation happens all the time throughout the body, and we have evolved some effective antioxidant systems (namely catalase, superoxide dismutase and glutathione) to prevent too much of this damage getting out of control. Furthermore, consuming ample levels of high-antioxidant foods (vegetables, fruits, nuts and seeds, dark chocolate, red wine, as will be detailed in Chapter 4) and antioxidant supplements (such as vitamin E, CoQ10, beta-carotene and lycopene) can help mitigate some of the damage. It's also extremely convenient that HDLs can remove some of the damaged cholesterol and take it back to the liver for recycling.

Your cholesterol processing system has evolved to expect a certain range and quality of dietary fat, protein, carbohydrate and antioxidants, as well as a certain level of exercise (to help promote insulin sensitivity in the muscles and maintain high levels of HDL) to provide appropriate gene signals and avoid artery disease. And because HDL particles are very small, they can get into the spaces between arterial wall cells and clean up the oxidised cholesterol. That's why pharmaceutical companies have tried – so far unsuccessfully – to create an effective drug to raise HDL and address existing atherosclerosis (some physicians prescribe the combination of prescription fibrates and over-the-counter niacin to raise HDL, but this treatment can be problematic and is not widely used).

The cholesterol processing system has served humans and most other mammals well for millions of years – until recently. As mentioned previously, oxidised small, dense LDLs are small enough that they can get trapped in the spaces between endothelial cells lining the artery (sometimes called a gap junction). Even if they are not oxidised to begin with, once trapped, they can oxidise in place because they are sitting there continually exposed to oxygen passing by while attached to haemoglobin in the red blood cells. Either way, this oxidation eventually causes injury and inflammation to the arterial wall, prompting the body's immune system to send macrophages (scavenging white blood cells) to gobble up the oxidised LDLs at the site where the first particles were trapped.

The immune system tries hard to do its job, but the macrophages are now overwhelmed by absorbing so much oxidised LDL. The consumption of oxidised LDLs causes certain genes to convert these macrophages into foam cells that attach to the arterial lining, laying the foundation for future trouble. The lesion prompts more macrophages to come to the rescue. They try to gobble up more and more oxidised LDLs which are floating by, increasing the severity of the lesion over time. This is the familiar saga of plaque accumulation on the arterial wall. The plaque grows and eventually compromises the inner diameter of the artery. If allowed to continue, it can eventually occlude blood flow or break off as a clot, preventing blood – and oxygen – reaching a vital organ. This describes your classic heart attack or stroke.

The oxidation of these small, dense LDLs most likely happens for a variety of reasons that have to do with modern dietary habits more than anything else: a high intake of unstable polyunsaturated fatty acids (PUFAs) from vegetable oils in the diet (PUFAs incorporated into the lipid layer are much more prone to oxidation than are saturated fats); a reduced intake of natural antioxidants in the diet, which would otherwise mitigate oxidation; the presence of fewer HDL particles to remove oxidised lipids (low HDL cholesterol readings may be partly caused by high-carbohydrate diets); and the fact that small, dense LDL particles do not bind as easily to the normal LDL receptors on muscle and fat cells. Unable to release their cholesterol load and with typically fewer HDL particles to gobble them up, these small, dense LDL particles linger longer in the oxygen-rich bloodstream until they oxidise. By the way, the reason atherosclerosis occurs in the arteries and not the veins is because venous blood has very little oxygen.

Note that the oxidation and inflammation process described has little or nothing to do with your total cholesterol or even your total LDL cholesterol levels. In most cases, atherosclerosis is a result of the oxidation of a small fraction of the total amount of LDL in your blood – the small, dense LDL particles. If you have little or none of these in your blood, your risk for heart disease drops dramatically. Also, if your HDL is high, it's very unlikely that you'll encounter a problem, because HDL does a great job of scavenging the oxidised cholesterol from LDL in the bloodstream.

Unfortunately for some of us, poor diet, lack of exercise, stress, certain drug therapies and, yes, family genetic history can all contribute to the increased production of the dangerous small, dense LDL particles. Your doctor can test for them if you ask, but most common blood tests don't yet distinguish between the benign 'fluffy' forms of LDL, sometimes called pattern A, and the small, dense particles, called pattern B. A comprehensive lipid blood panel such as the Berkeley Heart Lab test will typically provide values for total cholesterol, HDL, LDL, VLDL and triglycerides and indicate relative particle sizes.

A physician will generally dispense medication if your total LDL levels exceed a certain figure (this varies by doctor and individual patient profile), knowing your body will respond to the statins with a quick overall reduction regardless of particle size. This will indeed lower all forms of LDL (including both the good stuff and the bad stuff), but it's a much more sensible – and safe – option to simply alter dietary and exercise habits and minimise insulin production, thereby preventing excess accumulation of triglycerides in the blood and allowing the cholesterol system to work as intended. In fact, the combination of low carbohydrates and good fats in primal foods will generally raise HDL and lower both triglycerides and small, dense LDL. Meanwhile, compelling evidence suggests that Primal Blueprint-style eating and exercising will allow you, regardless of your genetic predisposition, to essentially have no participation in this heart disease saga whatsoever. If you feel any hesitation here, go get a 'before' blood panel, eat Primally for 21 days, and then get another panel. It's virtually certain you will see an impressive alteration of unfavourable numbers, giving you the motivation and clarity you need to plunge whole-heartedly into Primal eating.

> 'HDL does a great job of scavenging the oxidised cholesterol from LDL in the bloodstream ... if your HDL is high, it's much less likely you'll encounter a [heart disease] problem.'

STATIN STATS STINK!

Isn't it ironic, then, to discover that statins and other cholesterol-lowering meds do not have any ability to influence LDL particle size and can only lower total LDL by reducing both the good and the bad versions? The fact that some people taking statins experience a dramatic reduction in total cholesterol or in LDL means very little in the context of the true oxidation and inflammation nature of heart disease. To be clear, statins do slightly reduce the risk of additional heart attacks among men under the age of 65 who have had a prior heart attack. However, many doctors now believe that these benefits are independent of their 'cholesterol-lowering' properties and instead come from an anti-inflammatory effect that addresses the more proximate cause of heart disease. A cheaper and more effective anti-inflammatory effect can be achieved by eating foods high in omega 3, taking fish oil supplements, or popping a small dose of aspirin daily.

By simply adopting the Primal Blueprint laws, you can enjoy superior results without the perilous side effects and huge expense of drug therapy. In the case of statins, known side effects include muscle pain, weakness and numbness, chronic fatigue, tendon problems, cognitive problems, impotence and blood glucose elevations. These side effects are believed to be due in large part to statins' interference with the normal production of a critical micronutrient known as coenzyme Q10 (CoQ10). CoQ10 is essential to healthy mitochondrial function (energy production) and defending your cells against free radical damage. Statin therapy is believed to lower

CoQ10 levels by up to 50 per cent. Ironically, CoQ10 plays a particularly important role in the healthy function of the cardiovascular system, and heart attack patients show depressed levels of CoQ10! Some researchers suggest that statins' depletion of CoQ10 may nullify any potential benefits of statin therapy.

So why are millions of people being misguided to take dangerous, powerful drugs when lifestyle intervention is more effective, less expensive and has no side effects? Perhaps we like to search for easy answers with quick results, and statins produce a graphic and quick decline in blood cholesterol levels. Like other elements of conventional wisdom, there are billions of dollars invested and powerful market forces pushing us in the direction of swallowing drugs and their side effects, while the full story is lost amidst the hype of 'lower your numbers quick!'

If you are currently taking statins or other medications, I realise that asking you to reject conventional wisdom and the specific recommendations of your trusted physician can put you in a very uncomfortable position. I strongly urge you to engage in lifestyle modification (after all, there are no side effects or potential compromises to your drug regime when you improve your diet), while concurrently addressing the possibility with your doctor of gradually reducing your dependence on medication based on the ensuing favourable blood test results.

HOW TO SNEEZE AT HEART DISEASE

The catch-all term *Metabolic Syndrome* is used to describe an assortment of heart disease risk factors widely attributed to today's prevailing poor dietary and exercise habits. The highly respected Cleveland Clinic states that 'the exact cause of Metabolic Syndrome is not known … [but] many features are associated with insulin resistance.' Five markers are universally used as reliable indicators of Metabolic Syndrome. If you have three or more of these markers, you are diagnosed as having the condition. Here are the five markers:

- **Elevated fasting blood glucose of** 100 mg/dl or greater
- **Blood pressure of** 130/85 mm Hg or greater
- **Waistline measurement of** 40 inches or more for men and 35 inches or more for women.
- **HDL of** less than 40 mg/dl for men and less than 50 mg/dl for women.
- **Triglycerides of** 150 mg/dl or greater.

The US Government and other sources report that some 47 million Americans have Metabolic Syndrome – about one in five Americans. It's a chronic condition that develops and worsens over time (with no immediate discernible physical symptoms except that expanding waistline …) unless you take dramatic steps to alter your lifestyle. The Cleveland Clinic and *Journal of the American Medical Association* report that more than 40 per cent of Americans in their 60s and 70s have the condition. Dr Richard Feinman, one of the most often published and highly regarded researchers in the fields of nutrition and metabolism, has suggested that 'Metabolic Syndrome may be defined by the response to carbohydrate restriction' (that is, if you restrict carbohydrates, the symptoms subside).

A routine physical examination and blood panel will give you an indication of your Metabolic Syndrome status. Many experts recommend a few additional blood tests to assess overall health and risk factors, including:

- **C-Reactive Protein:** High sensitivity–C-reactive protein (hs-CRP) is produced by your liver as part of an immune system response to injury or infection. In the absence of other acute infections, high levels of hs-CRP in your blood are associated with an increased risk of heart attack, stroke and sudden cardiac death. Because atherosclerosis is primarily a disease of inflammation, some researchers contend that hs-CRP is a strong predictor of your heart disease risk. Given that cholesterol tests have become less reliable in predicting risk, especially among those with normal or low cholesterol levels, hs-CRP seems to be a good alternative.

- **Lp2A:** Another key inflammation marker associated with small, dense LDL particles.
- **A1c (estimated average glucose):** A1c measures how much glucose is attached to a haemoglobin molecule, a reliable marker for the dangers of elevated blood glucose levels over an extended time period. This is a superior test to the more common blood glucose readings (something commonly tracked by diabetics with a portable machine) that vary throughout the day and are strongly influenced by meals.
- **Fasting Blood Insulin Levels:** High-fasting insulin levels are indicative of pre-diabetic conditions.

DIET AND EXERCISE PREVENTION TIPS

If you are diagnosed with or on the borderline of Metabolic Syndrome, following the Primal Blueprint for 30 days can turn four of the five Metabolic Syndrome markers around (it might take a bit longer to get your waistline back in the safe zone) and cause your heart disease risk to plummet – even if you have a family history of obesity, high cholesterol and heart disease. Here are some specific recommendations and corresponding benefits of following the Primal Blueprint:

- **Balance omega 6:omega 3 Ratios:** Minimising consumption of omega 6 polyunsaturated fats gives you a greater surface area of saturated (and therefore protected) fats in lipoprotein lipid layers and fatty membranes. Increased consumption of omega 3 oils helps control the inflammation that is the precursor for athero-sclerosis and virtually all other metabolic diseases.
- **Exercise Primal Blueprint Style:** Regular exercise helps lower LDL and raise HDL.
- **Increase Antioxidant Intake:** If your antioxidant intake is appreciable (eating your vegetables?), it's likely that you'll help your natural defences against oxidation. Supplements are a great idea if you lead a stressful life (who doesn't?), your diet falls short from time to time, or you are at an increased risk of heart disease.

- **Reduce Carbohydrate Intake:** This will help lower your production of triglycerides, raise HDL, lower LDL and dramatically lower the small, dense LDL (because it is high levels of triglycerides that prompt small, dense LDL production).

PUT INFLAMMATION AT EASE WITH OMEGA 3s

A major feature of Primal Blueprint eating is that it provides high levels of healthy saturated and unsaturated fats. While conventional wisdom generally positions saturated fats as something to diligently restrict, they are an excellent energy source and offer a variety of nutrients critical to health. Consuming ample amounts of saturated fat helps prevent oxidative damage to your cells (saturated fat is an integral part of cell membranes). While your eyes might bug out at this statement, it's virtually irrefutable and proven by many respected long-term studies that you should:

> *Eat (healthy) fat and help prevent cancer and heart disease. Avoid fat and increase your risk of cancer, heart disease and even obesity.*

Fortunately, omega 3 polyunsaturated fatty acids don't have an image problem and are universally regarded as healthy. Adequate omega 3 consumption supports healthy cardiovascular, brain, skin and immune function. By turning on genes that improve blood circulation, reducing inflammation and supporting healthy cholesterol and triglyceride levels, omega 3s help reduce the risk of high blood pressure, blood clots that cause heart attacks, arthritis, autoimmune disorders and cognitive problems such as depression, Alzheimer's and even ADHD. The important role of omega 3s in supporting cognitive function is made even more evident by the fact that half the brain consists of fat, including concentrated levels of the omega 3 docosahexanoic acid, DHA. The benefits of adequate omega 3 intake and optimum fatty acid balance are strikingly evident from data on cultures that consume substantial amounts of fat but have markedly reduced heart disease rates compared to Westerners, such as the *traditional* Japanese diet (i.e., for those who frequent sushi bars instead of the 3,598 McDonald's in Japan) centred around fish and vegetables.

Another form of polyunsaturated fats called omega 6 plays a vital role in our health as well, but its extreme prevalence in the Standard American Diet – from vegetable oils, animal fats, bakery items (doughnuts, cookies) and processed snacks (the highly offensive trans and partially hydrogenated fats are classified as omega 6) – leads to a dangerous imbalance of excessive omega 6 and deficient omega 3. The ideal omega 6 to omega 3 balance is 1:1 or 2:1, ratios that Grok likely met with ease. Even 4:1 is okay today, but the typical modern eater has a ratio of 20:1 or worse! It's also interesting to note that imbalanced fatty acid intake can exacerbate the insulin resistance problem discussed earlier. Omega 6 fats (particularly arachidonic acid) suppress the expression of the major insulin receptor gene GLUT4 (promoting more fat storage), while omega 3 fats increase the expression of GLUT4 (promoting insulin sensitivity and less fat storage).

Once again, your genes are only doing what they are told to do by the signals you give them. The imbalance of fatty acids in the typical modern diet triggers a genetically programmed inflammation response throughout the body. Under normal circumstances, inflammation is your body's highly desirable first line of defence against pain, injury and infection. Inflammation processes detect and destroy toxic material in damaged tissue before it can spread to the rest of the body. Consider examples like a bee sting, taking an elbow to the face, or turning an ankle on a hiking trail – the reddened skin, black eye and ballooned ankle help your body quarantine the damage from the trauma to the inflamed areas, instead of letting toxins run wild through the bloodstream. Unfortunately, an out-of-control, body-wide inflammation response (also known as systemic inflammation) – which results from stress and imbalanced dietary and/or exercise habits – confuses your body into thinking it's under assault from destructive, infectious foreign agents or that a major trauma has just occurred. That's when the disease process begins.

In my own athletic example, the extreme stress of my Chronic Cardio training regime and my highly inflammatory grain-based diet led to excessive and prolonged inflammation throughout my body. What I should have been seeking was a more desirable temporary state of moderate inflammation (pumped muscles, elevated heart rate, oxygenated lungs, etc. – factors that enhance peak performance), from a Primal Blueprint-aligned training regime and plenty of recovery time and good food choices for my body to return to homeostasis. The systemic inflammation I experienced from overtraining tore down my muscles, joints and immune system. Interestingly, after extreme endurance events such as a marathon or ironman race, blood levels of CPK (creatine phosphokinase; it leaks into the bloodstream when muscle, heart or brain tissue is traumatised) can be elevated for weeks afterwards. In fact, if you ran a marathon and then immediately headed over to a hospital emergency room, a doctor might think you were suffering from a heart attack! In my case, when I adjusted my diet and training habits, virtually all my inflammatory and immune-suppressing conditions vanished.

We know that most forms of systemic inflammation have a strong dietary component and can usually be resolved with a few dietary modifications. Nevertheless, conventional wisdom within the medical community has recommended fighting our widespread inflammation-related health problems with corticosteroids, COX-2 inhibitors such as Vioxx and Celebrex, and other non-steroidal anti-inflammatories (asthma medications work on a similar chemical pathway). I have a nonscientific name for this approach: digging a hole to install a ladder to wash the basement windows. As you might imagine, because these medications interfere with normal hormone pathways and gene expression, they almost never address the underlying cause of inflammation. They simply mask the pain in the short term – if they mask it at all. Dietary modification (and exercise modification if you are overdoing it) is almost always a superior method of treatment and protection against pain and serious diseases triggered by systemic inflammation.

The Primal Blueprint eating style, with its emphasis on high omega 3 foods (such as oily, cold water fish, pasture-raised animal meats and eggs, and leafy green vegetables) and its aversion to processed foods and excessive omega 6 oils, provides an ideal dietary fatty acid balance without you really having to worry about it. When you combine healthy eating with the other Primal Blueprint laws, you can naturally avoid the systemic inflammation that is now believed to be the root cause of the major health problems affecting modern humans.

'I have a nonscientific name for this approach: digging a hole to install a ladder to wash the basement windows.'

CONTEXT IN, CALORIES OUT – UNDERSTANDING THE MACRO NUTRIENTS

While you likely have a basic understanding of what carbohydrate, protein and fat do in the body, it's important to examine the role of each nutrient further in the context of how they support the Primal Blueprint. This is particularly true in the light of the massive misinformation, distortion and confusion presented by opposing camps on this issue.

Most popular daily diets (and fitness programmes) follow the 'calories in, calories out' conventional wisdom approach towards weight loss, failing to understand the importance of context when making this otherwise literally accurate edict. Your body uses macronutrients for a variety of different functions, some of which are structural and some of which are simply to provide energy (as calories) – immediately or well into the future. Moreover, the body acts as either a fuel storage depot (and as a toxic 'waist' site) or a supplier of energy (calories), depending largely on the hormonal signals it gets from your lifestyle behaviours. Because your body always seeks to achieve homeostasis (balance), the notion of you trying to zero in on a precise day-to-day or meal-to-meal eating plan is generally fruitless, not to mention practically impossible and incredibly frustrating.

To figure your true structural and functional fuel needs (and, hence, to achieve your body composition goals), it's important to understand how the three major macronutrients work in the body – or should work – when you eat in a manner aligned with optimal gene expression.

PROTEIN

Most nutrition researchers are in agreement that protein is essential for building and repairing body tissues and for overall healthy function. Intake recommendations among doctors and nutritionists vary, with most falling in the range of 0.5 to 1 gram of protein per pound of lean body mass per day. There were days when Grok and his family probably obtained two or three times that amount, so if you happen to overdo your protein significantly on any given day or aren't the type to obsess about such things, you'll almost certainly be well within safe guidelines.

To calculate or estimate lean body mass, you must first determine your total weight and percentage of body fat. You can do this using any of the numerous methods ranging from costly water tank tests to the easier fat scales, skinfold calipers, or online calculators using certain body measurements. Most good gyms can help you with this, or you can just estimate roughly for these purposes, knowing that the average moderately fit male and female carry about 15 per cent and 22 per cent respectively. Multiply your total weight by your percentage body fat to attain your 'fat' weight, and then subtract that figure from your total body weight to obtain your lean body mass. For example, a 155-pound woman with 25 per cent body fat has a lean body mass of 116 pounds (155–39=116).

At a minimum you need 0.5 gram of protein per pound of lean mass per day to maintain your 'structure' and healthy body composition. If you are even moderately active, you need closer to 0.7 grams, and if you are an active athlete (or are under a fair amount of stress) you need as much as 1 gram of protein per pound of lean mass. That's at a minimum, but it's on a daily average. So, our 155-pound moderately active woman with 116 pounds of lean mass (25 per cent body fat) needs an average of 82 grams of protein per day (116 x 0.7). If she gets 60 or 70 some days and 110 on others, she'll still be in a healthy average range. She could even fast a day or two occasionally and, provided she has been regularly eating Primally and doesn't overexercise on fasting days, easily preserve her muscle using the body's tendency to burn fat and retain protein stores in the short term. On the other hand, if she exceeds the 110 grams, it's also no problem if she's eating Primally because the excess protein will convert to glucose, which will reduce her effective carbohydrate needs (see next section). At 4 calories per gram, her daily average of 82 grams is only 328 calories per day in protein.

This formula works with kilograms as well. The minimum protein requirement would be around .25 grams of protein per kilo of lean mass; moderately active persons would require around .33, and very active folks around .5 grams per kilo. Again, I'm not concerned with you counting or even meeting this requirement every single day. You'll find yourself intuitively arriving at a comfortable number or range of protein grams within a week of Primal Blueprint–style eating. You will discover that it's quite easy to eat one gram of protein per pound of lean body mass without a lot of planning, and pretty difficult to eat much more than two grams per pound without forcing yourself to. You simply aren't as hungry when you moderate processed carbohydrate intake and avoid insulin crashes and sugar cravings.

If you have ample stored glycogen in your muscle tissues and liver (not a problem for most people unless you are engaged in high-volume, high-stress endurance training or severely restricting your carbohydrates à la the Atkins Diet) and your body is getting the rest of its energy efficiently from fats, it's likely that the protein you consume will go first towards the repair or building of cells or enzymes. Proponents of the 'a calorie is a calorie' conventional wisdom will pipe in here that excess calories are always converted or stored as fat, regardless of their original ingested state. This is true, of course (remember, the Primal Blueprint doesn't like to upset scientists!), and when we eat a high-carbohydrate, high-insulin-producing diet, those excess calories indeed are stored as fat. But we must then ask what excess fat calories do when there is not a lot of insulin in the bloodstream (given that they cannot easily be stored as fat without insulin giving them a ride). No problem; the body will respond by raising metabolic rate (to burn more calories at rest) and by increasing the production of ketones, which may be burned or excreted (more on this shortly).

In summary, if you are the type to enjoy and observe details in your macronutrient intake, I suggest you strive to obtain your protein requirements first, in the activity-level-influenced range discussed previously. Focus on quality sources of protein such as the pasture-raised or organic animal products that will be detailed in the next chapter.

CARBOHYDRATES

If you've forgotten everything you ever learned in biology, just remember this and own it: *carbohydrate controls insulin; insulin controls fat storage.* Carbohydrates are not used as structural components in the body; instead they are used only as a form of fuel, whether burned immediately while passing by different organs and muscles or stored for later use. All forms of carbohydrates you eat, whether simple or complex, are eventually converted into glucose, which the brain, red blood cells and nerve cells generally prefer as a primary fuel. For reference, a little less than one teaspoon of glucose dissolved in the entire blood pool in your body (about five litres in the case of a 160-pound male) represents an optimal level of blood glucose. In most healthy people, glucose that is not burned immediately (exercising muscles prefer glucose, if it is available, but don't absolutely require it unless they are working at high intensity for long periods) will first be stored as glycogen in muscle and liver cells. When these sites are full, glucose is converted into fatty acids and stored in fat cells. It's insulin's job to take glucose out of the bloodstream and put it somewhere fast.

Unless you deplete lots of muscle glycogen every day, there is no physiological reason for you to consume high levels of carbohydrates. In fact, carbohydrates are not required in the human diet for survival in the way that fat and protein are. The body has several backup mechanisms for generating glucose internally: from dietary fat and protein, as well as from proteins stripped from muscle tissue (all done via gluconeogenesis). Some researchers have estimated that the body manufactures up to 200 grams of glucose every day from the fat and protein in our diet or in our muscles. This is a good thing, because entire civilisations have lived for thousands of years on 50 or fewer grams of dietary carbohydrates a day.

> '*There is no biological requirement for dietary carbohydrate in the human diet.*'

That said, the Primal Blueprint is not designed to be an extremely low-carbohydrate diet, because this strategy would restrict your intake of some of the most nutrient-dense foods on the planet – vegetables and fruits. I don't even characterise the Primal Blueprint as a 'low-carb' diet, as much as it is an 'eliminate bad carbs' diet. I don't advocate portion control or even diligently counting your macronutrient intake. You may want to journal now and then to establish benchmarks and reference points (visit paleotrack.com or FitDay.com and input a day or two of foods you eat, and it will generate a breakdown of macronutrients and calories), but you don't need to. It's really easy to stay in the optimum range of 100 to 150 grams per day of carbohydrates even when you eat a ton of colourful vegetables and fairly liberal servings of fruit – as long as you stay Primal and consume no grains or legumes. For example, a huge salad, two cups of Brussels sprouts, a banana, an apple, a cup of blueberries and a cup of cherries totals only 139 grams of carbohydrates.

Note: Perhaps you are familiar with the concept of 'net carbs' when measuring macronutrient intake. This is a calculation that subtracts fibre, because fibre is usually not digested and moderates the blood glucose impact of a carbohydrate food. For the sake of simplicity (and to assert the Primal Blueprint philosophy that you don't need many carbohydrates, nor any additional fibre from grain foods), all the calculations and zones in this book represent *gross* total carbohydrate grams.

THE CARBOHYDRATE CURVE – WHAT'LL IT BE? THE 'SWEET SPOT' OR THE 'DANGER ZONE'?

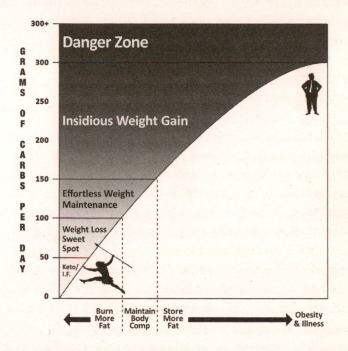

The Primal Blueprint Carbohydrate Curve illustrates how carbohydrates impact on the human body and the degree to which we need them, or don't need them, in our diet. Carbohydrate intake is the decisive factor in your weight-loss success or failure, and excessive carbohydrate consumption is arguably the most destructive modern lifestyle behaviour. Eliminating grains and sugars from your diet could be the number one most beneficial thing you ever do for your health!

0 to 50 grams per day
Ketosis and Accelerated Fat Burning

Acceptable for occasional one- to two-day Intermittent Fasting efforts towards aggressive weight loss (or longer term, for medically supervised weight-loss programmes for the obese and/or type 2 diabetics), provided adequate protein, fat and supplements are consumed. Excellent catalyst for quick, relatively comfortable weight loss and not at all dangerous. (Grok relied heavily on fat metabolism and ketosis to account for the difficulty in obtaining appreciable amounts of carbohydrates in daily life.) Not recommended as a long-term practice for most people due to likely deprivation of high-nutrient-value vegetables and fruits.

50 to 100 grams per day
Primal Sweet Spot for Effortless Weight Loss

Minimises insulin production and accelerates fat metabolism. By meeting average daily protein requirements, eating nutritious vegetables and fruits and staying satisfied with delicious high-fat foods (meat, fish, eggs, nuts, seeds), you can lose one to two pounds of body fat per week in the 'sweet spot'. Delicious menu options that land in the sweet spot are detailed in Chapter 8.

100 to 150 grams per day
Primal Blueprint Maintenance Range

Allows for genetically optimal fat burning, muscle development and effortless weight maintenance. Rationale supported by humans eating and evolving in this range or below for millions of years. Dietary emphasis on vegetables, fruits, nuts, seeds and animal foods, with grains and processed sugars eliminated. A prior history of heavy carbohydrate intake may result in a brief period of discomfort during the transition to Primal Blueprint eating. Adequate consumption of satisfying foods (high-water-content fruits and vegetables, high-fat snacks like nuts and seeds and meals emphasising animal foods) helps protect against feeling deprived or depleted.

150 to 300 grams per day
Steady, Insidious Weight Gain

Continuous insulin-stimulating effects prevent efficient fat metabolism and contribute to widespread health conditions. This zone is the de facto recommendation of many popular diets and health authorities (including the USDA Food Pyramid) despite the clear danger of developing Metabolic Syndrome. Chronic exercisers and active growing youth and those with physically strenuous jobs may eat at this level for an extended period without gaining fat, but eventually fat storage and/or metabolic problems are highly probable. This 'insidious' zone is easy to drift into, even by health-conscious eaters, when grains are a dietary centrepiece, sweetened beverages or snacks leak into the picture here and there, and obligatory fruits and vegetables are added to the total. Recall that Wendy Korg's trip to the juice bar for a healthy afternoon snack resulted in 187 grams of carbohydrates ingested at one sitting. Starting your day off with a bowl of muesli cereal, a slice of wholewheat toast and a glass of fresh orange juice might seem right from the heart-healthy menu at the luxury spa – but the numbers start racking up (that's 97 grams right there!), and the disastrous insulin-spike/sugar-craving cycle is set in motion. Despite trying to do the right thing by cutting fat and calories, many frustrated people still gain a pound or two of fat per year for decades as a result of the carbohydrate intake in the insidious range.

300 or more grams per day
Danger Zone!

The zone of the average American's diet, and in excess of official USDA dietary guidelines (which suggest you eat 45 per cent to 65 per cent of calories from carbohydrates), thanks to stuff like fizzy drinks tipping the scales over. Extended time in the danger zone results in almost certain weight gain and Metabolic Syndrome. The danger zone is the primary catalyst for the obesity and type 2 diabetes epidemics, as well as numerous other significant health problems. Immediate and dramatic reduction of grains and other processed carbohydrates is critical.

Carbohydrate Curve Variables

The 50-gram/200-calorie variation within each range on the curve attempts to account for individual energy disparities: a light, moderately active female will observe the low end of the range, while a heavy, active male with subscribe to the high end. If you are insistent on doing Chronic Cardio, you will likely have to increase carbohydrate intake to account for regular depletion of stored liver and muscle glycogen and an elevated metabolic rate. You can experiment with consuming 100 additional grams of carbohydrates for every hour of vigorous exercise and notice how your body responds. However, I'd prefer that you simply adjust your training programme to conform to Primal Blueprint guidelines and thus reduce your need for dietary carbohydrate.

FAT

I've already discussed how the common admonition to keep dietary fats low is truly unfounded in most credible research. As far as I'm concerned, fat is your friend. Consuming healthy fats from animal and plant sources supports optimal function of all the systems in your body. Furthermore, ingesting fat helps you feel full and satisfied in a way that carbohydrates cannot. Because fat has little or no impact on blood glucose levels and insulin production and takes far longer to metabolise than carbohydrates, you will feel a deep and long-lasting satisfaction from consuming ample amounts of fat in your diet.

> *'The Nurses' Health Study (90,000 nurses, two decades) showed no statistically significant association between total fat intake (or cholesterol intake) and heart disease.'*

I understand that this is a controversial topic that will be met with some opposition. Please take it upon yourself to gain a clear understanding of the issue, learn to distinguish healthy fats from unhealthy, and sort out misleading conventional wisdom that frowns upon the food staples that drove human evolution. The highly respected Nurses' Health Study tracked the dietary habits of 90,000 nurses over two decades. It is the largest epidemiological study of women in history, which led to the publication of 265 scientific papers in leading journals. The study showed no statistically significant association between total fat intake (or cholesterol intake) and heart disease. Many other studies have attempted to establish a firm connection, yet none have demonstrated that a high-fat diet by itself causes heart disease. So how can it be that low-fat eating became the conventional wisdom? I believe that the otherwise well-meaning, well-educated folks in the low-fat camp are influenced by a few factors that lead them to the party line conclusion that a high-fat diet is unhealthy.

- **Failure to distinguish between good fats and bad fats.** The skyrocketing rates of obesity, heart disease and cancer from eating a diet high in both processed carbohydrates and chemically altered fats have unfairly implicated all fats as dangerous. As I discussed earlier and will cover further in the next chapter, the typical modern diet is grossly imbalanced between omega 6 fats and omega 3 fats. We ingest way too much of the former (from processed foods, polyunsaturated oils and grain-fed animal products) and way too little of the latter (from oily, cold-water fish, free-range eggs and meat and omega 3 capsules).

  Furthermore, we consume excessive amounts of the highly toxic partially hydrogenated fats and trans-fats (they are not quite the same but are closely related and both evil). These 'Frankenfats' are created by heating and chemically treating vegetable and seed oils to become a solid. Solidifying fats effectively extends their shelf life and improves the flavour of processed foods. These fats are easily oxidised to form free radical chain reactions that damage cell membranes and body tissue, and compromise immune function. Because your brain, nervous system and vascular system are primarily composed of membranes, any dysfunction in these critical areas can be devastating. Research confirms that consumption of trans-fatty acids and partially hydrogenated fats may promote inflammation, ageing and cancer. The *New England Journal of*

Medicine reviewed numerous studies and reported a strong link between trans-fat consumption and heart disease.

"Which came first, the chicken or the egg?" In this case, neither – it's the carbs that make you fat.'

- **Carbohydrates making fat 'look bad'.** Fat is calorically dense at nine calories per gram. If you consume excessive carbohydrates (150 to 300 grams or more per day), produce a high level of insulin, and eat any appreciable amount of fat along *with your* high-carbohydrate diet, your fat intake will contribute directly to making you fat. You know the saying 'Which came first, the chicken or the egg?' Well, in this case, it's neither the chicken nor the egg making you fat – it's the carbohydrates! The carbohydrates cause high levels of insulin which steer both carbohydrates and fat (and protein) into your fat cells.
- **Propaganda and flawed science manipulated into conventional wisdom.** The machinations of public policy bureaucracy often leave rational thinking in the dust in favour of protecting and promoting corporate interests and the reputations of politicians. While I am all in favour of capitalism, it's unsettling how much decision-making power is controlled by corporations that spend billions of marketing dollars moulding and shaping conventional dietary wisdom in the direction of profits, with little regard for health.

The story of how saturated fat came to be vilified should mention the work of American scientist Ancel Keys. Keys was an eloquent and dynamic early promoter of the link between saturated fat intake, cholesterol levels and heart disease – a driving force in the origination and promotion of the lipid hypothesis of heart disease mentioned earlier. Keys received notoriety in the 1960s for his efforts to move the public away from saturated fats to replacements such as polyunsaturated oils or low-fat eating in general. It has taken decades, at a dawdling pace, to recognise the folly of his health suggestions. For example, Keys didn't even connect obesity to heart disease risk, and the foundation of his work was compromised when he was criticised for hand-picking examples (comparisons of fat intake and heart disease rates among different cultures) that supported his hypotheses. In fairness, Keys also did some great work helping to popularise the Mediterranean diet (highlighted by the liberal intake of healthy fats), even spending his last few decades living in a small town in Italy and studying the residents' dietary habits.

On a bureaucratic level, the US Government has time and again shown a penchant for doggedly defending the status quo and vigorously squashing voices opposing conventional wisdom. A shining example of the influence of power and money on the development of public policy is found in the FDA's so-called imitation policy, passed in 1973 (without Congressional approval, thanks to some clever legal manoeuvering). The legislation relieved food manufacturers from having to use that pesky 'imitation' designation on labels of foods created with artificial ingredients (coffee creamers, imitation egg mixes, processed cheeses, whipped cream and hundreds more), as long as manufacturers added synthetic vitamins to their concoctions to approximate the benefits of similar wholefoods.

Mary Enig, PhD, a renowned nutritionist, lipid biochemistry expert and author of *Know Your Fats*, from the University of Maryland, has spent a career battling conventional wisdom's position on fat intake and heart disease. In the 1970s she was a central figure in challenging the corruption and misinformation dispensed by the USDA and the US Senate's McGovern Committee (headed by former presidential candidate George McGovern). Influenced by highly questionable and lobby-influenced testimony, the committee published its report (many believe McGovern was hoodwinked by subordinates to buy into flawed conclusions) directing Americans to replace saturated fat with polyunsaturated fatty acids and to limit fat intake in general which was then disastrously replaced with excessive carbohydrates.

On the heels of these cultural turning points, ensuing government-funded research tends to fall in line with the committee recommendations. The notion that fats are bad gained momentum, became adopted into conventional wisdom and is still going strong! The discussion of the food propaganda topic is compelling enough to fill entire books (check out *Fast Food Nation*, *Food Politics*, *Appetite for Profit* and *Good Calories, Bad Calories* for fascinating and detailed examinations of the topic), so we'll finish here by asserting the point that it's clearly unwise to blindly trust conventional wisdom when it comes to fat and to dietary habits in general.

KETONES – THE FOURTH FUEL

By now you know that we evolved to burn primarily fats and a little glucose. We can also burn protein, when certain amino acids enter the energy pathways through a part of the glucose cycle (as happens when we run out of glucose or glycogen during a long workout or during starvation). Protein can also be converted to glucose in the liver.

While most cells in our body can easily burn both fats and glucose, there are a few select cells that function only on glucose (some brain cells, red blood cells and kidney cells, for example). Without glucose, those cells would cease to function and we would not last very long. The minimum daily glucose requirement to keep those systems running has been estimated at between 150 and 200 grams per day, but recent research shows that after a little adaptation, some of these cells can operate effectively on a fuel known as ketones, dramatically reducing your overall glucose requirement.

Ketosis was crucial to our evolution. As we have already discussed here, our ancestors rarely had steady access to carbohydrates like we do today. In fact, they may have gone weeks or months without appreciable carbohydrates, so they had to evolve a system whereby the liver could take protein either from the muscles or directly from the diet and convert it into glucose through gluconeogenesis. This system worked to keep Grok alive during short periods of starvation or longer periods when meat (protein and fats) was plentiful but plants (carbohydrates) were not. Today we can tap into this same system and prompt our genes to speed up the process of fat loss when we cut carbohydrates while still consuming adequate dietary protein. In this scenario, we never have to sacrifice lean muscle in pursuit of fat loss (the unfortunate story of traditional calorie-restriction weight loss) if we eat Primally.

Manufacturing glucose from protein requires its own source of energy, so liver cells happen to use fats (fatty acids, really) to fuel this conversion. When liver cells are involved in gluconeogenesis they are unable to completely burn off those fats to the final end products of carbon dioxide and water. Consequently, they produce an energy-rich by-product known as a ketone (also called a ketone body). Ketones are very safe, desirable, energy-efficient forms of fuel. They are quite literally the fourth fuel. In fact, when you become well adapted to burning fats on the Primal Blueprint, one of the side benefits is that you will also become keto-adapted. That means that over a few weeks of reducing carbohydrates (and, hence, decreasing insulin) and increasing the relative amounts of healthy fats in your diet, you will send signals to your genes that result in an increased production (an up-regulation) of the metabolic 'machinery' used to effectively and efficiently burn ketones throughout your body.

Many cells actually prefer ketones over glucose, given the choice between the two. Cardiac muscle, skeletal muscle and even certain brain cells thrive on the 4½ calories per gram delivered by ketones. After a little keto-adaptation, the brain can do very well, getting 75 per cent of its energy from ketones. The fact that we can so easily convert to this alternative energy plan may be the best proof that Grok didn't always have access to lots of carbohydrates.

A 2004 article in the *Journal of the International Society of Sports Nutrition* referred to numerous studies suggesting that a low-carbohydrate intake and the resulting mild ketosis may offer many benefits, including reduction of body fat, minimised damage from insulin resistance and free radicals (caused by metabolising a high-carbohydrate diet) and a reduction of LDL cholesterol.

So what exactly is ketosis then? Ketones can't be stored conveni-ently the way fats (and excess glucose) can be stored in fat cells or the way glucose can be stored as glycogen. Ketones simply circulate in the bloodstream where they are available to be picked up by any cells that want and need the energy they provide. *Ketosis* is the scientific name for a relative condition in the body where ketones start to accumulate in the bloodstream to a point beyond which they can all be picked up for energy. There is nothing wrong with being in ketosis; it is a natural, normal part of human energy production and metabolism. You have probably been in mild ketosis whenever you have fasted or skipped a couple of meals in a row.

If you haven't yet become keto-adapted, as is the case with most people who eat a moderate- to high-carbohydrate diet and then decide to fast, the ketones aren't yet able to be burned as efficiently. Ketones happen to be somewhat acidic, and because the body works hard to maintain a slightly alkaline (non-acidic) state, unused ketones are excreted in urine, stool or even breath. Some describe the smell of ketone breath as that of overly ripe apples or acetone. If you are new to Primal eating, you will require a few weeks to reprogramme your genes to become more efficient at burning ketones. As your body adapts to a genetically optimal, low-carbohydrate eating pattern, you will burn ketones effectively and excrete less, thereby further reducing your glucose requirements.

Some people – including some misinformed doctors – maintain an unnecessarily dim view of ketones and ketosis. I believe these criticisms arise because the diets in question allow for only 20 grams or less of carbohydrates per day, a level that does not allow for the plentiful intake of nutrient-rich vegetables. While we are not meant to run predominantly on carbohydrate energy, we do depend heavily on the nutrients offered by vegetables and most fruits. Other people may be mistaking ketosis for ketoacidosis, a very different (and potentially deadly) condition that affects insulin-dependent diabetics and alcoholics.

In the normal Primal Blueprint maintenance zone you rarely even get to a state of ketosis (but you will still burn lots more fat and produce more ketones than high-carbohydrate people), because 100 carbohydrate grams a day seems to be the cut-off point above which ketosis is reduced. The recommended range of 100 to 150 grams per day of vegetable- and fruit-based carbohydrates is plenty to fuel the glucose-/glycogen-dependent systems, while the majority of our energy comes from fat.

On the Primal Blueprint accelerated fat-loss programme (detailed in Chapter 8) you will eat in what I call the 'sweet spot' – a level of mild ketosis – by consuming 50 to 100 grams of carbohydrates per day. There, the protein needed for gluconeogenesis comes from your diet (not your muscles) and you will have plenty of fat to meet your daily fuel requirements.

By understanding how the metabolic processes work for protein, fat, carbohydrates and ketones, and knowing that you can control the rates at which each one burns by improving your diet and exercise habits, you needn't agonise over day-to-day calorie counting. As long as you are eating Primal foods you will be able to maintain your personal ideal body composition and mitigate your risk of diet-related health conditions and diseases.

> 'My doctor told me to stop having intimate dinners for four. Unless there are three other people.'
> ORSON WELLES

EATING WELL

The Primal Blueprint is about enjoying a healthy, happy, balanced lifestyle. As Dr Andrew Weil said in describing the title of his book *Eating Well for Optimum Health*, 'eating well' refers not only to choosing natural, nutritious foods but also to enjoying the experience as one of the great pleasures of life. It's likely that Grok appreciated food much more than we do today, because he had to work so hard for his meals and was never assured of success. Throughout history, food has represented a centrepiece of cultural celebration – let's not kill the momentum now! The key to eating well is to eliminate distractions and negative influences to your eating, which will allow the physical sensations of hunger and the simple pursuit of pleasure to have the predominant influence on your dietary habits.

THE 'OH, POSITIVE' DIET

If you wish to succeed with healthy dietary habits, it's important that you discard any negative emotions you have towards eating and embrace each meal as an opportunity to enjoy yourself. I strongly recommend that you give yourself permission to eat as much as you want, whenever you want, for the rest of your life. While this suggestion might scare the heck out of you, releasing yourself from restriction and deprivation enables you to become more connected with your physical nutritional needs rather than being driven by emotional triggers.

Take notice of that point in every meal where you have attained satisfaction and feel comfortable stopping – not the point at which you are full, but the point at which you are no longer hungry for the next bite – knowing that you can eat again whenever you like. If you wish to enjoy a treat once in a while (hopefully Primal-approved, but hey – maybe not!), do so with full attention and awareness to the pleasure that every single savoured bite gives you. Reject feelings of anxiety, guilt or rebellion connected to your food choices and replace them with the idea that you deserve to eat the most delicious, nutritious foods possible.

When it comes to specific meal choices, I prefer to let my taste buds guide me to the most enjoyable and nourishing diet within the broad guidelines of the Primal Blueprint. Forget the scientifically unproven admonitions to eat certain food-type combinations at certain times, or to align your food choices with your racial heritage, body shape or blood type (I can't remember if my blood is O positive or O negative, but when I eat my Primal salad most afternoons, my brain always thinks, 'Oh, positive!').

Humans have evolved on widely differing diets from settlements all over the globe. I do understand that some people have genetically predisposed grain or dairy allergies; however, Primal Blueprint foods have been shown to satisfy and nourish everyone, regardless of where the last 5 or 500 generations in your bloodline lived or what they ate. Essentially, my goal is for you to become a modern forager with a keen sense of what you need to do (or not do) to thrive day in and day out. When you understand this basic concept, the resulting sense of personal power you will gain is tremendous. When you eat Primal Blueprint style, there is no city you can't travel to, no restaurant you can't negotiate with, no grocery store you can't shop in and no family holiday you can't endure!

EATING ON GROK'S CLOCK

Ever notice how some people freak out if they miss a meal or can't find exactly what they want on a menu? They become irritable and start complaining about being light-headed – as if their world might stop if they don't inhale some calories right away. Ironically, other than a lifetime of cultural socialisation and a metabolism they've built to depend on ingested carbohydrates instead of fat, there is no reason why skipping a meal should be a big deal. Our ancestors ate sporadically – with continually varied mealtimes and food choices. Given the variables of the seasons and hunting success or failure, they didn't always have enough food or a varied diet. Our genes thrive on intermittent scarcity and can even handle occasional excess. In fact, they expect it.

Our genetic ability to thrive on intermittent eating habits is an important concept to retain because it unburdens you of having to eat every meal on a set schedule, to balance food groups (meat with starch, grains with protein, etc.), or to align your foods with time-of-day traditions (cereal for breakfast, sandwich for lunch, etc.). Skipping meals, fasting briefly and simply freeing yourself from an obsessive need to eat three square or six small meals a day when the clock strikes a particular hour might actually benefit your body. Doing so will align you more closely with your historic genetic experience. Unburdened by the strict and ill-advised 'rules' of conventional wisdom, eating becomes much simpler and more enjoyable.

> *'By eliminating sugars, grains and legumes from your diet and emphasising Primal foods, you will experience more consistent energy levels and a comfortably diminished appetite.'*

On this topic, it's interesting to note that your need to consume calories on a regular schedule will diminish substantially when blood glucose levels are moderated and you start burning fat and ketones more efficiently through low-insulin Primal Blueprint dietary choices. By contrast, if you eat the typical Western diet of 300 to 500 grams of carbohydrates per day (instead of the 100 to 150 from plant sources as suggested by the Primal Blueprint), you are going to experience significant blood glucose fluctuations and corresponding cravings for quick-energy, high-carbohydrate foods. This is perhaps the single quickest and most exciting revelation for converts to the Primal Blueprint eating style. By eliminating sugars, grains and legumes from your diet and emphasising Primal foods, you will experience more consistent energy levels and a comfortably diminished appetite.

These benefits will be long lasting, but they might take a bit of time to realise. Every once in a while, people commenting on MarksDailyApple.com mention difficulties with energy level swings during the first three weeks of their transition to a Primal eating style. During this transition period, your body expects sugar as fuel (which it's getting less of) but hasn't rediscovered how to get the most out of your fat reserves. Don't worry, it will. By limiting carbohydrates (and, hence, lowering insulin) you are sending a new series of hormonal signals to your genes. In turn, they are down-regulating their sugar-burning systems and up-regulating their keto-burning machinery.

While you may experience a few episodes of light-headedness during the transition, rest assured that the shift will be complete in a few weeks and energy levels will dramatically improve. Meanwhile, grab a handful of macadamia nuts or a cold drumstick to munch on if you get hungry for a snack (I'll detail some of my favourite snack choices in Chapter 4). You should always satisfy your cravings with abundant amounts of approved foods instead of suffering through them with willpower and other flimsy, short-duration weapons. Don't worry, these Primal food choices will totally satisfy you without bringing about a sugar crash later, as will happen when you reach for a bagel. This is due to the high caloric density and slow-burn rate of foods high in fat and/or protein (such as meat, fish, poultry, eggs, avocados, butter, coconut products, nuts, and seeds, olives and high-fat dairy products) and the high water and fibre content of vegetables and fruits.

Because modern life is all about schedules, we often find it convenient and enjoyable to eat regular meals. This is fine. I'm simply suggesting you pay more attention to your hunger levels than the clock. For example, I eat breakfast on most days, but in a wide range of food choices and total calories – based on my appetite, activity level and the day's schedule. Frequently I will have a huge omelette with four to five eggs, cheese, chopped mushrooms, peppers, onions and tomatoes and topped with some bacon and avocado. On other days I will grab some macadamia nuts or make a Primal smoothie to have on the go. Then again, on many days I simply skip breakfast altogether, with no accompanying guilt, hunger pangs or low blood glucose. As long as you are eating Primally most of the time, it all works well.

When you can be flexible with your food choices and eating schedules, your diet becomes more psychologically pleasing and less stressful to follow. However, the key is to make informed choices that minimise your exposure to toxic foods and, when you indulge or get off track, to allow your body to return quickly to balance. If you enjoy a decadent dessert or a weekend away from healthy food options, simply eat a few low-insulin-producing meals in a row and return to regulated energy levels and optimal metabolic function. Even a short walk after a big meal and rich dessert can mitigate the insulin response by diverting some of the glucose from your bloodstream into working muscles.

ONE SMALL SCOOP FOR MANKIND

When you eat Primal Blueprint style, the consequences of your food choices become crystal clear. Eat right and you have discernibly more energy and better health. Stick with it and your body composition goals happen effortlessly. Slide a little bit and you might get halfway to your goal (or less, owing to the vicious cycle of insulin-driven sugar crashes and cravings), have a little less energy and maybe catch an extra cold or two due to compromised immune function.

Every once in a while, I'll have a lapse in judgement and indulge in something like a small scoop of gourmet ice cream. It tastes delicious for the four minutes it takes to eat it (but not quite on a par with a bowl of fresh blueberries and raspberries with home-made whipped cream), but invariably I experience bloating and gas in the ensuing hour as well as a bit of a sugar crash. Because these lapses are out of my normal habit pattern, I am highly sensitive to the consequences of choices like these.

Understand that I enjoy the taste of ice cream as much as anyone, but I will assert my position that after eating Primally for some time, even the occasional treat that's not Primal Blueprint approved – for me – is *just not worth it*. I don't mean to come off as a Food Nazi here – I assure you that I'm tempted frequently and in the future will certainly indulge in a non-Primal manner again (and again after that…) – I'm merely trying to illustrate how, once you're sensitised to the negative effects of unhealthy choices, it gets easier to turn down what used to seem impossible to resist. This is especially true when you clearly understand the consequences of each and every food choice that you make, whether they are aligned with your primal genes or not.

When you use defence mechanisms like 'Everything in moderation', 'You only live once' and the like, you disguise the fact that over years and decades those little ice-cream outings can add up literally to hundreds of pounds of ingested substances that are toxic to your body. Furthermore, as unhealthy food choices ingrain themselves (pun intended) into your daily life, I believe you become desensitised to the negative effects they have on your health. This concept is illustrated by heavy tobacco or caffeine users who are able to function somewhat normally (that's not saying much) with volumes of chemicals in their bloodstream that would floor the casual user or teetotaler.

The complete lack of regimentation or caloric deprivation in the Primal Blueprint eating style (I refuse to use the word *diet* because it implies regimentation) is the secret to its long-term success. You don't have to force yourself to go hungry or to feel deprived or negative about eating. Simply make sensible choices by welcoming the abundant selection of delicious foods whenever you want, and move away from habitually consuming foods that may taste great for a brief moment but make your body feel bad or create long-term metabolic stress.

DEALING WITH THE (MAYBE RADICAL) CHANGE TO PRIMAL BLUEPRINT EATING

If you argue that life will never be the same without your bowl of Raisin Bran® or a heaping plate of pasta and garlic bread, see if these suggestions can ease your transition:

- **'80 Per Cent Rule':** Do the best you can, taking your transition step by step at a comfortable pace and relieving yourself from the pressure of perfection. Be sure that your indulgences are sensible, as I detail in the next chapter. Over time, you will naturally and comfortably become more compliant, particularly with the restriction and elimination of grains, sugars and legumes from your diet.
- **Build Momentum:** As you continue to go hungry or to make progress eating the way you were designed to eat, you will notice a heightened sensitivity to how food affects your body, both positively and negatively. During my years as an athlete, I thought my recurrent digestive bloating and post-meal fatigue were due to my hard training regime or simply the end of a long day – not from subclinical allergic reactions to excessive processed carbohydrates and/or dairy products.

Can you relate to that hyper, racing heart sensation that comes after consuming a sugary dessert? It's probably something that we've been aware of since childhood – a little annoying but no big deal, right? It was only when I started to aggressively clean up my diet a decade ago that my sensitivity went to the next level. What a pleasure it was to leave the dinner table feeling totally satisfied, yet alert and energetic – and not having to unbuckle the belt a notch or two! Passing on dessert took a little getting used to, but I noticed that the sacrifice of a few moments of instant gratification paled in comparison to not having to deal with sugar highs and sugar crashes. Plus, as you cut out simple carbohydrates, you begin to lose your craving for them. Hence, you escape the vicious cycle that befalls even those with tremendous willpower trying to do the right thing but eating the wrong stuff.

- **Five Favourite Meals Strategy:** Pick your five favourite Primal Blueprint-approved meals and rotate them for the first three weeks of your transition to Primal Blueprint eating. Maybe it's grilled salmon and steamed broccoli, lamb chops with grilled zucchini and summer squash, rotisserie chicken (with the skin – preferably organic) and a large steamed vegetable. As much colourful, creative salad as you want. Liberal snacking on Primal Blueprint-approved snacks. Yes, you are removing the baked potato, corn on the cob, Cheerios®, baguettes and other beige staples from the picture, but the discomfort of a habit change can be greatly assuaged when you can look forward to as much as you want of your favourite Primal foods during the crucial transition period to the Primal Blueprint eating style.

- **Never Struggle, Suffer or Go Hungry:** Surround yourself with Primal Blueprint-approved foods and enjoy them as much and as often as you like. Always have a Primal snack nearby to help you through the transition period. That said, pay close attention to your hunger levels and eliminate emotional triggers that negatively influence healthy eating. The key is to stop eating not when you are full – by then you've had too much – but when you are no longer hungry.

- **Substitute:** Consider whether you can switch some of your old favourite meals, snacks and even treats for interesting new Primal Blueprint options. I used to be a big blueberry pancakes and granola guy, but whatever deprivation I might have felt at first in eliminating the 'stack' from my life was more than made up for by a dozen bites of a delicious Primal omelette. Consider the overall impact of your current favourite foods on your body and if they are all truly worth it.

CHAPTER SUMMARY

- **Primal Blueprint Foods:** The essence of the Primal Blueprint eating style is to eat nutritious plants and animal products (the meat, fish, poultry, eggs, nuts, seeds, vegetables and fruit that have driven human evolution for two million years) and avoid processed foods, creating a more calorically efficient, nutrient-dense diet. Benefits of Primal Blueprint eating include enhanced cellular function, improved immune and antioxidant function, optimal development and repair of muscle tissue, enhanced fat metabolism and weight management, a reduction in disease risk factors and a stabilisation of daily appetite and energy levels. While the Primal Blueprint advocates restriction of processed carbohydrates just as some popular diet programmes do, it does not restrict most nutritious natural carbohydrates. The Primal Blueprint is no mere diet – it is a comprehensive lifestyle approach.
- **Insulin is the Master Hormone:** Perhaps the most important health benefit of eating Primally is moderating the wildly excessive insulin production of the Standard American Diet. Eighty per cent of your ability to achieve body composition goals is determined by your diet. When you moderate insulin production so you access and burn stored body fat for energy, while preserving or building muscle. The regulation of carbohydrate intake and, thus, insulin production is perhaps the most impor-

tant takeaway message of the Primal Blueprint. It is the key to maintaining ideal body composition and preventing obesity, heart disease, cancer and inflammation-related health problems.

When the delicate insulin balance is abused by consuming too many carbohydrates for too long, havoc ensues: cells become insulin resistant, excess glucose is present in the bloodstream, more fat is stored and it becomes increasingly difficult to mobilise that fat for an energy source. This sets the stage for the development of serious conditions such as Metabolic Syndrome, type 2 diabetes and heart disease. Synthesis of important hormones, including thyroid hormones, testosterone and human growth hormone are also hindered by excessive insulin production, creating an accelerated ageing effect that has more to do with your breakfast choices than chronology. While the long-term effects of excess insulin production are dire, there are also serious immediate drawbacks to consuming high-carbohydrate snacks or meals. The sugar high-insulin release-stress response cycle causes problems with fatigue, mental focus, mood swings and jitters, resulting in burnout.

- **Cholesterol:** Cholesterol is critical to healthy cell structure and numerous metabolic functions. Conventional wisdom's lipid hypothesis of heart disease is a flawed and narrow perspective on the actual chain of events and risk factors that contribute to heart disease. The direct connection between cholesterol and heart disease has been refuted in recent years by the Framingham Heart Study and many other respected studies and experts.

The true risk factors are best characterised by the common health condition of Metabolic Syndrome. In many cases, only small, dense LDL causes problems in the arteries, and only when triglycerides are high and systemic inflammation is present. These risk factors are typically a consequence of excessive insulin production, a poor omega 6 to omega 3 ratio, and poor exercise habits (either sedentary or too stressful). Furthermore, sufficient levels of HDL – generated by healthy eating and exercise habits – can often mitigate any potential threats from small, dense LDL. Conversely, the primary function of statin drugs – lowering cholesterol levels – does not directly address these risk factors. Statin's purported anti-inflammatory benefits can be easily achieved through diet, exercise and supplementation, saving the expense and harmful side effects of prescription statin therapy.

- **Healthy Fats:** Primal Blueprint eating provides high levels of the highly touted omega 3 polyunsaturated fatty acids, which support healthy cardiovascular, brain, skin and immune function, and of saturated fats, which promote cellular health and dietary satiety. The optimum ratio of omega 6 to omega 3 intake is dangerously out of balance in the modern diet. Efforts should be made to minimise omega 6 intake and bump up omega 3 intake. Balancing your omega 6:omega 3 ratio helps keep the inflammation response under control and protects against serious disease conditions resulting from uncontrolled inflammation.

- **Macronutrients:** Understand the 'context of calories' to see a bigger picture than the overly simplistic 'calories in, calories out' concept of weight loss. Obtain between 0.7 and 1 gram of protein per pound of lean body weight (range based on activity level) per day to ensure healthy metabolic function and preserve lean muscle mass. Limit carbohydrate intake to an average of 100 to 150 grams per day (or 50 to 100 grams per day if you seek accelerated fat loss), which will happen automatically when you enjoy plenty of vegetables and fruits and avoid grains, sugars, legumes and processed carbohydrates. The Carbohydrate Curve summarises how various levels of carbohydrates impact on your health and weight management success.

  With protein intake in an optimum range and carbohydrate intake strictly controlled, fat becomes your main caloric energy variable. This allows you to enjoy deeply satisfying high-fat foods whenever you are hungry, knowing they will more likely be burned as energy than make you fat – if you moderate insulin production. Although fat has been maligned by conventional wisdom for years, this prejudice comes from mistakenly attributing the negative effects of processed fats to all fats. Ketones are known as the fourth fuel because they provide an efficient energy source when carbohydrate intake is low. They are a by-product of gluconeogenesis in the liver. Achieving an occasional state of mild ketosis during weight-loss efforts is a safe strategy to burn off excess body fat more rapidly.

- **Eating Well:** Eating well means enjoying one of the great pleasures of life without deprivation, restriction, emotional stress or other negativity. Choose the foods that you enjoy most from the broad list of Primal Blueprint-approved choices and don't obsess about calories, nutrient ratios, regimented mealtimes or food combinations. Eat until you feel satisfied instead of habitually stuffing yourself until you are full. Realise that your genes evolved to easily handle sporadic eating habits without energy lulls or metabolic slowdowns and can do so now, provided you take 21 days to reprogramme them and become a fat-burning beast! We have complex mechanisms in the body to balance energy levels. Your need to consume calories on a schedule will diminish relatively quickly when insulin production is moderated on the Primal Blueprint plan.

- **Moving to The Primal Blueprint:** When adjusting to the Primal Blueprint eating style, discover desirable substitutes (you can rotate them over and over if desired) to avoid feelings of deprivation from discarding old meal choices. Have plenty of Primal Blueprint foods available for snacks and meals so you don't suffer or feel depleted. Follow the 80 Per Cent Rule by being compliant 80 per cent of the time and not stressing about perfection. Notice your heightened sensitivity to how foods affect your body and use that awareness to keep on track with high-energy, effortless weight management and optimal gene expression with Primal Blueprint foods.

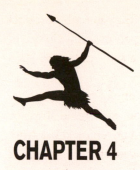

CHAPTER 4

LAW NUMBER 1: EAT LOTS OF PLANTS AND ANIMALS

(BUT DON'T LET THEM EAT YOU)

'If we're not supposed to eat animals, how come they're made out of meat?
TOM SNYDER

IN THIS CHAPTER

Here I will reveal the health benefits of eating Primal Blueprint style and how to choose the best products in the food categories of animal foods (meat, fish, poultry and eggs), vegetables, fruits, macadamia nuts, herbs and spices, moderation foods (coffee; high-fat dairy; other nuts, seeds and nut butters; supplemental carbohydrates, water), sensible indulgences (red wine, dark chocolate), and certain high-quality nutritional supplements (multivitamin/mineral/anti-oxidant formula, omega 3 oil, probiotics and protein powder).

Locally grown, pesticide-free or certified organic vegetables and fruits are the most nutritious and safest you can eat. They are packed with antioxidants and micronutrients that support health and help prevent disease. Some moderation is warranted with fruit to emphasise locally grown, in-season, high-antioxidant fruits, such as berries, and avoid excessive year-round consumption. Local, pasture-raised or certified organic animal foods are healthy and nutritious and will help you reduce excess body fat and build lean muscle. They are free from the offensive ingredients (hormones, pesticides and antibiotics) and processing methods found with mass-produced foods. Eggs, too, are healthy and nutritious; they have been mistakenly maligned due to the flawed assumption that their high cholesterol content is a heart disease risk factor. The budget increase for buying local or organic plant and animal products pales in comparison to the importance of leading a healthy life and avoiding disease risk factors.

If you are trying to memorise the most important, life-changing sound bites from the Primal Blueprint, here's another one: animals (meat, fish, poultry and eggs), plants (vegetables, fruits, nuts, seeds and herbs and spices) should represent the entire composition of your diet. While vegetables, fruits and herbs and spices don't provide a ton of calories, they should represent your main source of healthy carbohydrates and micronutrients (vitamins, minerals, antioxidants, anti-inflammatory agents and thousands of other phytonutrients). Animal foods are calorically dense, stimulate

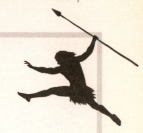

PRIMAL BLUEPRINT FOOD PYRAMID

for effortless weight loss, vibrant health, and maximum longevity

Herbs, Spices, Extracts
High-antioxidant/ nutritional value

Sensible Indulgences
Dark chocolate, red wine

Supplements
Multi, omega-3, probiotics, protein/meal powder, Vitamin D

Moderation Foods

Fruits – locally grown, in-season, high-antioxidant (berries, pitted fruit)
High-Fat Dairy – Raw, fermented, unpasteurised
Starchy Tubers, Quinoa, Wild Rice - Athlete's carbohydrate option
Other Nuts, Seeds and Nut Butters - Great snack option

Healthy Fats

Animal fats, butter & coconut oil (cooking)
Avocados, coconut products, olives & olive oil, macadamias (eating)

Vegetables

Locally grown and/or organic. Abundant servings for flavour, nutrition, and antioxidants.

Meat • Fish • Fowl • Eggs

Bulk of dietary calories: saturated fat (energy, satiety, cell & hormone function)
and protein (building blocks, lean mass). Emphasise local, pasture-raised or certified organic.

Revisions to pyramid since 2009 hardcover:

Macadamia nuts: Elevated above other nuts and seeds due to concerns about moderating omega-6 intake. Other nuts and seeds have unfavourable O6:O3 ratios.

Meat, Fish, Fowl, Eggs: Moved to base as primary calorie source. 'Emphasise local, pasture raised': Local is superior to organic since organic animals likely have grain supplemented diets (more popularity, more mass production elements), lowering nutritional value versus a pastured animal.

Vitamin D: Added to supplements to respect the challenges of obtaining adequate sunlight year-round outside the tropics.

Other: Quinoa added as supplemental carbohydrate (it's a chenopod, not a grain; good nutritional value, no anti-nutrients). More attention for avocado, coconut, and olives. Less emphasis on fruit (easy to overdo it, especially when trying to reduce fat).

minimal insulin production, offer the best forms of healthy protein and fat, and should represent the bulk of your caloric intake.

In Grok's time, the bulk of calories in the human diet (estimates range from 45 to 85 per cent, depending on geography) came from eating a variety of animal life, including insects, grubs, amphibians, birds, their eggs, fish and shellfish, small mammals and some larger mammals. In general, those living closer to the Equator consumed more plants and less animal food, while those at colder latitudes with fewer plant options consumed more meat. These meat sources provided significant amounts of protein and all types of essential fatty acids and vitamins. Grok often ate as much as 300 or 400 grams of protein and up to 200 or more grams of fat in a day during times of plenty – and yet maintained a svelte physique. Of course, he also ate very limited amounts of carbohydrates, produced moderate levels of insulin and excelled at using stored fat as fuel. These macronutrient breakdowns allowed him to build or preserve muscle and provided ample fuel for both long treks and short bursts of speed.

Animal foods are healthy and nutritious and will help you reduce excess body fat, build lean muscle and generally promote peak performance. While I highly respect those who have philosophical objections to consuming animal flesh, I want to dispel conventional wisdom that eating a diet high in animal foods leads to obesity and heart disease or that vegetarianism is somehow healthier. Like it or not, our bodies have evolved for two million years on animal foods, ever since meat eating became a survival factor and a trigger to population expansion on earth (our ability to migrate to the higher latitudes depended on us developing 'meat-adaptive' genes).

The fact remains that no culture or society has ever survived for an extended period of time on a meatless diet. While it would seem to be much easier to live and evolve without having to run around and kill animals, the truth is that we need concentrated, nutrient-rich energy sources like meat to support accelerated brain development – our distinguishing feature that brought us to the top of the food chain. Remarkably, about 500 calories a day are required just to fuel the human brain (both primitive and modern). Anthropological evidence strongly suggests that it was protein and omega 3 fatty acids from animal foods that provided both the raw materials and energy necessary for the human brain to grow larger over the course of evolution. Our ability to hunt and catch animals and cook their meat (cooking makes meat easier to chew, swallow and digest) was critical in our branching up and away from our mostly vegetarian ape cousins.

> *'My favourite animal is steak.'*
> FRAN LEBOWITZ, *AMERICAN AUTHOR AND HUMOURIST*

At this point in our discussion, it's important to acknowledge that over the past decade some studies about red meat consumption have prompted alarming headlines that 'excessive' consumption of red meat may be associated with a slightly increased risk of cancer and heart disease. In all such studies to date, however, there has been no distinction or separation between groups who consumed local, pasture-raised or certified organic red meat versus the vast majority of participants who ate the standard hormone-laden, grain-fed, antibiotic-laced, mass-produced by Concentrated Animal Feeding Operations (CAFO). Nor has there been any evaluation of the negative effects of excessive carbohydrate intake in the Standard American Diet when it comes to how we metabolise meat (remember that carbohydrates *and* fats consumed together increase triglyceride production in the liver). Furthermore, most of these studies (in which participants self-report their dietary intake) include in the general red meat category all manner of popular processed meats (hot dogs, breakfast sausage, bacon, salami), which generally contain preservatives that act as potential carcinogens. These agents have been shown to accelerate the formation and growth of cancer cells throughout the body. Of course, the Primal Blueprint suggests that you generally avoid those meats entirely.

Authors of these studies also offer another possible explanation for the increased risks: overcooking of meat. You may have heard that some forms of seared, burned or overcooked meat may contain heat-altered chemical byproducts called heterocyclic amines (or

HCAs) which may be carcinogenic if consumed frequently over long periods of time. Since mankind has been cooking with fire for hundreds of thousands of years, it's apparent that we have developed a host of natural genetic adaptations to allow us to eat most properly cooked foods without problems. Furthermore, some studies indicate that consuming antioxidant-rich foods (such as vegetables, fruits, herbs and spices, and even red wine and dark chocolate) along with cooked meats can essentially neutralise any potentially harmful by-products of overcooking. Of course, the Primal Blueprint would argue that eating only 'clean' meats, avoiding nitrosamine-laden processed meats, using appropriate cooking techniques (like slow-roasting, undercooking or using crock pots), enjoying a variety of different forms of animal foods, eschewing deep-fried or high-heat barbecued meats, or eating certain forms of meat raw (sushi, tartar, etc.), will likely eliminate any possible risk altogether.

While it's indisputable that our bodies thrive on the rich and unique nutrients provided by animal foods, it is possible – albeit pretty darn difficult – to be healthy and enjoy a nutritious diet without consuming meat. However, it will be a real challenge to obtain sufficient protein and fat – or simply enough calories – to fuel an active lifestyle while also avoiding grains, sugar and legumes, foods that by choice or default constitute a high percentage of calories for vegetarians and vegans. If you consume moderate to high amounts of grains in an effort to make up for the absence of meat, you are probably going to encounter a host of possible health challenges, as I will explain in the next chapter.

Animal fats used in cooking (e.g., butter, chicken fat and lard) have long been maligned by conventional wisdom in the movement towards polyunsaturated fatty acids (PUFAs) that has spanned the last few generations. However, saturated fats (solid at room temperature, unlike PUFAs) are the most beneficial fats with which to cook. While they are not teeming with micronutrients and so you may wish to limit them somewhat in favour of more densely nutritious calorie sources (such as the meat or vegetables you might be cooking!), they are not at all bad for you, as we've been conditioned to believe. In contrast, PUFAs become easily oxidised when heated, contain too much omega 6 and are a strong contributor to the oxidation and inflammation conditions detailed in Chapter 3. The sidebar 'Primal-Approved Fats and Oils' later in this chapter lists my favourite fats and oils, as well as which ones to avoid.

Brightly coloured fruits and vegetables supply high levels of antioxidants that are critical to good health. The flavonoids, carotenoids and myriad other important phytonutrients found in these foods can serve as a powerful first line of defence against oxidative damage from ageing, stress and inflammation. Moreover, antioxidants and other phytonutrients appear to contain cancer-fighting properties, support immune function, aid in digestion and help preserve muscle mass – a critical longevity component for those of advanced age.

While leading a healthy, balanced lifestyle will activate the genes that make our built-in antioxidant systems (catalase, superoxide dismutase and glutathione) fight hard against cellular and DNA breakdown, research suggests that we may require additional antioxidant support from foods and supplements. Of course, most processed foods and starchy carbohydrates are devoid of antioxidants, while vegetables, fruits and nuts are the best sources of these natural antioxidants.

Recall from Chapter 3 the discussion of oxidation as a central heart disease component; antioxidants protect against oxidative damage in the body, it therefore follows that if you want to be healthy and prevent disease, vegetables (and fruits with a bit of moderation and selectivity we'll discuss shortly) must play a prominent role in your diet. It is also apparent that modern food-processing methods, which include growing produce in soil bereft of important minerals and the widespread use of pesticides, may further hamper our efforts to get enough antioxidants.

Consequently, many people may benefit from a prudent supplementation programme.

'Animals (meat, fish, poultry and eggs) and plants (vegetables, fruits, nuts, seeds and herbs and spices) should represent the entire composition of your diet.'

For a quick primer, red plants (pomegranates, cherries, watermelon, etc.) have been shown to help reduce the risk of prostate cancer as well as some tumours. Green fruit and vegetables (avocados, limes, green beans, zucchini, etc.) are high in carotenoids that have a powerful anti-ageing effect and are especially helpful for vision. Yellow and orange produce (bananas, papayas, carrots, butternut squash, pineapple) offer beta-carotene for immune support as well as bromelain, which has been shown to aid in digestion, joint health and the reduction of inflammatory conditions. Cruciferous ('cross'-shaped, with a branch and leaves) vegetables, including broccoli, Brussels sprouts, kale, arugula, turnips, bok choy, horseradish and cauliflower, have demonstrated specific anti-cancer, anti-ageing, and anti-microbial properties. Nuts and seeds provide high levels of beneficial monounsaturated and omega 3 fatty acids, fibre, phyto-nutrients, antioxidants (e.g. vitamin E and selenium) and a host of essential nutrients (e.g., manganese, magnesium, zinc, iron, chromium, phosphorous and folate).

Plant foods also naturally promote a beneficial balance between acidity and alkalinity (also known as 'base', or non-acidic) in your bloodstream. Almost all cells prefer a slightly alkaline environment to function properly, but many metabolic processes, including the normal production of cellular energy, result in the release of acidic waste products. The buildup of acidic waste is toxic to your body, so it works very hard at all times to preserve a slightly alkaline environment, measured by the familiar 'pH' levels.

While we have evolved several highly refined buffering systems to balance our pH, ingesting acid-producing foods makes it that much more difficult to achieve pH homeostasis. As you might guess, consuming heavily processed foods, sugars, grains, deep-fried foods, alcohol, caffeine, cigarettes, carbonated drinks, artificial sweeteners and many recreational and prescription drugs are acid-forming in the body, a precursor of many health problems and diseases. In contrast, by emphasising alkaline-forming foods – vegetables, fruits, nuts and seeds – in your diet, you optimise your acid/base balance and improve metabolism to burn fat, build muscle and reduce your susceptibility to environmental and dietary toxins. Meat and dairy products also happen to be acid-producing, making it essential to balance the intake of these foods with sufficient vegetables and fruits that support alkalinity.

MEAT AND POULTRY

Many of the conventional wisdom health objections to eating animal foods can easily be countered by eating local, pasture-raised, 100 per cent grass-fed, or certified organic sources of meat. This suggestion is highly recommended due to the generally poor quality of much of today's mass-produced feedlot animals, which typically contain hormones (to grow them bigger more quickly and therefore increase profits), pesticides (ingested from their own inferior food sources; vegetarian advocates claim that 80 to 90 per cent of your total dietary pesticide exposure comes from eating meat, although that's disputed by the EPA) and antibiotics (to prevent widespread illness result-ing from consuming immune-suppressing feed and living in filthy, cramped feedlots and coops). Hormones, pesticides and antibiotics: these three stooges can really mess up your efforts to eat healthily.

Furthermore, today's feedlot cattle, chickens and other animals are usually fed a diet of fortified grains, which have a similar effect on their bodies as on humans! Purchase your meats at a supermar-ket (excluding the organic section), and there's a good chance you'll end up eating a malnourished, insulin-resistant and quite possibly diseased animal whose meat is higher in omega 6 fats – a far cry nutritionally from Grok's fresh, lean, wild kills. Finally, humane reasons compel many to avoid meat. The animals we typically dine on consume half of our crop harvest; their waste pollutes air, rivers and streams; and many claim they are subjected to horrifying treat-ment at unsanitary production facilities (as detailed in such books as *Fast Food Nation*, *The Omnivore's Dilemma*, *Diet for a New America*, and even *Skinny Bitch*).

For these reasons, I strongly urge you to look for local sources of pasture-raised meat whenever possible – typically found at farm-ers' markets or your local butcher. If local, pasture-raised meats are not available, the next best alternative is certified organic. Clearly, there is a continuum here where you can find options that are various degrees away from ideal. While the ultimate meat would be a wild animal with lots of lean mass, little fat and a nutritious, high omega 3 natural diet, there aren't many of them running around the continent these days. Beyond local, pasture-raised meats) from small farms or USDA-certified organic animals, there is minimal regulation in this industry, and assorted other descriptors such as 'free-range' and 'all of-natural' have only minimal significance (more details in the 'Meet and Greet For Your Meat' panel).

Fortunately, the popularity of eating locally and/or organic is skyrocketing, so you should be able to find healthier animal products in your area quite easily. If not, you can have a look on the Internet to find local, registered organic suppliers.

Besides being free of hormones, pesticides and antibiotics, pasture-raised animals offer higher levels of healthy omega 3 and monounsaturated fats than feedlot animals. If, for reasons of budget or availability, you find yourself eating a less-than-ideal source of meat, always choose the leanest possible cuts and simply trim the excess fat. This will significantly limit your potential exposure to these toxins. Of course, you can add back some delicious fat by cooking the now leaner meat in butter!

A LITTLE MEET AND GREET FOR YOUR MEAT

Following are brief descriptions of common labels on meat products to help you make informed purchasing decisions. Many of the terms have no official designation or are not regulated in a meaningful manner. For further insights, *The Omnivore's Dilemma*, by Michael Pollan, is a highly regarded book that offers extensive commentary on the subject of eating meat in a healthy way.

Local, Pasture-Raised: This is the premier choice for meat, whether or not your local farmer is large enough or has otherwise gone to the trouble and expense of applying for organic status. A locally raised animal from a small farm represents the ultimate in sustainability and minimal carbon footprint. A chicken, cow or lamb grazing in the open pasture consumes a variety of grass, grubs, worms and bugs that are rich in nutrients such as omega 3 fatty acids and assorted vitamins and minerals that are deficient in CAFO animals.

Organic: To be labelled as 'organic', foods in the UK must adhere to set EU standards that include restrictions on pesticide, fertiliser and additive use; banning the use of genetically modified organisms; and promotion of animal welfare and farming sustainability. This is regulated by the Department for Environment, Food and Rural Affairs (DEFRA), which oversees a number of organic certification bodies. These bodies inspect farms and other production facilities to be sure regulations are adhered to. The food label must carry the name (or at least the code number) of the body that carried out the certification for DEFRA. The EU sets the minimum standards that must be met for organic certification; however, a number of UK organisations set significantly higher standards to achieve a more rigorous certification. One of the best known is the Soil Association. Some supermarkets also have their own organic label, which must also meet EU regulations. While not organic, the LEAF Marque (Linking Environment and Farming) is used to indicate foods produced with an emphasis on sustainable and environmentally responsible farming principles. In practice this means the promotion of wildlife habitats and recycling and limitations on pesticides and fertilisers. It requires an audit of farm practices and an independent inspection of the property.

Organic meat may not be locally raised (and in fact may have travelled a great distance to your market or supermarket) and has possibly received grain-based feed to supplement calories obtained from free-ranging on the pasture. This results in a slightly-to-significantly less optimal nutritional profile than a 100 per cent pasture-raised/grass-fed animal.

Certified: Meat labels may include information on the way an animal is reared, its age or maturation, the region or the breed. For example, it could be labelled as Orkney lamb or

Aberdeen Angus Beef matured for 21 days. Producers must apply for approval to use these terms, provide evidence to back them up, and submit to inspections.

Conventional: Absent any special label designations, you are likely buying a mass-produced animal raised on grains containing pesticide residues. Such animals are often treated inhumanely.

Country of Origin: The law specifies that meat must be labelled with where the animal was raised, slaughtered and processed. British produce may be indicated with the Union Jack flag. As with produce, local products are preferred.

EU Protected Food Names: These may be found on meat from certain geographical areas, such as Welsh lamb, and are a good way to know that your meat was locally produced. This label requires a strict verification process and inspection scheme to guarantee the origin.

Free-Range (chicken): This term is usually applied to poultry, indicating that the animals are given 'access' to the outdoors. In the UK, it's further broken down into 'Free Range', 'Traditional Free Range', and 'Free Range – Total Freedom', all with increasing access to roam outdoors. However, the term does not guarantee the quality of the feed given to the birds. Note: if not you're not buying free range chicken, you could consider the more humanely raised indoor chickens, which may be labelled as 'Extensive Indoor' or 'Barn Reared'.

Fresh: This label implies that the meat has not been frozen (internal temperature dropping below -3 degrees Centigrade) prior to sale. It does not pertain to how the animal was raised, fed or slaughtered, and it is not third-party verified.

Grass-fed (beef): This label may only be applied to meat from animals that have been fed mainly on grass or silage. The producer must apply to use the label, be able to verify the information, and be inspected by a government-recognised organisation.

Humane Designations: These include a variety of labels from different organisations promoting higher levels of animal welfare. It is important to check the details of individual schemes because standards very widely. For example, the most common label, Red Tractor, designates farms that meet legislative standards and in some cases go further, but tends to be less stringent than some other welfare assurance marques. However, it also focuses on areas such as hygiene and environmental aspects. Freedom Foods, the RSPCA's assurance marque, requires significantly higher welfare standards. The Soil Association's marque is only applied to meat produced under even more stringent welfare levels, and also guarantees the food is produced to high organic standards.

Humane certified animals are probably a suitable choice in the absence of local or USDA-certified organic meat.

Kosher or Halal: Meats with this label have been prepared under strict religious guidelines, and must be labelled as such according to EU law. Because animals are killed without stunning, this is considered to be less humane by groups such as the RSPCA.

Outdoor bred, outdoor raised, free range (pork): These terms indicate how much access pigs have had to the outdoors while being raised. Free range pigs are the best option, and live their lives outside. Outdoor reared have outdoor access for about half their lives, and outdoor bred only until they are weaned. Although this is a voluntary scheme, most major supermarkets and many food outlets have signed up. This does not indicate what quality of feed the animals have been provided with.

FISH

Fish offer a rich source of omega 3 fatty acids (particularly the important omega 3 fractions known as DHA and EPA that are not present in most other foods), complete protein, B complex vitamins, selenium, vitamin D, vitamin E, zinc, iron, magnesium, phosphorous, antioxidants and other nutrients. A 2006 study by the Harvard School of Public Health indicated that regular consumption of fish helps dramatically reduce the risk of heart disease and that the benefits (particularly the omega 3 content) outweigh the potential risks of ingesting toxins from polluted waters. Regular consumption of fish has been shown to exert a strong anti-inflammatory effect, reduce risk of heart disease, help protect against asthma in children, moderate chronic lung disease, reduce the risk of breast and other cancers by stunting tumour growth, and ease the symptoms of rheumatoid arthritis and certain bone and joint diseases. Nursing and pregnant women enjoy a host of benefits from fish consumption, including support for fetal and early childhood brain and retinal development and a lowered risk of premature birth.

While the benefits of eating fish are substantial, you should learn to choose wisely to avoid fish that have possibly been tainted with environmental toxins, and to steer clear of certain farmed species that you should never eat (some farmed species are fine; we'll cover the particulars shortly). The risk of ingesting fish tainted by environmental contaminants (heavy metals such as mercury, polychlorinated biphenyls [PCBs], dioxins and other toxins) can be countered by emphasising fish caught by domestic operations in remote, pollution-free ocean waters. The healthiest sources of fish are small, oily, cold-water fish, such as wild-caught Alaskan salmon, sardines, herring, anchovies and mackerel.

Certain fish at the top of the marine food chain, such as swordfish and shark, should be limited or avoided due to their tendency to accumulate concentrated contaminants. However, the popular refrain to limit fish intake due to mercury poisoning concerns has been exaggerated. The Western Pacific Regional Fishery Management Council, based in Hawaii, asserts that almost every Pacific Ocean fish except sword and shark contain substantially high enough levels of selenium (a potent antioxidant) to negate concerns about mercury toxicity. 'Our favourite fish are more likely to protect against mercury toxicity than cause it,' according to the Council.

The reason why you should avoid some species of farmed fish is that they are often raised under unsanitary conditions similar to those of ranch animals, and are exposed to high levels of dangerous chemicals, such as dioxins, dieldrin, toxaphene and other pesticides or toxic residue. These chemicals (from contaminated sediments in their fish meal) are easily absorbed into fat cells. Farmed fish may be routinely exposed to their own waste and are often fed artificial dyes (to match colour with wild varieties; e.g. wild salmon derive their pink colour from the healthy carotene astaxanthin in their natural diet) and antibiotics to ward off the high risk of infection and disease from living in cramped farms. The waste from a large salmon farm is estimated to equal the sewage from a city of 10,000 people. A 2004 report in the popular journal *Science* warned that farmed salmon contained 10 times the amount of toxins of wild salmon and should be eaten rarely – once every five months – due to their high cancer risk. Hey, *Science*, how about never?

While wild salmon offers 19 to 27 per cent of its total fat in omega 3s, the farmed Atlantic salmon (by far the most common farmed species) contains significantly less omega 3s and much higher levels of omega-6 fats (obtained from their commercial feed, unlike the omega-3-rich algae that nourishes wild fish). Of additional concern is the estimated three million salmon that escape from their pens into the ocean each year, contaminating and genetically diluting nearby wild salmon (farmers' daughters sneaking out to fool around with wild boys from out of town – what else is new?).

Use discretion and look for wild Alaskan salmon, even if your budget requires that you choose less expensive frozen fish at times. You can also look for farmed coho salmon as a healthy, budget-friendly alternative, especially from freshwater tanks. Avoid Atlantic farmed salmon (ask your waiter; sorry, it's probably Atlantic) due to concerns about industrial and environmental contamination and inferior nutritional value.

Having warned you of the risks of some types of farmed fish, I can also assert that there are certain other categories of farmed fish with minimal toxin levels and superior nutritional profiles that make them acceptable to consume. You just have to do a little home-work. If you do choose to eat farmed fish, insist on domestic sources to alleviate the risk posed by polluted waters and lax chemical regulations in high-producing countries such as China. Barramundi, catfish, crayfish and tilapia from domestic farms have impressive nutritional profiles and minimal toxin risks. Farmed trout from the United States or Canada is nutritionally comparable with wild trout, with minimal contaminant concerns, making it another sensible choice. Farmed shellfish are okay because they don't eat artificial foods and have similar living circumstances as wild shellfish – that is, they are attached to a fixed object. However, make a strong effort to eat fresh over frozen shellfish.

If you are wild about salmon and willing to endure the trade-off of a big carbon footprint and substantial expense to get a quality product, you can do your shopping online.

For smart shopping, cultivate a relationship with a local dedicated fish market or farmers' market vendor. Fish from a specialty vendor is more likely to be fresh than grocery store fare. Take aggressive, close-up sniffs of the offerings. Odour should be nonexistent for freshwater fish and perhaps a faint ocean smell for saltwater fish. Bad fish will have the unmistakable smell of, well, bad fish. Inquire about the source of the fish and stay away from Chinese or Asian imports, both farmed and wild-caught.

Finally, be advised that the safety, quality and sustainability of fish are in constant flux. Check resources such as the Marine Stewardship Council, Monterey Bay Aquarium Seafood Watch (montereybayacquarium.org) and the Environmental Defense Fund (edf.com) for up-to-date information.

> *'Most farmed fish should be avoided because they are raised in unsanitary, waste-infested waters; have dangerous chemical additives in their diets; and offer much lower levels of omega 3s than their wild counterparts.'*

EGGS

Eggs can be freely enjoyed as an excellent source of healthy protein, fat, B complex vitamins and folate. Be sure to obtain local, pasture-raised or organic chicken eggs, which contain up to 20 times more omega 3s than factory-produced, grain-fed chicken eggs. The popular conventional wisdom 'heart-healthy' concept of discarding the yolk to avoid cholesterol is misguided, as the yolk is one of the most nutrient-rich foods you can find – laden with omega 3s and the other aforementioned nutrients. In contrast, egg whites, besides being a good source of complete protein, have otherwise a rather low nutrient content. Furthermore, and contrary to conventional wisdom, there is no proof that eggs have anything to do with blood cholesterol or your risk for heart disease.

A Harvard Medical School study of 115,000 subjects over the span of 8 to 14 years demonstrated no correlation between egg consumption and heart disease or stroke. A 2008 study published in the *International Journal of Obesity* suggests that eating two eggs for breakfast (not just the whites, the whole deal) is healthier than eating a bagel. Your local farmers' market should be teeming with pasture-raised eggs. Otherwise, most quality grocers, health-food shops and major supermarkets stock abundant sources of organic eggs.

'Eliminating processed or packaged foods and bottled beverages and growing your own fruits and vegetables can reduce your budget and improve your dietary quality.'

GOING PRIMAL ON A BUDGET

I understand that buying organic animal products can be cost-prohibitive. I will accept criticism that the distinctions I elaborate here could characterise the Primal Blueprint eating style as elitist in the eyes of some. I'll discuss this philosophical issue with great enthusiasm and detail in Chapter 9, but for now I'll proudly stand as an advocate for healthy living and getting your priorities straight, including budgeting for the best foods you can afford – even if this means your diet potentially (but not necessarily, if you do a little legwork) becomes more expensive and cumbersome for you than for other families you know.

If you sharply cut back or eliminate processed carbohydrates from your diet, you avoid the vast majority of the high-cost (and high-profit), low-nutritional-value products in the store. Shifting from bottled waters, juices and all manner of sweetened beverages to a simple water-filtration system in your home can save money and improve dietary quality. Shifting from designer foods such as synthetic energy bars and meal replacements (Kelly Korg spends about 70 bucks a month on her twice-daily Slim-Fast shakes) to such basics as trail mix or farm-fresh eggs can also reduce your budget while improving dietary quality.

Consider growing your own fruits and vegetables in your backyard garden or rent a patch in a community garden if your urban environment is short on soil. Part-time employees at many food stores enjoy a purchase discount. Perhaps there is even a co-op or farmers' market in your area where you can trade time for food? One popular post on MarksDailyApple.com detailed the concept of 'cowpooling' – chipping in with other families to purchase and divide up all or part of a butchered cow, typically raised locally and naturally. A concerted effort to follow these simple tips will likely get you very close to break even with your 'before' Primal Blueprint grocery expenses compared to your 'after' expenses.

Even the most vocal complainers about high-priced organic food might benefit from examining their discretionary purchases and moving healthy food up the priority list. You have the right and also the obligation – to yourself and your loved ones – to pursue the absolute highest dietary quality possible. Yes, it may require more time, energy and even expense, but the payoff here is arguably greater than from any other lifestyle change you ponder (new TV, new car, new clothes, vacation, etc.). And not to sound trite, but an investment in your health today pays dividends far greater and far longer than you might ever see in any health or national insurance contributions you make.

Now that I've climbed down off my soapbox, let's admit that real-world concerns may have you falling short here and there of the ideal spelt out in these pages. It's important to default back to the big-picture view that the Primal Blueprint is a way of life, not a boot camp. If you are agonising over which fruit stimulates less insulin or you find yourself eating conventional hamburgers at the company picnic yet are diligent enough to toss the buns in the garbage before you dig in, congratulations are in order for the momentum and awareness you have already created. When it comes to health and fitness, there is always a higher standard to strive for, but the Primal Blueprint allows for enough deviation from 'ideal' such that you need not compromise your enjoyment of today. Every step you take towards living Primally puts you that much closer to your health and fitness goals – and makes you more adept at righting the course when the inevitable deviations happen.

VEGETABLES

It is preferable to select locally grown, in-season, organic vegetables whenever possible. The shiny, buffed-up vegetables on display in our local supermarkets are typically cultivated in an objectionable manner – sprayed with pesticides, picked too early (and then artificially ripened by exposure to ethylene gas), jet-lagged from their distant origins (thumbs-down from a green perspective) and even genetically modified to grow bigger and more colourful, albeit at the cost of being less nutritious and flavoursome.

It may take some acclimatisation to centre your diet around vegetables, as we are so accustomed to reaching for packaged, high-carbohydrate snacks as a first option. Don't follow the example of restaurants that serve skimpy vegetable portions seemingly just for decoration; serve yourself heaped portions that crowd everything else on your plate! Enjoy vegetables raw, steamed, baked or grilled – even slathered in butter, if you like.

Cook or slice up extra portions for easy preparation or snacking the following day. Reject your attachment to cultural meal traditions centred on starches or grains and get wild and colourful with your meals! Have some steamed carrots and beets with your eggs for breakfast, or kale, squash and chicken for lunch. Try some of the many delicious vegetable-focused recipes at MarksDailyApple.com, *The Primal Blueprint Cookbook*, or the *Primal Blueprint Quick and Easy Meals*. Grab some stuff you've never tried before and ask your grocer about the best preparation methods.

While virtually all vegetables offer excellent nutritional value, some offer particularly high levels of antioxidants. One of the best objective resources to determine the antioxidant power of any vegetable, fruit, herb or other food is the USDA's ORAC (Oxygen Radical Absorbance Capacity) report. I like to aim for at least 10,000 ORAC units a day, which is easily obtained from a few servings of the top fruits and vegetables (the USDA recommends a much lower number, between 3,000 and 5,000 per day).

Here (in alphabetical order, not point value order; but don't worry – they're all gold-medal winners) is a list of some of the highest antioxidant vegetables. Make a special effort to include these regularly in your meals:

Aubergine
Avocado
Beets
Broccoli
Brussels sprouts
Carrots
Cauliflower
Garlic
Kale
Onion
Red bell pepper
Spinach
Yellow squash

If, for reasons of budget or availability, you decide to eat non-organic produce, note that there are varying levels of residue exposure risk depending on the item. Be particularly careful to avoid conventional sources of vegetables that have a large surface area (leafy greens, including spinach and lettuce, are treated with some of the most potent pesticides) or a skin that is consumed (peppers are perhaps the most pesticide-tainted vegetable; also avoid conventional celery, cucumbers, green beans, winter squash and carrots). If you do find yourself purchasing these, be sure to soak and/or rinse them with soap or a 'fruit and vegetable wash' solution, which you can find in any health food store. On the other hand, conventional broccoli (also a good source of omega 3s), asparagus, avocados, cabbage, onions and other vegetables with an easily washable or non-edible skin have minimal pesticide exposure risk.

MACADAMIA NUTS

Macadamia nuts earn a distinction above other nuts and seeds because of their superior nutritional value. They are predominantly monounsaturated fat (84 per cent – more than any other nut or seed), which is less likely to be stored as fat and helps raise HDL and lower LDL. They have the most favourable O6:O3 ratio of any nut (actually with minimal amounts of both).

Macadamias contain all of the essential amino acids, various forms of healthy fibre, high levels of vitamins, minerals and plant nutrients, and only trace amounts of carbohydrate. The flavenoids and tocopherols in macadamia nuts offer excellent antioxidant properties. They have a rich and satisfying taste, making them a great snack. Macadamia nut butter is hard to find, but worth the effort and additional expense. Check out ArtisanaFoods.com for 100-per cent raw, organic macadamia/cashew nut butter, and many other nut butters and natural products that are delicious.

COCONUT PRODUCTS

Integrating coconut products (oil, milk, butter, water, flakes and other derivatives) into your diet provides a variety of health benefits and can conveniently replace Standard American Diet (SAD) foods such as milk, flour and polyunsaturated cooking oils that can compromise your health. Coconut is an excellent source of a special type of fat – medium-chain fatty acids – that are difficult to find even in a healthy diet. While all vegetable oils are comprised of some ratio of monounsaturated, polyunsaturated or saturated fatty acids, there is another classification based on molecular size or length of the carbon chain within each fatty acid. Nearly all oils we consume are classified as long-chain fatty acids. Coconut's distinctive medium-chain composition has been shown to offer protection from heart disease, cancer, diabetes and many other degenerative illnesses, to improve immune function and fat metabolism, to protect against liver damage from alcohol and other toxins, and to deliver anti-inflammatory and immune-supporting properties.

Nearly one-third of the global population has had coconut as a dietary centrepiece of their traditional diets for centuries. Of particular note are Polynesian cultures with heavy coconut intake and high saturated fat diets in general that are remarkably free of heart disease. Asia Pacific cultures love the healing properties of coconut and use it extensively in their traditional medicine, particularly for skin and digestive conditions since it offers potent antimicrobial properties.

Due to its high saturated fat content, coconut oil is especially resilient to oxidation and free radical formation, even when heated to high temperatures during cooking. Unfortunately, coconut has been maligned along with other saturated fats for several decades, beginning with the SAD's migration over to polyunsaturated oils in the 1960s. Coconut is indeed the most saturated of all vegetable oils; 92 per cent saturated, it's solid at room temperature but will liquefy in hot weather. While it may seem like a minor issue, cooking and preparing recipes with coconut oil instead of polyunsaturated oils can be one of the healthiest dietary changes you can make. *The Primal Blueprint Cookbook* and *Primal Blueprint Quick and Easy Meals* have extensive recipes featuring coconut or substituting familiar ingredients (flour, milk, PUFAs) with coconut products.

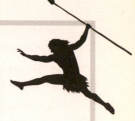

MARK'S FAVOURITE PRIMAL SNACKS

Celery: Enjoy with cream cheese or macadamia nut butter. Celery offers that satisfying texture and is a great vehicle to carry these and other low-carbohydrate toppings.

Cottage Cheese: Enjoy with nuts, berries, balsamic vinegar or other creative toppings.

Dark Chocolate: Any lingering sweet tooth issues relating to your transition to Primal eating can be assuaged with a couple of squares of dark chocolate (look for 75 per cent or greater cocoa content).

Fish: Canned tuna or sardines (yes, packed in oil) can easily replace a full meal for nutrient intake and satiety.

Fresh Berries: Raspberries, blueberries, blackberries, strawberries – all are Grok-like, nutritious and very satisfying. Add some heavy cream for a good dessert option.

Hard-Boiled Eggs: Sprinkle some salt, spices and a little olive oil in a ziplock bag and then roll the peeled egg around in the bag for a tasty snack.

Macadamia Nuts: Best Primal health value due to high mono-unsaturated content (and great taste!).

Other Nuts and Seeds: Almonds, pecans, pumpkin, sunflower, sesame seeds, nut butters (except peanut butter). Enjoy with some moderation due to 06:03 ratio goals.

Olives: Great source of monounsaturated fatty acids.

Trail Mix: Emphasise nuts and seeds. A little dried fruit or even some dark chocolate chips are okay, but avoid yogurt-covered raisins, M&Ms, other high-carbohydrate ingredients and peanuts.

Look at the website for more ideas, MarksDailyApple.com has hundreds of postings for snack and recipe ideas, including some creative make-your-own Primal snacks. We also have dozens of our ever-popular 'top 10 lists' for everything you can think of relating to meat, vegetables, fruits, seasonal favourites, recipes, foods to avoid and healthy dietary habits.

To get started on the coconut bandwagon, grab a jar of coconut oil at a health-food store or elite market and use it for pan frying. Get some coconut milk and use it as a liquid base for smoothies or for replacing dairy milk. Get some coconut flakes and enjoy them in smoothies, sprinkled on salads or with nuts as a trail mix. On those special occasions when you need a carbohydrate drink during or after exercise, coconut water is a great choice. Try some coconut manna as a delicious spread on vegetables or dabbed onto some squares of dark chocolate (find at a health-food store or specialist grocer). Visit MarksDailyApple.com and review the many posts on coconut (including some amazing desserts) as you explore this wonderful new dietary centrepiece.

FRUITS

While fruits are outstanding sources of fibre, vitamins, minerals, phenols, antioxidants and other micronutrients, some moderation is warranted for a few reasons. First, modern cultivation and chemical treatments have resulted in fruits that are large, brightly coloured, uniformly shaped and extra sweet, with much less micro-nutrition than the small, varied, highly fibrous, deep-coloured, less sugary and less insulin-stimulating fruits that Grok foraged for.

Second, these overly sweetened beauty queens are available year-round thanks to modern growing and transportation methods. Third, fructose, the predominant carbohydrate form contained in fruit, can cause significant metabolic problems when consumed in excess – as can easily happen with year-round availability. This is particularly true when combined with the wildly excessive intake of grains and sugars in the Standard American Diet.

When fructose is consumed, it's converted in the liver not only into usable carbohydrate in the form of glucose, but also into triglycerides (fat). For heavy exercisers who regularly deplete muscle glycogen, fruit is a great choice to efficiently reload their liver glycogen. On the other hand, if your glycogen stores are already full, as happens when we don't engage in regular short bouts of intense exercise, that Sunday brunch strawberry could just as easily convert into fat in the liver, and then get dumped into the bloodstream.

High blood triglycerides interfere with the function of the hormone leptin, causing you to want to overeat rather than rely on your stored body fat for energy. Possibly one-third of the population is fructose intolerant to some degree, evidenced by digestive symptoms such as flatulence, cramps, bloating, irritable bowel syndrome and diarrhoea. Excessive fructose consumption is also linked to fatigue, insulin resistance, diabetes and high blood pressure.

Yep, eating too much fruit can make you fat – even more so than eating too much fat, since at least fat will make you feel full! It's not my desire to scare you away from eating fruit, but simply to get you to recognise that it *is* a source of sugar and should generally be consumed in moderation. The most simple and sensible approach is to try and emulate Grok by eating fruits grown locally during their natural local ripening seasons (exceptions granted if you live in a fruit-challenged climate), especially if you are trying to shed excess body fat.

CHOOSING THE BEST FRUITS

The three major categories that affect fruit quality are growing methods, nutritional value (antioxidant levels as well as how much the sugar content affects your metabolism) and the risk of pesticide exposure. The 'Fruit Power Rankings' chart in this section details which types of fruits to enjoy in abundance, which to eat in moderation, and which to strictly avoid. Regarding growing methods, organic fruit (or fruit grown locally without the use of pesticides) offers vastly superior nutritional value to conventionally grown fruits. Some experts estimate that organic fruits are 10 times richer in key micronutrients than their conventional counterparts! Organic fruits must manufacture high levels of antioxidants to defend themselves against pests – something conventional fruits don't have to worry about, thanks to their treatment with synthetic herbicides and pesticides.

Organic is not always the be-all and end-all, however. Organic fruits from distant lands are less tasty and nutritious because of their premature picking and long transit time to market. Even if local fruit is not certified organic, your local farmer likely uses less offensive growing methods than large commercial operations, and the optimum picking time means the fruit has matured to be bursting with great nutrition and flavour. Those living in progressive areas with thriving farmers' markets and food co-ops might even encounter fruits designated as 'wild'. As the term conveys, these fruits are as good as it gets – if you can find them. If you are so inclined, visit your local garden centre or go online and find a fruit and vegetable nursery so you can choose your own seeds or plants and grow your own wild-variety fruit trees, berry bushes and vegetable plants.

> *'Year-round availability of overly sweetened fruit can lead to excessive intake, and rapid conversion of fructose (the carbohydrate form in fruit) into fat.'*

Be strict (particularly with children, due to their substantially higher risk of harm from pesticides) about avoiding conventionally grown fruits with a soft, edible skin that is difficult to wash, such as berries. You can be less strict on fruits with tough, inedible skins that peel; they offer a protective barrier against chemical ingestion. If you must eat conventional fruits, wash your fruit thoroughly with soap or a special solution. Avoid genetically modified fruit, a concept that elicits serious health and philosophical concerns and is about as far away from Grok as you can get. Genetically modified organisms (GMOs) have insufficient research to guarantee their health and safe ingestion.

Almost all fruits offer a host of nutritional benefits, but some (detailed on the chart) are relatively low in antioxidant values while having a high impact on your blood glucose/insulin production. Paleo Diet author Loren Cordain, PhD, ranks common fruits according to a 'Total Metabolic Fructose' (TMF) to take this factor into consideration. Fruits with high TMF scores (sometimes referred

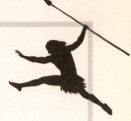

FRUIT POWER RANKINGS

You can be more selective by considering a fruit's growing methods, pesticide risk and glycemic/ antioxidant values (high-antioxidant, low-glycemic fruits being the best) and TMF scores. Each list is ranked in order of best to worst.

GROWING METHODS

Wild: Difficult to find – plant your own or scour the farmers' market!

Local organic: Superior choice for nutritional value, taste and safety.

Local conventional: Superior to remote organic due to freshness and ideal picking time. Wash thoroughly with soap or vegetable solution.

Remote organic: Ranks below local conventional due to negative effects of transportation and premature picking.

Remote conventional: Avoid due to diminished nutritional value and pesticide risk. (*Hint*: if it's out of season in your area, don't eat it!)

GMO fruit: Don't even think about it. Instead, ask yourself, 'What would Grok do?' 'Nuff said.

NUTRITIONAL VALUE

Outstanding: High-antioxidant, low-glycaemic fruits, including all berries and stone (pitted) fruits (cherries, prunes, peaches, apricots), avocado, casaba melon, lime, lemon, tomato and guava.

Great: Lower-antioxidant, higher-glycaemic, medium-TMF fruits, including apples, bananas, cherries, kiwi and pomegranates.

Exercise some moderation: Low-antioxidant, high-glycaemic fruits, including dates, dried fruits (all), grapes, mangoes, melons, nectarines, oranges, papayas, pineapples, plums and tangerines.

PESTICIDE RISK

Low risk: Fruit with tough, inedible skin, including bananas, avocados, melons, oranges, tangerines, mandarins, pineapples, kiwis, mangoes and papayas.

High risk: Fruit with soft, edible skin, including apples, apricots, cherries, grapes, nectarines, peaches, pears, raisins, raspberries, strawberries and tomatoes.

---

to as 'high-sugar' or 'high glycaemic' fruits) warrant moderation, particularly if you are trying to reduce excess body fat.

In light of the popularity of juicing, it's important to note that whole fruits are vastly superior to juice – even the most nutritious, freshly squeezed glass. Juice is generally higher in sugar and lower in many other micronutrients than its produce sources, because juicing eliminates the nutrient-rich skin and fibre and provides a more concentrated, less filling source of carbohydrates than whole foods. Recall that Kelly Korg's 24-ounce Strawberry Surf Rider smoothie contained 71 grams of sugar! That's like eating 51 large strawberries! (Can you say, 'Cool Hand Luke?'). I strongly suggest passing on juice in favour of whole foods.

If your eyes are bouncing up and down the page sorting out which fruits are good and bad, relax! If you've junked sugars, grains, legumes and PUFAs to become preoccupied with prioritising your fruit choices you're progressing nicely. I'm certainly not advocating sitting forlornly off to the side at a family picnic, watching others eat sausage rolls, quiches, corn on the cob and watermelon. By all means enjoy the watermelon guilt-free (just forget the former three and smuggle in your own smoked wild salmon for a main course!). Simply use a bit of restraint for fruits on the moderation list, particularly if you are pursuing ambitious fat-reduction goals.

MARK'S TOP 10 FAVOURITE FRUITS

Naturally, everything on this list assumes an organic, locally grown variety. Consult the three previous sections to ensure your pesticide risk is minimised and you otherwise choose the best fruit possible – and avoid problematic fruits. These are in my personal rank order, but again, anything on this list is superior.

1. Blueberries, strawberries, raspberries, blackberries and nearly all other berries
2. Cherries
3. Prunes
4. Apples
5. Peaches
6. Pears
7. Figs
8. Grapefruit
9. Kiwis
10. Apricots

HERBS AND SPICES

No discussion of healthy eating would be complete without the inclusion of herbs and spices. Although these tasty additions provide minimal calories, they are packed with significant amounts of important micronutrients. Extensive evidence suggests that herbs and spices support cardiovascular and metabolic health, may help prevent cancer and other diseases, and will improve mental health and cognition. Some of the highest antioxidant values (from ORAC scores) among all foods can be found in herbs and spices. Certain marinades and herbal preparations are so powerful in their antioxidant capacity that they have been shown to mitigate or eliminate potential issues that may arise from overcooking meat.

Herbs are generally green plants or plant parts used to add flavour to foods. Herbal extracts have been used for thousands of years in Eastern medicine and continue to enjoy widespread popularity today, for their powerful immune and health-supporting properties. Spices, on the other hand, are typically dried seeds, fruits and plant parts. Spices are used to enhance flavour, add colour, or help prevent bacterial growth on food.

You can bet that Grok surely partook of the many varieties of plants he encountered. Throughout history, herbs and spices have played a large role in the human diet and even in culture as a whole. During the Middle Ages, spices were a currency that had substantial economic value. Their popularity to enhance flavour and preserve food was a catalyst for the fervent exploration of the globe by such explorers as Marco Polo, Columbus and Magellan.

The specific health properties of individual herbs and spices could fill an entire book. A couple of headliners that are easy to integrate into everyday meals include curcumin (offers potent anti-inflammatory effects and high antioxidant value) and cinnamon (regulates blood sugar and demonstrates high antibacterial, anti-inflammatory and antioxidant values). Visit MarksDailyApple.com for extensive coverage of numerous herb and spice benefits.

MODERATION FOODS

While they may not be exactly what our ancestors ate, moderate consumption of the following foods can add some nutritional bene-fit to your diet without negative consequences, provided they are not overemphasised. Furthermore, I want to make the Primal Blueprint as accessible and enjoyable to as many people as possible. If you are pursuing ambitious fat-reduction goals, you will probably want to eliminate some of these from the picture.

COFFEE

Coffee is fine in moderation, as long as you avoid using caffeine as a crutch to raise energy levels. Proper diet and exercise should enable you to wake up feeling refreshed and energised each morning and will avoid the afternoon blues caused primarily by high-carbohydrate eating habits. Make an effort to drink organic coffee, as many big coffee-producing countries don't regulate chemical and pesticide use.

Research is divided on the effects of caffeine on the body. Some studies suggest that caffeine can actually reduce risk of heart disease and cancer and enhance fat metabolism, particularly during exercise; other studies are inconclusive; while still others suggest that caffeine is harmful to the cardiovascular system, does not enhance fat metabolism, and stresses the adrenal glands as an artificial central nervous system stimulant. It seems reasonable to assume that it's unhealthy to habitually ingest a beverage that can keep you cranking at warp speed when what you really need is a nap; however, it appears that a cup or two a day won't hurt. I myself enjoy coffee, especially after adding heavy cream and a pinch of sugar (yes, a pinch won't hurt). It's a warm and comforting element to my morning routine, especially on those freezing cold winter mornings in Malibu …

HIGH-FAT DAIRY PRODUCTS

Raw dairy products retain more nutritional value due to their minimal processing. Some purists in the paleo-diet world totally eschew dairy of any kind; however, I have concluded from extensive research that certain forms of dairy are suitable for some people and not for others. Truth is, Grok probably did not consume much in the way of dairy products. He certainly didn't go around milking wild beasts; that phase of agriculture didn't start until about 10,000 years ago at the earliest. On the other hand, since he ate most parts of the animals he killed, Grok also very likely consumed the milk in mammary glands he ate on occasion (along with kidney, liver, heart, lung, intestines, bone marrow and brain), so it's not accurate to say he completely avoided dairy.

Dairy does not need to be an essential part of anyone's diet and many of us might be well served never having dairy again. But if you are one who exhibits no acute problems (lactose intolerance or casein sensitivity) and have a desire to keep some dairy in your diet, certain dairy products can offer a decent source of nutrition and be acceptable under the Primal Blueprint. Just be sure to select carefully to minimise potential problems and obtain maximum nutrient benefit.

The best dairy choices are raw, fermented, unpasteurised, unsweetened and high-fat options such as ghee, butter, full cream, aged cheese, cottage cheese, cream cheese, Greek-style full-fat yogurt, half and half, kefir and raw whole milk. Stick to pasture-raised/grass-fed, or organic dairy products to avoid the hormones, pesticides and antibiotics common in commercial dairy products. Eliminate fruit-sweetened yogurt, frozen desserts and other high-carbohydrate dairy offerings. Stay completely away from regular pasteurised, homogenised, two-per cent and skimmed milk.

Fermented dairy products may help you avoid the immune system issues and allergenic reactions that many have towards the lactose and casein in cow's milk. They also offer a good source of probiotics (healthy bacteria for your intestines). Raw dairy products undergo the least processing, increasing their nutritional value. High-fat dairy products have low levels of the objectionable casein protein, which I will discuss shortly. And how can you not love an eating style that lets you have butter and heavy cream? As a last allowable choice, organic products protect (both of which are almost entirely comprised of healthy saturated animal fat).

Cheese does have broad appeal and can play a minor role in a healthy diet. Play it snooty and go for the high-quality, aged stuff. Aged cheese is a fermented food, so it contains little to no lactose (for those with intolerance concerns). Cheese offers high-quality fats and proteins, as well as many other essential nutrients, with a satisfaction level that's just as important as the aforementioned health benefits. For a change of pace, try some raw, non-pasteurised cheese that is loaded with good nutrition.

Having offered possible options of what might constitute acceptable dairy, let's now look at why milk doesn't necessarily 'do a body good'. Lactose is a carbohydrate in milk that is difficult to digest for the many people who stop producing lactase (the enzyme that helps digest lactose) after age three or four. This is in alignment with our genetically programmed transition away from breastfeeding in early childhood (breast milk contains significant lactose). The incidence of lactose intolerance varies wildly by ancestral heritage – something that is believed to be a rare example of recent genetic change through selection pressure in the manner of evolution (I discuss this topic at length in the Q&A appendix at MarksDailyApple.com). People of herder ancestry (and, hence, high dairy consumption), such as the Swedes and Dutch, are generally quite lactose-tolerant. Other ethnic groups, such as those of African or Asian descent, have high rates of lactose intolerance. If you carefully examine your dietary habits, you may discover incidences of bloating, gas, cramping, or diarrhoea in conjunction with consuming milk products – all indications that you have some level of lactose intolerance and should avoid milk and other lactose-heavy dairy products, including ice cream.

> *'Milk doesn't necessarily "do a body good". At least the usual storebought kind. The calcium benefits are overstated, and it often contains agents such as lactose, casein, hormones, pesticides and antibiotics.'*

Casein is a protein that can have autoimmune-stimulating properties and can initiate very serious allergic reactions in some people, particularly those who have experienced 'leaky gut' syndrome as a result of a concurrent intolerance to grains. Casein is believed to contribute to or exacerbate conditions such as coeliac disease, Crohn's disease, irritable bowel syndrome, asthma and possibly autism in some people. Success has been reported treating these conditions holistically with a wheat- and dairy-free diet. *Paleo Diet* author Loren Cordain notes that a substance known as epidural growth factor (EGF) in milk and other dairy products can increase cancer risk and tumour progression and also suggests that milk and other dairy products worsen acne cases.

These negatives do not even address the consequences of consuming the hormones, pesticides and antibiotics contained in commercial milk and dairy products (which was discussed at length in the context of commercial animal meats). Fortunately, the dangers and objections of the commonly used recombinant bovine growth hormone (rBGH – a treatment given to cows to increase their milk production) are well publicised, leading some forward-thinking nations to ban its use and sophisticated consumers to steer clear of milk made with rBGH.

Milk's modern processing methods also present health objections. Milk that is homogenised and pasteurised is certainly free of dangerous bacteria, but it is also devoid of beneficial bacteria, vitamins and enzymes due to the heating process. Furthermore, the homogenisation process alters the otherwise healthy milk fats by reducing the size of the fat globules, interfering with their digestibility. Bottom line: even if you don't have any acute symptoms, it's sensible to conclude that, during the first couple years of life, milk consumption should be limited to mother's milk. From there, it's a matter of choosing your dairy wisely and not making it the foundation of your diet.

For those who recoil at the suggestion to limit intake of milk, let's examine further why some of the conventional wisdom about dairy is flawed. Yes, most dairy is an excellent source of calcium, but we don't need nearly as much calcium as we have been led to believe. The United States and other Western nations with high dairy intake also have high rates of osteoporosis, suggesting that calcium is not the be-all and end-all for bone health. Experts are in agreement that magnesium, vitamin D, vitamin K, potassium and other agents are also extremely important. Furthermore, just as with omega 3 and omega 6 fatty acids, these agents need to be obtained in proper balance to provide optimal bone health benefits, an area where the average Western diet falls short. Today, we generally consume too much calcium, largely from heavy use of dairy products. This hampers our ability to absorb magnesium because they compete on the same absorption pathways.

To make matters worse, many of us don't consume enough magnesium (found in leafy greens, nuts, seeds and fish) nor synthesise enough vitamin D (from sun exposure, as I will explain in Chapter 7). Many experts believe that vitamin D intake might be more critical than calcium to bone health. Furthermore, chronic stress may play a huge role in osteoporosis, since the stress hormone cortisol inhibits calcium uptake by bones, rendering ingested calcium less effective. How about that? Taking a break from your busy day to bag some rays in your lounge chair might be better for your bones than drinking a glass of milk or swallowing a bunch of calcium pills!

Since we've discussed the importance of promoting an alkaline environment in the body, it should be noted that dairy foods are acid forming – a reality that actually hampers calcium absorption. For your calcium needs, you will better off consuming easily assimilated, high-calcium, alkaline foods, such as leafy greens, nuts, oranges, broccoli and sweet potatoes, or calcium-rich fish, including wild salmon and sardines. All told, it would be preferable to push dairy aside in favour of the Primal Blueprint stalwarts of meat, vegetables, fruits, nuts and seeds. That said, when you look at the spectrum of foods from best to worst, the previous list of allowable dairy is still a preferred choice over grains, if you are going to depart from the Primal Blueprint now and then.

APPROVED FATS AND OILS

Many fats and oils offer significant health benefits, but they are generally high in calories with minimal vitamin and mineral values. Obviously, Grok didn't press oils in his day, but his omega 3 intake was quite high from animal and plant sources. Today, we need all the help we can get towards optimum essential fatty acid balance. Many oils offer a way to boost your intake of omega 3s and other healthy monounsaturated and saturated fats. I'd advise moderation in this category because I'd rather enjoy the delicious taste of fatty whole foods, such as avocados, coconut, macadamia nuts, oily, cold-water fish, olives, meat and eggs to obtain my fat calories.

For cooking, animal fats (butter, ghee, lard, recycled bacon grease and tallow and coconut oil) are great choices, because they are temperature-stable, even under high heat. The best oil to consume with meals is domestically grown, extra-virgin, first cold press only olive oil (yes, a mouthful; I'll explain the importance of these distinctions shortly). Olive oil, the most monounsaturated oil, offers proven cardiovascular benefits (raises HDL and lowers LDL cholesterol) and has powerful anti-inflammatory and antioxidant properties. It's very good for cooking at low heat, but be careful because excessive time at high temperatures can compromise the health benefits of any oil.

As you probably know, various processing methods dramatically affect the health quality of olive oil, with extra virgin designated as the purest form. The use of the 'extra-virgin' moniker is loosely regulated, and there is a tremendous disparity in quality between local extra-virgin olive oil and imports from Greece, Italy or Spain (which comprise the vast majority of products on the market). The additional distinction 'first cold press only' suggests that the olives have been pressed only once and bottled immediately, instead of being repeatedly pressed for maximum crop yield (this is the most common method, particularly with the large bottle–low price imports). You may have to contact the manufacturer to determine whether your bottle is indeed first cold press only.

You'll notice the difference with a single taste of a locally grown, first cold-pressed extra virgin olive oil in comparison with a much blander, duller-tasting extra virgin import. The aroma and taste are incredibly powerful – the high level of tocopherols (a potent antioxidant) may actually sting the back of your throat! In my estimation, nothing beats a Primal Big Ass salad with a generous drizzling of olive oil.

High omega 3 oils are a good way to bump up your omega 3 intake if you don't eat a lot of oily, cold-water fish. Omega 3 fish oil capsules are a convenient daily supplement, or you can get bottled omega 3 oils at a health food store or fine market. These oils are extremely delicate and easily suffer damage from exposure to heat, light, oxygen and the vagaries of time. Thus, you'll often find them refrigerated in small containers.

Look for something other than flax oil. While flax is the most common offering and is high in omega 3, recent research suggests that the predominant type of omega 3 found in flax oil, alpha-linoleic acid (ALA), is difficult to assimilate in the body. It must be enzymatically

MARK'S PRIMER ON FATS AND OILS

Approved Fats and Oils

This list (in alphabetical order) contains a variety of saturated and unsaturated types, with different ideal uses. The saturated fats listed here (animal fats, butter, coconut oil and palm oil) are great choices for cooking because they are temperature stable (they won't oxidise under high heat). Review the list carefully, stockpile your fridge, and be sure to stick to the best intended use for each.

Animal fats: Chicken, duck or goose fat; lard (aka pork fat); beef or lamb tallow; and other animal fats are excellent for cooking because their saturated composition makes them temperature stable.

Butter: An excellent choice for cooking or enhancing the taste of steamed vegetables, butter is a good source of vitamins A and E as well as selenium.

Coconut oil: Temperature stability and numerous health and immune-supporting benefits make it an excellent choice for cooking. Find an organic brand and try it in the Primal Energy Bar or Primal Chocolate Mousse recipes you will find at MarksDailyApple.com!

Dark roasted sesame oil: This oil's intense flavour makes it a great choice for cooking vegetables or meat in a wok, or for salads. Some alternative healers promote its antibacterial properties to heal wounds and prevent infection.

High omega 3 oils: These delicate oils are a great addition to salads or protein shakes for an omega 3 boost. Choose borage, cod-liver, krill, salmon, hemp seed, hi-oleic sunflower or safflower seed oils (not to be confused with their unhealthy polyunsaturated derivatives) as alternatives to flax.

Marine oils: Typically delivered in capsule or soft-gel supplement form, these fish or krill oils are an excellent source of omega 3s.

> **Olive oil:** Choose locally or domestically grown, first cold press, extra virgin and savour the flavour! It is best not to cook with olive oil due to its temperature fragility. If you must, use the lowest heat you can.
>
> **Palm oil:** The unprocessed variety (not to be confused with widely used partially hydrogenated palm oil) is great for cooking.

converted into the more useful omega 3 fractions: docosahexanoic acid (DHA) and eicosapentanoic aicd (EPA). Even then, there's still no guarantee that your body will handle that conversion efficiently. Some alternative offerings you might find are borage, cod liver, krill, salmon and hemp seed. Always compare the expiration dates on a few bottles within the same brand and buy the one with the most amount of time left on it.

It's best to store oils (all kinds, but especially high omega 3s) in the refrigerator and use them quickly – usually within six weeks of opening. Remember, while omega 3 oils are healthy, they are still subject to rancidity and, when exposed to air, they will oxidise a bit. If you detect a slightly rancid smell in any oil or if it's been on the shelf for more than six months, discard the product immediately.

OTHER NUTS AND SEEDS AND THEIR DERIVATIVE BUTTERS

Nuts and seeds are concentrated foods that represent an energy source (some might call it a 'life force') for future generations of their plant – packed with protein, fatty acids, enzymes, antioxidants and abundant vitamins and minerals. You can conveniently carry and eat nuts and seeds anytime, anywhere. They stimulate minimal insulin production and will keep you satisfied for hours until your next meal.

Numerous respected studies (Iowa Women's Health Study of 40,000 women, Harvard School of Public Health's Nurses' Health Study of 127,000 women and Physicians' Health Study of 22,000 men are among the most prominent) suggest that regular consumption of nuts significantly reduces the risk of heart disease and diabetes.

Nevertheless, some moderation is warranted with nuts due to concerns about O6:O3 ratios and caloric density. Most nuts except macadamia contain multiples more omega 6 than omega 3 fatty acids. For example, walnuts are lauded for being a great source of omega 3s – the highest of any nut or seed – but they are five times higher in omega 6 than omega 3. What's more, some people who move over to a Primal eating style tend to overdo nuts as they try to fill the void left by ditching grains, sugars and legumes. If you are used to frequent, perhaps even absent-minded, snacking to get through the day, and you switch from carbohydrates to nuts, you may eat enough extra calories over the short term to compromise fat loss efforts. Understand that with nuts and other high-fat foods, a little goes a long way. A handful of nuts will satisfy hunger and provide fatty acids to burn for hours afterwards. Unlike carbohydrate snacking, you don't experience the insulin crash leading to cravings for more snacks in the ensuing hours.

Almonds, hazelnuts, pecans, pine nuts, pistachios, walnuts, flaxseeds, chia seeds, pumpkin seeds (best O6:O3 ratio among seeds – 'only' 2:1) and sunflower seeds are all nutritious and satisfying – great for salads or as snack fodder. The ever-popular peanuts should be avoided. Peanuts are technically a legume, not a nut; they are highly allergenic and also can contain dangerous moulds that produce aflatoxin, a potent carcinogen. Obviously, avoid nuts that have been processed with sugary or oily coatings or other offensive ingredients.

Use a mini food processor to grind nuts and sprinkle onto salads, over baked vegetables, or even into omelettes. Whole nuts (in the shell) will last up to a year without spoiling. Shelled nuts have less shelf life, and sliced nuts less again. Store nuts in the refrigerator (or freezer, if longer than six months) to prolong freshness. If your nuts have a rancid, oily smell or any discolouration, fleckings or signs of mould, discard them. Concerns about pesticide exposure from nuts is minimal due to protection offered by shells. Don't worry about looking for organic nuts; less than one per cent of US tree nut farmland is certified organic anyway.

Nut and seed butters offer a versatile and great-tasting way to spread your intake of nuts and seeds over different meals and snacks. Take care to choose cold-processed butters that are simply ground up (at low temperatures and free of added ingredients – except salt, which is fine) and refrigerate them at all times. Many health proponents claim raw nuts, seeds and butters have superior nutritional value to those that have been roasted, so by all means choose raw products if you can find them. Almond butter is believed by many to be the best butter choice besides macadamia. Almonds have the highest protein content of any nut (20 per cent of total calories) and are high in antioxidants, phytonutrients, vitamins, minerals and plant sterols that support health and lower disease risk.

SUPPLEMENTAL CARBOHYDRATES

Sweet potatoes (the orange variety are typically called yams), quinoa and wild rice are the best choices for heavy exercisers who require additional dietary carbohydrates to replenish frequently depleted muscle glycogen. These select few folks who fall into the 'need supplemental carbs' category are effortlessly maintaining ideal body fat levels, and train so heavily that bonking (a sudden and severe drop in energy) and delayed recovery are occasionally concerns – think Tour de France cyclists, NBA basketball players or high-school cross-country runners.

If you decide that you need supplemental carbohydrates, sweet potatoes and yams are superior to the more starchy white, russet, red or new potatoes. Quinoa is technically not a grain, but a *chenopod* – closely related to beets, spinach and tumbleweeds. Vegetarians or Primal enthusiasts looking for a grain-like taste or recipe base laud quinoa for being a complete protein (containing all nine essential amino acids, with 12–18 per cent of total calories as protein) and free from gluten. Wild rice is also not a true grain, but an aquatic grass. It offers a better nutritional value than grains, a nearly complete profile of essential amino acids (14 per cent protein calories) and is gluten-free. Categorise these supplemental carbohydrate foods as an indulgence. They may be enjoyable, but are likely unnecessary – especially if you are trying to reduce excess body fat.

WATER: OBEY YOUR THIRST, IT'S NOT TOO LATE

'Drink eight glasses of water a day to ensure good health.' 'By the time you're thirsty, it's too late.' We've heard these adages our entire lives as part of conventional wisdom's 10 (or 20, or whatever) commandments to be healthy – right up there with 'Drink milk to get your calcium', 'Eat your grains for fibre', 'Stay out of the sun to prevent skin cancer', 'Cut down on fat intake to lose weight' and other fables. While adequate hydration is paramount to good health, there is absolutely no scientific evidence to support the age-old rule of thumb that you should drink eight glasses of water per day.

Dr Heinz Valtin, former chair of physiology at Dartmouth Medical School and one of the world's foremost experts on kidney function, after conducting research for 11 months with the assistance of a professional librarian, discovered no conclusive studies about drinking eight glasses of water per day. Valtin believes that the myth originated in the 1940s when the National Institute of Medicine first issued recommendations for dietary nutrient intake, including water. Their suggestion to consume about two litres of water per day (this equals about eight 225-millilitre glasses) for optimum hydration contained the long-forgotten comment that 'much of this can be gained from the solid food we eat.'

Indeed, raw milk is 90 per cent water, chicken 54 per cent, minced beef 53 per cent, pizza 50 per cent, white bread 30 per cent (but, of course, we wouldn't be eating any pizza or bread, right?) and so on. Caffeine and alcohol, which constitute a significant portion of total fluid intake for many adults, have long been thought of as diuretics that dehydrate you by increasing urine flow. While this is true when you drink them in excess, your daily cup of coffee, bottle of beer, or glass or two of wine will actually contribute to hydration levels and not lead to any appreciable fluid loss.

When you experience such variables as hot weather and increased activity levels, your thirst mechanism works wonderfully to dictate how much you need to drink each day. This is a mechanism that has evolved over millennia to prevent dehydration, which is one of the quickest ways in which you can die. To date, there is no archaeological evidence that Grok carried litres of water around with him during his extremely active life, but he did just fine scooping water out of streams, licking the dew off leaves and maintaining adequate hydration incidentally through his diet.

Even when your water intake fluctuates significantly, your kidneys and endocrine system work very efficiently to promote optimum fluid levels in your bloodstream. When you experience even a slightly higher than normal concentration of your blood volume, an agent known as antidiuretic hormone goes to work, increasing the absorption of water from the kidneys and returning it to the bloodstream. According to Dr Valtin and other experts, if your blood becomes concentrated by about 2 per cent, your thirst mechanism will kick in big time, telling you to consume additional fluids. It is only when your blood becomes concentrated by 5 per cent that the medical concerns about dehydration present themselves. Dr Valtin further asserts that while dark urine indicates a need to drink perhaps a glass of water, there is no validity to the idea that your urine needs to be clear to indicate that you are adequately hydrated.

Even with a wide variation in water intake, our bodies will do a great job at maintaining normal blood concentration. And yes, there is such a thing as too much water; hyponatremia is a serious and occasionally fatal condition where sodium levels become too diluted in the blood as a result of overconsumption of water. What's more, some believe that drinking too much fluid near or during meals can result in poor digestion and excretion due to the dilution of stomach acids that are critical to the digestive process.

As an alternative to the bottled water industry-influenced mantra, 'drink, drink, drink!' without regard to your thirst, I recommend consuming a sensible amount of fluid each day, using your thirst as a guide to maintain optimum hydration. Sometimes this might be eight glasses of water, sometimes much less than half that. Heavy exercise, hot temperatures, body weight and the water content of the foods you eat are obviously all significant variables. When in doubt, obey your thirst! (Finally, a marketing slogan with a ring of truth to it!)

> *'Forget love – I'd rather fall in chocolate!'*
> SANDRA J. DYKES

SENSIBLE INDULGENCES

The following indulgences can actually promote health when you partake sensibly. Moderation is the key here. With that in mind, here are a few items that Grok rarely or never enjoyed, but which can be added to a Primal lifestyle with little or no downside.

ALCOHOL

Red wine is the superior alcoholic beverage choice for its impressive antioxidant benefits. Recent studies have shown so many health-enhancing benefits from the resveratrol in red wine that red wine extracts have become very popular as supplements. Beer is marginal (after all, it's made from grain!), while hard liquor and mixed drinks using sweetened beverages are the most objectionable. Note that alcohol calories (at seven per gram) are devoid of nutritional value and are generally the first to burn when ingested, which means the burning of stored body fat is interrupted while you indulge.

Furthermore, studies have clearly shown that alcohol in excess of one or two glasses a day can increase the risk of cancer (as well as car accidents, divorces, bar fights and other tribulations), so let's be clear that I'm not advocating anything but extremely responsible alcohol consumption, with a clear preference for red wine.

DARK CHOCOLATE

Dark chocolate is rich in antioxidants and brain-stimulating compounds known as phenolic phytochemicals or flavonoids. The ORAC values of cocoa powder and dark chocolate are higher than those of virtually any fruit or vegetable! Chocolate is the most craved food in the world for a reason – a chemical called phenylethylamine. This is found to trigger a feeling similar to that of falling in love. Choose dark chocolate, eat moderate portions, and enjoy with total awareness and absolutely no guilt.

I must say that the oft-repeated advice to do it with 'full awareness' while feeling no guilt is a pretty elegant non-guilt way of saying watch out, but is a little passive-aggressive – 'Don't feel guilty but have full awareness that you are breaking my heart.'

Be sure to get the absolute highest-quality chocolate you can find, because not all chocolates are created equal, from both a taste and a health perspective. The higher the cocoa content, the more you'll enjoy the aforementioned health benefits. This means milk chocolate is a distant also-ran to dark chocolate. Commercial bars like good old Hershey's have diminished cocoa content and such additives as sugars and milk solids, (even in bars labelled as 'dark') agents that dramatically compromise health benefits. I recommend choosing chocolate that is 75 per cent cocoa or greater (anything with more than 50 per cent cocoa content is classified as bittersweet chocolate). However, as you get closer to 100 per cent cacao, the lack of sweetness will be make this indulgence tough to appreciate (85 per cent is perfect for me). It may take a bit of time, but once you attune to the rich taste of high cocoa content dark chocolate, you'll likely lose your affinity for milk chocolate, which will consequently seem too sweet.

Organic chocolate offers you the comfort of greater oversight along the growing, harvesting and processing procedures – important due to the fact that conventional cocoa beans have a high pesticide concern and commonly often arrive from countries with questionable growing regulations and safety standards.

FINALLY, A WORD ABOUT SUPPLEMENTS

Given the lack of certain critical nutrients in even the healthiest diets (refer to the discussion on the drawbacks of conventional animal, vegetable and fruit products) and the excessive stress levels of hectic modern life, using premium-quality supplements in a few key categories can be quite effective to keep you Primal-aligned and support general health. The fact that Grok didn't use supplements doesn't mean we can't benefit from using small doses of certain concentrated natural substances to assist us in achieving optimal health. As you may know, I own and operate a supplement company called Primal Nutrition, so I'm hardly an impartial observer on this issue. If you object to me covering stuff that I sell in this book, I invite you skip ahead to the next chapter on exercise!

While supplementation is a personal choice and sometimes a difficult budget expense to justify, I urge you to consider a bare minimum programme to stay Primal-aligned and promote optimal gene expression. If you lead an extremely active life and/or have elevated stress factors, you may wish to investigate a more comprehensive regime, with details available at primalblueprint.com. Following is an overview of some supplements that can address the major shortcomings in our modern eating and lifestyle habits.

MULTIVITAMIN/MINERAL/ANTIOXIDANT FORMULA

Eating, exercising and living according to the Primal Blueprint will help mitigate much of the oxidative damage modern humans sustain as a result of eating the Standard American Diet, chronic or insufficient exercise, inadequate sleep and sunlight and generally excessive life stress levels. Your internal antioxidant systems work quite well when you are healthy and stress-balanced. However, pushing the limits with sub-par meals, jet travel, emotional stress or chronic exercise can quickly compromise your digestive, immune and endocrine systems, and other aspects of general health.

We need a broad mix of antioxidants on a daily basis, because they work in different ways and in different parts of the cell. Too much of any single antioxidant (in the absence of others) has been shown to have potentially negative effects, as a few recent vitamin E-only studies delivering negative results have demonstrated. Unfortunately, many of the best sources of dietary vitamins, minerals and antioxidants historically have all but disappeared or have been rendered impotent by today's aggressive factory farming techniques. In the fruit industry, for example, obtaining the highest possible sugar content has replaced nutritional value as the focus.

When you take a quality broad-spectrum antioxidant formula (containing hard-to-get nutrients such as full-spectrum vitamin E [not just alpha-tocopherol], mixed carotenoids [not just beta-carotene], tocotrienols, n-acetyl-cysteine, alpha-lipoic acid, curcumin, resveratrol, milk thistle, CoQ10 and quercetin, to name a few), the agents can work synergistically to mitigate oxidative damage and then help each other recycle back to their potent antioxidant form after donating an electron to the antioxidant effort. For that reason, I take my high-potency Damage Control Master Formula multivitamin loaded with extra antioxidants every day.

OMEGA 3 FISH OIL

In Grok's day, virtually every animal he consumed was a decent source of vital omega 3 fatty acids. The fish he caught had eaten algae to produce omega 3 fatty acids rich in EPA and DHA (which helped build the larger human brain over a couple of hundred thousand years). The animals he hunted had grazed on plants that generated high levels of omega 3 in these meats. Even the vegetation Grok consumed provided higher levels of omega 3s than found in today's plants. In Grok's diet, the ratio of pro-inflammatory (bad) omega 6 to anti-inflammatory (good and healthy) omega 3 was close to 1:1.

Today, even a conscientious eater can fall short of ideal O6:O3 ratios and consequently exist in a constant state of mild systemic inflammation. Normalising your ratio is a matter of strictly minimising omega 6 intake and boosting omega 3 intake by eating lots of oily, cold-water fish and/or taking a daily dose of highly purified omega 3 fish or krill oil supplements. The research on fish oils is extraordinarily positive, showing such benefits as decreased risk for heart disease and cancer, lowering of triglycerides, improvement in joint mobility, decreased insulin resistance and improved brain function and mood. The drug companies are even starting to recognise the power of this 'natural' medicine and have begun promoting prescription fish oil (at four times the price of a comparable supplement, of course!). As healthy as my own diet is, I rarely go a day without taking a few grams of an omega 3 fish oil supplement.

PROBIOTICS

Grok ate dirt … all day, every day. Hey, when you never wash your hands, your food, or anything else for that matter, you pretty much can't avoid it. But with all that soil came billions of soil-based organisms (mostly bacteria and yeast) that entered his mouth daily and populated his gut. Most were 'friendly' bacteria that actually helped him better digest food and ward off infections. In fact, much of Grok's (and our) immune system evolved to depend on these healthy 'flora' living in us symbiotically. Grok also ate the occasional 'unfriendly' organisms that had the potential to cause illness, but as long as the healthy flora well outnumbered the bad guys, all was well. Several trillion bacteria live symbiotically in the human digestive tract – some good and some bad. Much of your health depends on which of the two is winning the flora war.

The problem today is that not only do we avoid dirt, but we pursue sterility to the extent that we virtually eliminate all forms of bacteria – even the healthy stuff – from our diet. Of course, given the germs that prevail in the civilised world, it's probably best that we do thoroughly wash or cook everything we eat. In most healthy people, exposure to routine germs doesn't usually present a problem. As long as there are some healthy gut bacteria present (healthy, natural foods contain these probiotics inherently, even if we wash them); as long as we don't get too stressed out (stress hormones can kill off healthy flora) or too sick (diarrhoea and vomiting are ways by which the body purges bad bacteria – but it also purges good bacteria along with them), eat too much processed food (sugar, grains, trans and partially hydrogenated fats and chemical additives support the growth of unhealthy bacteria and yeast, while choking out healthy flora), or take antibiotics (antibiotics tend to kill most bacteria, good and bad – that's their job); and as long as we are eating well, those healthy bacteria can flourish and keep us healthy.

Of course, the healthy bacteria balance in our intestinal tract gets compromised regularly in all the ways mentioned (even with generally healthy people), creating an opportunity to benefit from supplementation. You don't necessarily need to take probiotics every day, because once these 'seeds' have been planted in a healthy gut, they tend to multiply and flourish easily on their own. Rather, consider taking extra probiotics under times of great stress, when you have been sick or are taking (or have just taken) a course of antibiotics, when you are travelling (particularly to foreign countries, where unfamiliar bacteria – even good stuff from good foods – can overwhelm your digestive system), or when you detect any sign of compromised immune function (the digestive system is critical to immune function). The reversal of fortune from a few days of taking probiotics can be dramatic. Better than eating dirt, I always say.

PROTEIN POWDER/MEAL REPLACEMENT

Restricting your intake of processed carbohydrates often means being at a loss for quick, convenient snacks or small meals. We are so conditioned to reach for a bagel, an energy bar, crisps, crackers and other grain-based products or sweets for snacks, we often run short of convenient, transportable, nonperishable options for an afternoon pick-up snack or mini meal. While not exactly Primal, protein powders/meal replacements do combine the best of 21st-century technology with a true Primal intent: they get me a fast, good-tasting source of nutrients without too many carbohydrates or unhealthy fats. I prefer micro-filtered whey protein to obtain an impressive profile of all the essential and nonessential amino acids, and coconut milk solids to provide healthy fats that can be delivered in a powdered formula.

I also recommend finding a product that tastes great when mixed only with water (so you don't have to add sugary juices or milk just to choke it down). That way you can always throw in a piece of fruit if you like for added calories or flavour. If I am in a hurry and want a quick, high-protein start to my day, my morning smoothie shake takes less than a minute to make and covers the necessary bases. Adding some omega 3 oil covers you on two more critical Primal areas. Micro-filtered whey, while derived from dairy, has insignificant amounts of lactose, so it's fine for all most lactose-intolerant people.

VITAMIN D

Vitamin D supplements can be useful when you are unable to obtain enough direct sunlight to manufacture abundant stores of this agent (which is technically a precursor hormone, not a vitamin). Sunlight is by far the most plentiful source of vitamin D; even an excellent diet provides for only a fraction of your vitamin D needs. Following the basic strategy outlined in Chapter 7, adequate sun exposure should enable you to maintain a sufficient blood level of vitamin D year-round, since vitamin D can be stored in your fat cells for winter use.

Unfortunately, many modern citizens are vitamin D-deficient for a variety of reasons: indoor-dominant lifestyles, minimal intake of oily, cold-water fish (by far the most plentiful dietary source), consuming high levels of phytates (nutrient depletion increases vitamin D requirements), being obese (excess body fat inhibits vitamin D absorption), or avoiding sun exposure (or screening obsessively; are you listening, preschool mums?) due to misguided fears about skin cancer. Getting enough vitamin D is especially challenging for those living at latitudes above 49 degrees (Canada/US border, France, Germany, Russia) or those with dark skin pigment living outside of tropical latitudes.

Beyond those in the aforementioned high-risk categories, many of us can benefit from routine vitamin D supplementation in the winter months, when the sun's rays are of insufficient intensity to facilitate vitamin D production. In the Continental US, this is the case for 3–4 months per year. Those in Canada, Northern Europe and Scandinavia are inhibited for 7–8 months per year.

Expert vitamin D advocates recommend obtaining an average of 4,000 International Units (IU) per day of vitamin D. You can easily bag 5,000–10,000 IU during a single half-hour sunbathing session in the summertime. In the wintertime, I recommend supplementing with 2,000 IU of vitamin D per day. If you struggle to remember to take pills consistently, you can take a bunch of vitamin D at once with no ill effects. I am fair-skinned, live at 34 degrees latitude in Los Angeles, and get a ton of sun exposure during the summer, but I still supplement during the winter to be extra sure that my blood levels are adequate.

If you have even a hint of the aforementioned risk factors, consider obtaining a blood test for '25-vitamin D' or 'serum 25(OH) D'. Make sure you ask for these specific tests, since many doctors are uninformed about which tests are the most accurate. Your vitamin D goal range is 40-60 ng/ml. If your reading is under 40 ng/ml, take aggressive action to get more sunlight and/or supplement diligently. Even if you are not the pill-popping type, the recommendation to supplement with vitamin Ds should be strongly considered. Dietary sources for vitamin D are inadequate, supplements are inexpensive, and maintaining adequate vitamin D levels is critical to healthy cellular function and prevention of cancer, including melanoma.

The aforementioned categories represent what I believe to be the most useful products to consider for supplementation, but there are numerous other product categories and individual supplements that address more specialised needs. Among them are phosphatidylserine (PS), which improves cognitive function and moderates cortisol spikes in the bloodstream; and buffering joint compounds (glucosamine, chondroitin, MSM and enzyme cofactors), which support connective tissue and alleviate pain. A knowledgeable healthcare practitioner may recommend other products to address your particular needs.

SUPPLEMENT QUALITY

Regardless of what brand of products you choose, you should be extremely vigilant in an industry that is minimally regulated. Good manufacturers have a tightly controlled production environment where every single raw material that goes into the finished product is easily sourced and certified by the supplier. Contact your supplement manufacturers and ask them if they obtain 'Certificates of Assay' attesting to the source, potency and purity of each ingredient. Ask if their products are produced in a pharmaceutical-grade manufacturing environment and whether they adhere to the 'Good Manufacturing Practices' (GMP) overseen by the Food and Drug Administration. Notice how well products are sealed when presented for retail sale.

You will be able to quickly discern from email replies (or lack thereof) or phone conversations whether the manufacturer of the supplements you consume or are considering consuming has its act together. Examine labels and choose supplements that are free of common fillers and additives, such as colourings, waxes, preservatives and other chemicals, listed under 'inactive' or 'other' ingredients. You'll be surprised to discover just how prevalent these agents are in many of the leading vitamin brands and discount products available through retailers and in supermarkets and chemist shops. Understand that premium-quality supplements are considerably more expensive than the giant bottles found on the shelves of warehouse stores. The latter offer minimal potency and bioavailability (ease of digestion and utilisation by the body) and bring literal accuracy to the expression 'pissing away your money'.

CHAPTER SUMMARY

- **Meat and Poultry:** Choose local, pasture-raised animal products (or, next best, USDA-certified organic animal products) to avoid today's poor-quality, mass-produced feedlot animals fattened up with grains and laden with hormones, pesticides and antibiotics.
- **Fish:** Emphasise wild-caught fish from remote, pollution-free waters. Oily, cold-water fish (anchovies, herring, mackerel, salmon, sardines) have the highest level of omega 3 fatty acids.

Choose only approved farmed fish (coho salmon, shellfish, domestic trout and certain other domestic species), and avoid other farmed fish (including the popular Atlantic salmon), fish at the top of the food chain (shark, sword), fish caught by environmentally objectionable commercial methods, or imports from Asia (both wild-caught and farmed).

- **Eggs**: Should not be avoided based on the flawed assumption that their high-cholesterol content is a heart disease risk factor. Local, pasture-raised chickens deliver superior values of omega 3 and other nutrients than commercially raised chickens.

- **Vegetables:** Plant foods should play a central role in your diet and comprise the largest section of your daily 'plate'. Brightly coloured foods have high levels of antioxidants, phenols, fibre, vitamins, minerals and other micronutrients. Consuming vegetables and fruits helps naturally promote alkalinity in your body, boosting immune function and reducing disease risk. Dark leafy greens are an excellent choice to consume regularly as a base for any main course. Fresh berries offer excellent antioxidant and nutrient levels. Eating fruits and vegetables liberally, and seasonal fruits with some moderation and selectivity, will still result in a satisfactory average total carbohydrate intake of 150 grams or less per day.

  It's essential to select locally grown, preferably organic plant foods for maximum nutritional value and health safety. Be strict about going organic with fruits and vegetables that have a large surface area (leafy greens) or a soft open skin (bell peppers, carrots, winter squash, berries, peaches). You can be less strict with plants that have a tough, inedible skin (bananas, avocados, melons, oranges). Certain fruits with relatively high sugar, low antioxidant values should be consumed in moderation, respecting how different today's cultivated fruits are from Grok's more fibrous, less sugary wild fruits that were enjoyed only in narrow ripening seasons.

- **Macadamia Nuts:** Macadamias earn special distinction due to their superior nutritional profile of mostly monounsaturated fats, as well as phytonutrients, fibre, antioxidants and numerous vitamins and minerals. They are deeply satisfying – an excellent snack choice for appetite control – and have been found to minimise disease risk. Other nuts, seeds and their derivative butters are a healthy component of Primal eating, but some moderation is warranted due to their caloric density and a desire to regulate O6 intake.

- **Coconut Products:** Coconut's medium-chain fatty acids offer exceptional health benefits and are difficult to obtain, even in a healthy diet. Integrating coconut oil, milk, flakes and other derivatives can be great substitutes for offensive Standard American Diet ingredients. Coconut oil is excellent for cooking due to its high saturated fat composition.

- **Fruits:** Fruits offer an outstanding source of fibre, vitamins, minerals, antioxidants and other nutrients. Choose wisely by sticking to locally grown, in-season, pesticide-free fruits that are high in antioxidants. Some moderation is warranted with fruit due to year-round availability of highly cultivated modern fruits that are extra sweet. This is particularly true for those with fat-reduction goals, since fruit is easily converted into fat in the liver, so those with fat reduction goals should exercise.

- **Herbs and Spices:** Herbs and spices offer tremendous micronutrient value, *especially as they pertain to antioxidants*. Herbs and spices can enhance your enjoyment of meals and offer potential *benefits for certain health c*onditions.

- **Moderation Foods:** Certain foods that weren't around in Grok's day are acceptable today, provided they are not overemphasised. These include coffee, high-fat dairy products (preference for raw, fermented, high-fat dairy products), approved fats and oils, other nuts, seeds and their derivative butters, supplemental carbohydrates (sweet potatoes, quinoa, wild rice) and water (obey your thirst).

- **Sensible Indulgences:** Enjoy with full attention and awareness, and never feel guilty. Red wine and dark chocolate (75 per cent cacao or greater) offer numerous health benefits, making them superior choices to enjoy in a responsible manner.

- **Supplements:** Supplements can play a critical role in adapting Primal recommendations into the realities of hectic modern life. Supplements offer a convenient source of concentrated nutrition that helps account for nutrient deficiencies (e.g. depleted soil or objectionable conventional growing and production methods) in today's food supply. The following categories offer comprehensive protection and added support for even the healthiest of diets: multivitamin/mineral/antioxidant formula, omega 3 fish oil, probiotic formula, protein powder/meal replacement and vitamin D.

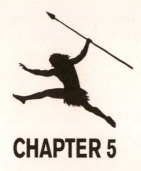

CHAPTER 5

LAW NUMBER 2: AVOID POISONOUS THINGS

'DROP YOUR FORK AND STEP AWAY FROM THE PLATE!'

'When you see the golden arches, you are probably on your way to the pearly gates.'
WILLIAM CASTELLI, MD, DIRECTOR OF THE FRAMINGHAM HEART STUDY

IN THIS CHAPTER

Here I will outline the health risks of eating 'poisonous things'. In Grok's day, poisonous plants could drop him on the spot. Today, our poisons are factory-produced items in bright packages that kill more insidiously over decades. In this chapter we will explore the cultural factors that create tremendous momentum towards unhealthy choices and consider strategies for resisting these manipulative influences.

I will pay particular attention to dispelling the conventional wisdom tenet that grains (wheat, rice, bread, pasta, cereal, corn, etc.) and legumes (alfalfa, beans, lentils, peanuts, peas and soy products) are healthy, countering these common assumptions with extensive research and details indicating the problems grains and, to a slightly lesser extent, legumes cause with their relatively recent introduction into the human diet. Grain and legume consumption offers minimal nutritional value and generates a high insulin response. The phytates in these foods inhibit the absorption of minerals. Glutens disturb healthy immune function and promote inflammation. Lectins inhibit healthy gastrointestinal function. Wholegrains are no healthier than refined grains and have a worse impact on health because they have more of these harmful agents.

Trans and partially hydrogenated fats, and excessive consumption of polyunsaturated fatty acids (PUFAs) wreak havoc at the cellular level, promoting inflammation, ageing and cancer. Also important to avoid are all sugary foods and beverages, and assorted other processed foods.

I'd like us all to reflect for a moment on our priorities and our vision of a long, happy, healthy, fit life. When the topic of food comes up in conversation with family, friends or casual acquaintances, it's fascinating to hear the litany of rationalisations, knee-jerk defence mechanisms, self-limiting belief statements and general confusion or ignorance from otherwise intelligent folks when it comes to eating healthily. But then again, conventional wisdom has often led even the best and brightest minds in nutritional science astray.

It's truly remarkable how successful Madison Avenue has been at indoctrinating lifestyles that produce huge profits for giant multi-national corporations – and devastating health consequences for consumers – into generations of society. The marketing messages are so pervasive in modern culture that it's difficult, even stressful, to take control of your health and swim upstream against such cultural norms as fast food, the all-American high-carbohydrate breakfast, post-meal desserts and the massive overconsumption of all manner of sweetened sodas, juices, energy drinks, teas and coffees. Even noble attempts to do the right thing miss the mark: mass-market 'health foods', such as nutritionally challenged meal replacements, energy bars and other heavily processed 'fuel' marketed to athletes, or purification/detox diets with clever ideas, such as eating nothing but brown rice for a week (talk about a long, hot insulin bath!). Finally, many of our eating habits are driven by cultural, social, emotional or stress-related triggers other than hunger.

While savouring the occasional moderate serving of a rich treat can be an acceptable element of enjoying life, it's an entirely different story to ingest junk food habitually and mindlessly. If you notice yourself treading in these waters (or, worse, repurposing the classic quote from Sir Edmund Hillary about why he climbed Mount Everest – 'Because it's there' – into an excuse), please give this topic some sincere reflection and take decisive action. Remember, your ancestors worked unimaginably hard to survive, thrive and create the amazing opportunities we have today for a healthy, happy, active and long life. As I say here often, your genes want you to be healthy and you deserve nothing less than the very best your genes have to offer.

The most common retort I hear on this thread is, 'Hey, everything in moderation.' Sage advice indeed, but Mark Twain best put this proverb in perspective when he said, 'Everything in moderation, *including moderation*.' As the Korgs prove dramatically, we live in a world where extreme measures are necessary just to avoid serious disease (remember, some three-quarters of today's American population will eventually die of heart disease or cancer), let alone enjoy optimum health, fitness, energy levels and body composition.

I support enjoying the occasional indulgence, but why not make it from the list of approved foods of the absolute highest quality? Take a glance at the label of a Milky Way or Snickers bar in comparison with some delicious high-antioxidant, organic dark chocolate bar with no additives, toxic chemicals, chemically altered fats or fillers (and check the disparity in carbohydrate count). This sensible and deeply satisfying indulgence can hardly be described as a sacrifice or compromise. You can walk past the candy machine without skipping a beat!

> "'Everything in moderation" is sage advice indeed, but Mark Twain best put this proverb in perspective when he said, "Everything in moderation, including moderation."'

GOING AGAINST THE GRAIN

Perhaps the most the most widely accepted and damaging element of dietary conventional wisdom is that grains are healthy – the 'staff of life' – as we've been led to believe our entire lives. While grains have indeed enjoyed massive global popularity for the last 7,000 years, they are simply not very healthy for human consumption. From two million years ago, when the first *Homo erectus* arose and steadily evolved into the first modern *Homo sapiens* between 200,000 and 100,000 years ago, and continuing until about 10,000 years ago, humans existed entirely as hunter-gatherers. Early *Homo sapiens* derived their food from 100 to 200 different wild food sources, including animal meats, fruits, vegetables and nuts and seeds. Grains were notably absent.

Around 10,000 years ago, forces conspired to create a dramatic shift in the human diet. The widespread extinction of large mammals on major continents coupled with increases in population forced humans to become more resourceful in obtaining food. Those living by water used boats, canoes, nets and better fishing tools to catch more bounty. On land, humans refined their toolmaking and hunting strategies to include more birds and small mammals in the food supply. Escalating competition for animal-sourced food led to agricultural innovations sprouting up independently in the most advanced societies around the world (Egyptians, Mayans, etc.). As wild grains (which were a very small part of some earlier diets but difficult to harvest for any significant yield) and much later, legumes became domesticated, humans derived more and more calories from these readily available high-calorie sources. This trend has continued to the present day – with dire consequences.

Loren Cordain, PhD, author of the 2002 best-seller *The Paleo Diet*, explains:

> *Cereal grains [meaning cultivated grains in general, not breakfast cereals] have fundamentally altered the foods to which our species had been originally adapted over eons of evolutionary experience. For better or for worse, we are no longer hunter-gatherers. However, our genetic makeup is still that of a paleolithic hunter-gatherer, a species whose nutritional requirements are optimally adapted to wild meats, fruits and vegetables, not to cereal grains. There is a significant body of evidence which suggests that cereal grains are less than optimal foods for humans and that the human genetic makeup and physiology may not be fully adapted to high levels of [cultivated] grain consumption. We have wandered down a path towards absolute dependence upon [cultivated] grains, a path from which there is no return.*

Culturally, the cultivation of grains is the key variable that allowed modern civilisation to develop and thrive. Families could successfully feed and raise more children. Large populations could now live permanently in proximity and labour could be more specialised, leading to continued exponential advancements in knowledge and modernisation. However, as Cordain elaborates: '[Grains] have allowed man's culture to grow and evolve so that man has become earth's dominant animal species, but this preeminence has not occurred without cost .... Agriculture is generally agreed to be responsible for many of humanity's societal ills, including wholescale warfare, starvation, tyranny, epidemic diseases and class divisions.'

Dr Jared Diamond, evolutionary biologist, physiologist and Pulitzer Prizewinning professor of geography at UCLA and author of *Guns, Germs and Steel,* goes so far as to say that agriculture was 'the worst mistake in the history of the human race' and that 'we're still struggling with the mess into which agriculture has tumbled us, and it's unclear whether we can solve it.'

Costs to the individual were also significant. The flourishing of agriculture paralleled a reduction in average human life span as well as body and brain size, increases in infant mortality and infectious diseases, and the occurrence of previously unknown conditions such as osteoporosis, bone mineral disorders and malnutrition. As cultural and medical advancements have eliminated most of the rudimentary health risks faced by early humans (infant mortality, predator danger, minor infections turning fatal, etc.), we can now live long enough to develop, suffer and die from diet-related diseases, including atherosclerosis, hypertension and type 2 diabetes (it used to be called adult-onset diabetes until millions of kids started developing it in recent years!).

> '*The wise man sees in the misfortune of others what he should avoid.*'
> MARCUS AURELIUS, ROMAN EMPEROR (121–180)

THE BASE OF THE DISEASE PYRAMID

Grains offer the great majority of their calories in the form of carbohydrate, so they cause blood glucose levels to elevate quickly. High-carbohydrate foods, such as sugar and grains (and to a lesser extent, legumes – which we'll discuss shortly), have been recently and suddenly introduced to the human food supply (that's right, even 10,000 years ago is 'recent and sudden' in evolutionary terms) and yet are consumed in massive quantities. These sugars and grains shock our delicate hormonal systems, which are better adapted to what today would be considered a low-carbohydrate, high-fat diet.

Please realise that mismanaging your *Homo sapiens* genes by consuming a high-carbohydrate diet occurs even when you take care to emphasise whole grains over refined grains. Yes, brown rice and wholewheat toast burn slower than soda, but your body still has to produce a requisite amount of insulin to deal with the wildly excessive level of daily carbohydrate intake that is typical today.

A grain-heavy diet stresses the all-important insulin regulation mechanism in the body. After consuming that bagel, scone, muffin, French toast or bowl of cereal (all derived from grains) and a glass of juice for breakfast, your pancreas releases insulin into the bloodstream to help regulate blood glucose levels. Even after the routine meal just described, many Americans technically become temporarily diabetic, with blood glucose levels soaring to clinically dangerous highs. You know the drill by now: after your meal, insulin is released into the bloodstream to promote the storage of glucose as muscle glycogen or direct its conversion to fat. Experience this often enough and you gain weight and develop insulin resistance and Metabolic Syndrome.

If, instead, you were to have a Primal Blueprint breakfast consisting of a delicious cheese-and-vegetable omelette with some bacon, you would enjoy a moderated insulin response, leading to balanced energy levels for the hours after your meal instead of a sugar high and insulin crash. Furthermore, with blood glucose levels balanced, you would be able to access and burn stored body fat for energy until your next insulin-balanced meal.

PHYTATES WE HATE

There is sufficient evidence that this overreliance on grains – as well as on simple carbohyrate and sugar products in general – leads to numerous vitamin, mineral and nutritional deficiencies. Most grains contain substances called phytates that easily bind to important minerals such as calcium, magnesium and zinc in the digestive tract, making them more difficult to absorb. Ironically, the unpro-cessed – and, therefore, supposedly healthier – 'whole' grains are typically the highest in phytates. Mineral deficiencies are common in underdeveloped nations that depend almost entirely on grain for their sustenance (bread accounts for 50 per cent of the total calories consumed in at least half the countries in the world; some people get up to 80 per cent of total calories from grain products).

Grains also interfere with vitamin D metabolism and in related deficiencies of vitamins A, C and B12. These nutrients are not present in grains (again, ironically, unless they have been processed and then 'fortified' by adding back the missing vitamins – albeit at a much-reduced nutritional value). Deficiencies of these basic vita-mins are prevalent mainly in third-world countries (see the recurring theme?); however, even Western eaters with more balanced diets, but who still rely too heavily on grains, miss out on eating more nutritious foods, such as meats, vegetables, fruits, nuts and seeds. In the US, 45 per cent of citizens consume zero daily servings of fruit or juice and 22 per cent eat no daily vegetables.

GLUTEN, LECTIN – IMMUNE AFFECTIN'

Certain grain (and also some legume and dairy) proteins mimic those found in viruses and bacteria, triggering an autoimmune (your immune system attacking healthy cells by mistake) response when ingested. Gluten – the large, water-soluble protein that creates the elasticity in dough (it's also the primary glue in wallpaper paste) – is found in most common grains, such as wheat, rye, barley and also in beans. Researchers now believe that as many as a third of us are probably gluten-intolerant or gluten-sensitive. That third of us (and I would suspect many more on a subclinical level) 'react' to gluten with a perceptible inflammatory response. Over time, those who are known to be gluten-intolerant can develop a dismal array of medical condi-tions: dermatitis, joint pain, reproductive problems, acid reflux and other digestive conditions, autoimmune disorders and coeliac disease. And that doesn't mean that the rest of us aren't experiencing some milder negative effect that just doesn't manifest itself so obviously.

Grains and legumes also contain high levels of mild, natural plant toxins known as lectins. Researchers have found that lectins can inhibit healthy gastrointestinal function by damaging delicate brush borders that line your small intestine. Brush borders (named for their resemblance to paintbrush bristles; also known as microvilli) are where most of the nutrients from the food we eat are absorbed. They contain digestive enzymes that help break down carbohydrates as the final component of their digestive process, and allow appropriate forms of nutrients (glucose, amino acids, fats, vitamins and minerals) to become absorbed into the bloodstream from the intestine (envision the dangling cloth strips applying soap to your car as it passes through a car wash).

Lectin damage to brush borders allows larger, undigested protein molecules to infiltrate the bloodstream. The ever-vigilant immune system sees these unfamiliar protein molecules (not necessarily lectins, but *anything* you ingest that was supposed to be fully processed in the digestive tract before entering the bloodstream) and sets up a typical immune response to deal with them. Unfortunately, these undigested protein molecules can resemble molecules that reside on the outside of healthy cells, leaving your immune system confused as to who is the real enemy. An autoimmune response ensues, something experts believe is the root cause of many common diseases. like rheumatoid arthritis, lupus, Hashimoto's thyroiditis, multiple sclerosis and a host of others.

The millions of folks who have been diagnosed with coeliac disease or gluten intolerance will not do well switching to a diet heavy in legumes or even so-called 'gluten-free grains'. They are simply exposing themselves to other kinds of lectins, and of course too much insulin production.

THE HOLES IN THE WHOLE GRAIN STORY

Many health-conscious eaters are well aware of the drawbacks of eating refined wheat flour, white rice, pasta and other grains that have been stripped of their natural fibre and other nutrients during the manufacturing process. While a refined grain product will (in most cases) produce a higher initial insulin spike response than a whole grain food (because fibre delays the absorption process and mutes the blood glucose effect), a whole grain might well be considered less healthy than its stripped-down cousin for many other reasons.

By definition, whole grains are those that have all three edible components intact: the endosperm (starchy), the bran (fibrous) and the germ (oily). As we learned earlier in this chapter, many whole grains contain harmful phytates, glutens and lectins that promote inflammation and offend your immune and digestive systems. While you also get that highly touted dose of fibre from your whole grains, this too can be seen as a negative. Contrary to conventional wisdom, excessive fibre intake (practically automatic when you emphasise whole grains) can increase appetite and interfere with healthy digestion, mineral absorption and elimination. (I detail the drawbacks of consuming too much fibre in the Primal Blueprint Q&A at MarksDailyApple. com.) You can obtain optimal amounts of fibre (and eliminate the risk of overdoing it) from emphasising vegetables, fruits, nuts and seeds à la the Primal Blueprint.

When you ingest a refined product, such as processed white breads, fizzy drinks or sweets you get empty calories and a big insulin hit – but that's all you get. Furthermore, the eventual total insulin production is the same for a slice of white bread as it is a slice of wholewheat bread. True, the wheat bread might burn a little slower, but you eventually produce the same amount of insulin to deal with the glucose load. The only thing in whole grain's favour is a very minimal amount of protein (and most of that is the offensive gluten) and a few micronutrients. However, the nutritional advantages of eating whole grains are insignificant – especially in comparison with any vegetable, fruit, nut, seed, or organic animal food with far more nutritional value calorie for calorie (and, unlike whole grains, they also taste good!) and which are also free from objectionable agents.

For purposes of weight control and preventing disease, a gram of carbohydrate from a whole grain is no better than a gram from a refined grain. I'm not suggesting that you choose refined grains over whole grains; I'm suggesting you ditch *all* grains in favour of Primal Blueprint foods. The next time you are faced with the option to eat grains and you rationalise that whole grains are a step up from processed white bread and fizzy drinks, be sure you understand the 'whole' story.

SAY GOODBYE TO FATIGUE, ILLNESS AND SUFFERING

Understanding that the long-term effects of chronic hyperinsuline-mia (high insulin levels in the bloodstream) are such conditions as general systemic inflammation, obesity, diabetes, heart disease and cancer should be enough to convince you that it is critical to pursue a more natural way of eating. Eating low-carbohydrate, grain-free meals will not only result in immediate gratification in the form of regulated energy levels, but it can help you succeed with long-term weight management and quite possibly save your life.

As a reminder, insulin is a 'master hormone' that regulates the metabolism of fat and carbohydrate in your body. The single most important requirement to improve your fat metabolism and succeed with long-term weight management is to reduce the total amount of insulin you produce. High insulin levels promote fat storage and disease. Moderated insulin levels (typical of Primal Blueprint eating) stimulate fat burning and good health. It's that simple.

At the risk of sounding overly dramatic or redundant on this position, we must understand that the reasonable, 'evolutionary' voice challenging conventional wisdom about grains is being battled by billions of dollars in corporate and government propaganda pushing us to conform to dietary habits that we are not suited for, that do not nourish us, and that are downright destructive to human health. As Professor Diamond reminds us, humanity is very far down a disastrous road, and righting the course is incredibly problematic.

If you are one of the fortunate folks who are less sensitive to glutens, lectins and phytates than most, you might take exception to my wholesale damning of foods that are a dietary centrepiece across the globe. Absent acute symptoms, I'll still argue that we are all genetically 'allergic' in some way to foods that are not aligned with the Primal Blueprint. Perhaps you can try eliminating grains for 30 or 60 days, taking note of any general improvements in your condition. I'll bet your energy will be more regulated after meals, your digestive and elimination will improve, the frequency of minor illnesses or inflammation conditions will subside and you will be more successful controlling your weight. There simply are no good reasons to base your diet on grains – and a lot of reasons never to eat most grains again.

> *'High insulin levels promote fat storage and disease. Moderated insulin levels (typical with Primal Blueprint eating) stimulate fat burning and good health. It's that simple.'*

> *'More die in the United States of too much food than of too little.'*
> JOHN KENNETH GALBRAITH

POLYUNSATURATED FATTY ACIDS (PUFAs)

Conventional wisdom has unwisely transitioned away from saturated fats to widespread consumption of PUFAs over the past several decades. PUFAs are easily oxidised and quickly go rancid (on shelf and *in your body!*) particularly when heated during cooking. Oxidised PUFAs have a pro-inflammatory effect on your system, leading to assorted health problems and a disruption in healthy immune and hormone function.

The endocrine system is especially vulnerable to the effects of PUFA ingestion, leading to symptoms such as a slowed metabolism, low energy levels and sluggish thyroid function. Heavy consumption of PUFAs in the modern diet is blamed as a leading contributor to insulin resistance, obesity, diabetes, heart disease, cancer, immune problems, arthritis and other inflammatory conditions. Strictly avoid the following categories of PUFAs, replacing them with the approved fats and oils discussed in the previous chapter.

- **Canola Oil:** Canola oil is touted as a great cooking and eating choice due to its high monounsaturated content. Unfortunately, canola oil is a heavily refined, genetically engineered product derived from the rapeseed plant. This plant is believed to be toxic to humans and animals – particularly harmful to respiratory function. Most canola oil is put through a deodorising process that converts some of its natural omega 3s into harmful trans fats. The popularity of canola oil today is a classic example of conventional wisdom taking facts (canola has a high monounsaturated content; monounsaturated fats are healthy) out of context or otherwise distorting them at the expense of our health.

- **Margarine:** Comprised of offensive ingredients and processed with chemical additives at high temperatures. While most all margarines today have the 'trans fat-free' distinction proudly adorning the label, the PUFAs that some margarines contain still potentially raise LDL, lower HDL and suppress immune function and insulin sensitivity. Research strongly suggests an increased risk of cancer and heart disease from margarine use.

- **Other Vegetable and Seed PUFA Oils:** Includes corn, safflower, sunflower, soybean, cottonseed and others. These oils, popular in packaged and frozen foods, as well as in bottles, are heavily refined in an offensive manner. They contain poor omega 6:omega 3 ratios and are believed to disturb endocrine function. They are a poor choice for cooking since they are highly vulnerable to oxidation when heated.

- **Vegetable Shortening:** Similar to lard in appearance but chemically produced to create a trans fat. Bad stuff – stay away!

TRANS AND PARTIALLY HYDROGENATED FATS

Perhaps the most overtly offensive and dangerous element of the modern diet is the widespread consumption of toxic processed fats: partially hydrogenated, hydrogenated and trans fats. *Note*: the three are not quite the same but are very similar – and all evil. Throughout the book, we use the term *partially hydrogenated*, because it is more widely used in food manufacturing and a more familiar term on food labels than plain *hydrogenated*. What's more, partially hydrogenated fats are actually more objectionable than fully hydrogenated fats.

These fats are found in almost every processed food product in the supermarket, including frozen dinners, breakfast foods, sweets and desserts; packaged snacks (e.g. crackers, crisps and biscuits); deep-fried foods; pastries and baked goods (e.g. doughnuts, croissants and cupcakes); and peanut butter, soups and even grain products (e.g. bread, cereal, pasta and rice mixes). A commonly cited estimate is that 40 per cent of all products in a typical supermarket contain partially hydrogenated oils.

Partially hydrogenated fats are easily oxidised to form free radical chain reactions that damage cell membranes and body tissue and that hamper immune function. Because your brain, nervous system and vascular system consist primarily of fat-based membranes, any dysfunction in these critical areas can be devastating. Trans are not recognised as foreign by the body, so they are incorporated into cell membranes and asked to function as natural fats. Of course, they don't function normally, they just take up space usually reserved for healthy fats and wreak havoc on homeostasis.

Many scientists consider the cell membrane to be the brain of the cell (as opposed to the more common assumption that the nucleus runs the show) because the membrane receives feedback from the outside environment (e.g. ingested nutrients such as glucose entering the blood-stream, the presence of a virus attacking healthy cells, or increased blood flow due to exercise stimulus) and takes consequent action (e.g. triggers the expression of certain genes or the release of certain hormones).

When you have cell membranes comprising natural molecules and you replace them with synthetic dysfunctional molecules such as partially hydrogenated fats, the intricate signalling system is compromised. Plain and simple, the routine and prolonged ingestion of these toxic agents is a major contributor to the alarming increase in not only diet-related cancers but many other diseases and adverse health conditions. Many experts believe there is a direct connection between consuming processed foods and obesity (beyond their direct contribution to caloric excess), theorising that insulin resistance could be exacerbated by dysfunctional fat molecules accumulating in cell membranes.

Research suggests that consumption of trans and partially hydrogenated fats promotes inflammation, ageing and cancer. The *New England Journal of Medicine* reviewed numerous studies and reported a strong link between trans fat consumption and heart disease (including the strong tendency for processed fats to significantly raise LDL cholesterol levels and lower HDL levels). Harvard Medical School estimates that partially hydrogenated fats may be responsible for as many as 100,000 premature deaths each year in the United States. The United States Academy of Sciences says that there is 'no safe level' of trans fatty acids in the American diet. The good news is that when you change your diet to eliminate these toxic agents, over time your cells will repair or replace these dysfunctional molecules with healthy ones.

OTHER FOODS TO AVOID

GRAINS ... OH, DID I ALREADY MENTION THEM?

Wheat, corn, rice, oats, barley, millet, rye, breakfast cereals, pastas, breads, pancakes, rolls, crackers and even 'natural' grains such as barley, millet, rye and the like. Buoyed by conventional wisdom, I consumed grains with reckless abandon as a major percentage of my dietary calories for some 40 years. It wasn't until I completely eliminated grains from my diet that some epiphanies occurred. Those occasional stomach cramps that I always attributed to stress? They were more likely due to wheat allergies (their severity triggered by stress, of course). That sluggish feeling I had after pasta dinners that I attributed to fatigue from a hard day training or working? It was actually my brain experiencing glucose depletion from the post-meal insulin flash flood in my bloodstream. The bloating that caused me to loosen my belt buckle after big meals that I attributed to eating big meals? This may have represented a mild allergic reaction to gluten. The mild arthritis in my fingers that I first began to notice on the golf course in my forties and chalked up to the ageing process? Likely due to the pro-inflammatory nature of the lingering amounts of grains still remaining in my diet. These routine tribulations that I had long considered a regrettable but inevitable part of life completely disappeared once my transition to a completely Primal diet took hold.

I've met very few people who eat a lot of grains, yet who also claim to enjoy ideal weight, experience perfectly satisfactory and steady energy levels and never feel digestive distress. At the very least, it's worth conducting a 21-day test to determine your sensitivity – and get a glimpse of your potential upside – from eliminating grains from your diet. Chances are, even if you are at a decent launching point now, you will experience a noticeable stabilisation of daily energy levels, improved immune function and a reduction in minor digestive distress from reducing or eliminating grains.

LEGUMES

Alfalfa, beans, lentils, peanuts, peas and soybeans. While legumes can serve as a passable source of protein, fibre, potassium and anti-oxidants, they also provide significant levels of carbohydrate and increase the overall insulin load of your diet. Furthermore, legumes contain those pesky anti-nutrients, lectins. As *Paleo Diet* author Dr Loren Cordain explains: 'Most legumes in their mature state are non-digestible and/or toxic to most mammals, when eaten in even moderate quantities.'

The fact that legumes need to be altered for human consumption through cooking, soaking or fermenting should be our best clue to avoid or strictly minimise their consumption (all truly safe fruits and vegetables can be eaten either raw or cooked). To tiptoe into a sensitive subject, the beans that are consumed liberally by many world cultures (kidney, pinto, black beans, lentils) come with the annoying by-product of flatulence, caused by the fermentation of indigestible carbohydrates.

While soy has achieved great popularity as a 'healthy' alternative to meat, unfermented soy products contain compounds that may interfere with thyroid hormone production and have demonstrated an estrogenic (feminising) effect in certain tissue. That said, some select soy products do have decent nutritional value and certain fermented products may be less objectionable (tempeh, natto, etc.).

There is simply no good reason to ever consume legumes. Well, except as a source of supplemental carbohydrates for that select group of mega calorie burners, without any excess body fat, who are not negatively affected by the lectins and who are looking for ways to replenish depleted muscle glycogen. I understand that many people have a strong affinity for legumes and that legumes enjoy a reputa-tion as a healthy food category – particularly among vegetarians, who otherwise have limited protein options. It will not be a disaster if you occasionally dip your vegetables in hummus at a dinner party, fry some tempeh with vegetables for a main course, or enjoy side dishes of peas, lentils or steamed beans. However, emphasising legumes in your diet is an inferior strategy to having vegetables, fruits, nuts and seeds and animal foods as your primary meal and snack choices.

PROCESSED FOODS

Anything with chemical additives or that's been heavily altered from its natural state requires little discussion. Realise that you have been pummelled with marketing messages your entire life to consume branded, boxed stuff that has contributed directly and tragically to the obesity, illness and death of those in your family and community. As important as knowing what our ancestors ate is knowing what they *didn't* eat: Grok never touched refined sugar, trans or partially hydrogenated fats, grains, legumes, desserts, processed foods or anything with hormones, pesticides, antibiotics, herbicides, fungi-cides, preservatives or other chemicals.

SUGAR

I recognise how addictive sweets are. After all, our genes were programmed to appreciate those rare sweet natural sugars our ancestors discovered on occasion. Unfortunately, today we are bombarded by sugar everywhere. Sugar products greatly stress your insulin sensitivity and reinforce an addiction to both sugar and all simple carbohydrates.

No discussion of sugar would be complete without mention of high fructose corn syrup (HFCS). Fructose has long been considered a superior sweetener to table sugar (sucrose), since it is the primary sugar in fruit and generates a lower insulin response (fructose must be converted into glucose in the liver before it can be utilised in the bloodstream, thus muting both the glucose and insulin spikes). Unfortunately, the fructose that sweetens most processed foods and beverages today – HFCS – is derived from corn, not fruit. This inexpensive and extremely sweet chemically processed agent is found in the vast majority of fizzy drinks, energy drinks, teas, juices, baked goods, desserts and snack foods in your grocery store.

It has been well established that HFCS is even more lipogenic (fat-promoting) than glucose, since it is readily converted into either glucose or triglycerides in the liver. Diets high in HFCS have been shown to substantially increase triglyceride levels, increase risk of obesity (particularly in kids, since their fizzy drink consumption is so excessive in relation to their body weight) and contribute to the development of serious health problems such as type 2 diabetes, Metabolic Syndrome and non-alcoholic fatty liver disease (NAFLD).

Many health-conscious consumers believe that honey or agave nectar are superior alternatives. Unfortunately, honey has a similar effect on blood sugar levels as table sugar, while agave has a higher fructose concentration than even HFCS (and thus prompts undesirable triglyceride production). There's no free ride here!

Artificial sweeteners are to be strictly avoided too, not only due to the health risks of ingesting chemically processed agents, but because they trick the brain into thinking you have just consumed a very sweet food or drink. As a result, your confused hormone response system stimulates an inappropriate insulin release, and the 'high-low, high-low' cycle begins. Some research suggests that your brain will seek even more 'replacement' calories in reaction to being tricked with a sweet food that provides no energy. Supporting this theory are the ever-increasing obesity rates despite widespread use of non-caloric artificial sweeteners in beverages and other foods (which, absent any other variables, should predict a collective decrease in caloric intake and obesity).

All forms of natural and processed sugars and sweeteners have a deleterious effect on your insulin system and general health. The less you eat sweeteners of any kind (yes, even the somewhat less objectionable stevia) the less you will crave them. Try cutting way back on sweets and fizzy drinks for even a couple of days and notice how your life improves immensely. See if you can maintain it for 21 days to begin to reprogramme your genes to not need or want these agents. If you can do away with sweet desserts altogether, you'll be well on your way to eliminating the addiction.

CHAPTER SUMMARY

Avoid the following:
- **Poisonous Things:** Make a sincere effort to reject the powerful manipulative influence of corporate advertising that is pushing you in the direction of poor food choices and the cultural traditions that favour unhealthy meal habits. Processed carbohydrates, including sugars, grains (wheat, rice, bread, pasta, cereal, corn, etc.) and even legumes should be eliminated or strictly moderated due to their effect on insulin levels and immune function and their inferior nutritional value to natural plants and animals.
- **Grains:** While grains (and legumes) have been presented as healthy staple foods for thousands of years of civilisation, our genes are maladapted to ingesting them because they elicit a high insulin response compared to the foods that have sustained human life for two million years: vegetables, fruits, nuts, seeds and animal products. The regular pattern of stimulating high

blood insulin levels from a diet of excessive grain and sugar products leads to difficulty burning stored body fat (hence, lifelong weight gain) and serious long-term health problems, including heart disease and diet-related cancers.

Grains offer minimal nutritional value in comparison to vegetables, fruits, nuts, seeds and animal products, ironically making grains a leading cause of nutritional deficiencies across the globe. Objectionable agents in grains compromise health mildly to severely, depending on your sensitivity. The phytates in grains can inhibit the absorption of minerals. Glutens can disturb healthy immune function and promote inflammation. Other lectins can inhibit healthy gastrointestinal function. Whole grains are no healthier than refined grains, and can have a worse impact on health in many cases due to higher levels of these three agents.

- **Polyunsaturated Fatty Acids (PUFAs):** We have unwisely moved over to these oils from saturated animal fats in recent decades. PUFA oils oxidise easily, particularly when heated during cooking. They are pro-inflammatory, have unfavourable O6:O3 ratios, hamper healthy immune and hormone function, lower HDL and raise LDL cholesterol, and are associated with obesity, diabetes, cancer and heart disease. Strict avoidance of canola, margarine, other vegetable and seed PUFAs and vegetable shortening is critical to health.

- **Trans and Partially Hydrogenated Fats:** These chemically altered molecules found in heavily processed foods are highly toxic to the body and are a major contributor to inflammation, accelerated ageing and many cancers. Trans and partially hydrogenated fats promote rampant oxidation and free radical damage in the body and disturb the healthy composition and function of cell membranes.

- **Other Foods:** Legumes are often incorrectly considered vegetables. While offering some nutrient value, they can stimulate a high insulin response, may also contain offensive lectins, and are best replaced with Primal foods. Sugary foods and beverages are devoid of nutrition, stimulate excessive insulin and are the leading factors in the modern decline of human health.

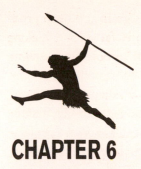

CHAPTER 6

THE PRIMAL BLUEPRINT EXERCISE LAWS

'HERE'S A HINT: WALK, LIFT AND SPRINT!'

'Those who think they have not time for bodily exercise will sooner or later have to find time for illness.'
LORD EDWARD STANLEY, THREE-TIMES PRIME MINISTER OF GREAT BRITAIN (1799–1869)

IN THIS CHAPTER

In the following pages I will outline the rationale and benefits of the three Primal Blueprint exercise laws: Law Number 3: Move Frequently at a Slow Pace; Law Number 4, Lift Heavy Things; and Law Number 5, Sprint Once in a While. Following these laws will enable you to approximate the active lifestyle of Grok and develop what I call Primal Blueprint Fitness. Primal Blueprint Fitness represents a versatile and diverse set of abilities that allow you to tackle varied active lifestyle or athletic challenges safely and competently. In contrast, many pursue narrow, specialised forms of fitness that are minimally functional and often compromise general health (endurance athletes and bodybuilders fall into this category). Following the Primal Blueprint exercise laws will also help delay the ageing process by preserving lean muscle mass, which correlates with enhanced organ function, a concept known as organ reserve.

In this chapter I will compare the benefits of Primal Blueprint Fitness exercise with the many drawbacks and health risks associated with conventional wisdom's fitness recommendations. Moving frequently at a slow pace is superior to an exhausting routine of Chronic Cardio. These workouts often lead to sugar cravings that compromise weight-loss efforts as well as hamper immune system and endocrine function. Lifting heavy things involves brief, intense sessions (lasting 10 to 30 minutes) that promote optimal hormone secretion and prevent the catabolic effects of prolonged sessions where muscles are worked until 'failure' and you leave the gym exhausted and depleted.

Few things are more Primal than Law Number 5 – running for your life once in a while! Brief, intense sprints (or other maximum efforts that are low or no impact for those interested) trigger optimal hormone balance, lean muscle development, accelerated fat metabolism and incredible fitness breakthroughs. I will discuss here the best strategic approach for conducting workouts for each of the three Primal Blueprint laws, including form pointers for running and cycling and the benefits of going barefoot. Specific workout suggestions for strength training and sprinting are provided online at MarksDailyApple.com, including a free downloadable ebook called *Primal Blueprint Fitness*.

The movements that dictated how our genes evolved were simple: squat, crawl, walk, run, jump, climb, hang, carry, throw, push, pull and more stuff we probably don't even have names for! This primal 'training programme' helped Grok survive the rigours of a hostile environment, explore new territories, track and exploit new types of food, build shelters and basically become ripped. Becoming super fit is as simple as blending lots of low-level work and intermittent bouts of higher-intensity efforts. There is little need for the incredible complexity of today's fitness scene – the outrageous gym equipment, obsessively detailed and regimented training programmes and fancy contraptions, such as cyclometers and GPS units and video analysis. This stuff, while possessing a high 'cool' factor, can also lead us astray from the benefits of having a simple, varied and intuitive approach to exercise. By the way, most young kids will employ many of Grok's movements (squat, crawl, walk, etc.) when left outside to play in a suitable environment.

Unfortunately, commuting, work, digital entertainment and modern comforts hinder our opportunities to enjoy spontaneous play and get fit naturally. Furthermore, conventional wisdom has brainwashed us to believe that a lean, fit body comes from either lucky genes or following a regimented, often overly stressful, exercise routine. It's no wonder that many well-meaning enthusiasts have become either exhausted or totally turned off to getting fit. Millions more endure with flawed approaches that leave them disappointed and discouraged when they fall far short of their ultimate peak performance potential and ideal body composition.

At the bare minimum, you can get extremely healthy and fit on two hours a week of walking around, one abbreviated strength workout a week lasting 10–15 minutes, one full-length strength workout a week lasting around 30 minutes, and a sprint session every 7 to 10 days lasting 15–20 minutes, with only a few minutes of accumulated hard effort.

That's less than three hours out of the 168 at our disposal each week. You don't have to endure the fatigue and exhaustion that so many have suffered when following conventional wisdom's recommendation to adopt a consistent and unnecessarily complex exercise programme. You don't even have to be consistent; in fact it's better if you are *inconsistent* with your workout routine. Heck, the old saying: 'All you need is a pair of shoes' doesn't even apply – you don't even need shoes! (See 'Happy Feet' on page 238.)

> *'Pursue challenges that turn you on instead of worrying about what the magazines say is the "best" workout or the marketing hype that glorifies extreme events.'*

While it's comforting to realise how well you can do with the bare minimum prescriptions, I'll assert that you can take the Primal Blueprint exercise laws all the way to the top. If you are a devoted gym rat looking to get ripped, if you dream of auditioning for a swimsuit ad, or if you are competing at the elite level in team or individual sports (yep, including endurance sports), a comparatively minimal time commitment of the Primal Blueprint approach can produce vastly superior results (and decreased risk of injuries and burnout) to a traditional approach of frequent, prolonged, strenuous workouts.

For example, an optimal week for a very devoted exerciser could include a two-hour hike, another easy cardio session of one hour, two full-body strength-training sessions lasting no more than 30 minutes each, another lasting just 10–15 minutes, a sprint session with an accumulated five minutes of maximum effort and a hard 'play' day (e.g. a pickup soccer, basketball or Ultimate game). This still only totals about seven hours of exercise. If you are currently racking up a dozen or more hours of Chronic Cardio each week, or hitting the gym almost every day for prolonged strength-training sessions isolating specific muscle groups, I encourage you to reframe your perspective from 'more is better' to 'intense is better'. If you find yourself bouncing off the walls with extra energy because your new Primal schedule is 'too easy', make your hard workouts *even harder*, not longer or more frequent. Remember, the goal is to trigger optimal gene expression, not to fill in all the blanks of your log book and teeter on the edge of injury and burnout.

For those interested in the effects of Primal exercise on weight loss, we must start with the critical assumption that 80 per cent of your body composition results are determined by how you eat. Reprogramming your genes through dietary signals to derive most of your energy from stored fat will continuously push you towards your ideal body composition, regardless of whether or not you work out hard. Also understand that low-level cardio sessions alone do not raise your metabolic rate significantly enough to stimulate significant fat reduction. However, low-level cardio workouts greatly enhance your ability to metabolise fat – both during exercise and at rest. Meanwhile, brief intense strength and sprint sessions elevate body temperature and stimulate an increase in your metabolic rate, not only during the workout but also for many hours afterwards.

Put everything together and you have a formula for successful long-term weight management: eating Primally and moving frequently at a slow pace (optimising your fat-burning system) and lifting heavy things and running really fast occasionally (stimulating lean muscle development and increasing metabolic rate). This 'round-the-clock' concept of reprogramming genes (through Primal Blueprint eating and exercise habits) for optimal expression is the true secret to natural, effortless, long-term weight loss and/or weight management. The story stands in sharp contrast to conventional wisdom's 'calories in, calories out' model, where you hope the 600 calories burned during your 50-minute step aerobics class will somehow lead to weight loss. (Recall that a depleted Kelly Korg consumed nearly double that on her quick visit to the juice bar!)

PRIMAL BLUEPRINT FITNESS

With a balanced regime patterned after Grok and designed to promote optimal gene expression, you will develop what I call Primal

Blueprint Fitness. This means you have a broad range of skills and attributes (strength, power, speed, endurance) that allow you to do pretty much whatever you want (or, in Grok's case, survive the various challenges of primal life) with a substantial degree of competence and minimal risk of injury.

By breaking free from the cycle of carbohydrates fuelling stressful, sugar-burning Chronic Cardio workouts, you can easily get into the ideal body fat percentage range of 8 to 15 per cent for men and 12 to 20 per cent for women. This is true no matter who you are or how plump your family tree is.

For women, a Primal Blueprint Fitness programme will tone your entire body – not just by lowering body fat levels but also by giving you some noticeable definition in your arms, legs and core. While many female exercisers are concerned exclusively with weight management and not inclined toward competitive athletic endeavours, you may surprise yourself – and gain some street cred with the neighbourhood kids – when you display your aptitude on the football field or in a race. When you expand your horizons beyond 'jogging at a strenuous pace for five songs on my iPod', your body will begin to show the effects all over, most notably by correcting the common trouble spots of excess bottom, hip, thigh and abdominal fat.

For the competitor, you can expect to branch out beyond your bread-and-butter skills to become a more complete athlete. Those who rely on bulk to hoist mucho plates or push forward in a scrum will become leaner and improve their power-to-weight ratio (how strong you are in relation to your body weight). This translates into more pull-ups, a higher vertical leap and more quickness on your first step. Those who tend to be slight of frame and lacking in power will add a bit more muscle and improve pure strength and explosiveness, expanding their repertoire not only to outlast the competition but to out-power them.

Power-to-weight ratio is a critical Primal Blueprint Fitness benchmark because it has a strong functional component. A skinny dude like the late Bruce Lee was by reasonable definition more powerful than Hulk Hogan because he had a superior power-to-weight ratio. Brian Clay, the American 2008 Olympic decathlon gold medallist, is the quintessential Primal athlete. At five feet eleven inches and weighing in at 174 pounds, Clay is smaller than many of his competitors but is capable of a stunning versatility in his athletic performances. While his physique is certainly impressive and looks great on the beach, it is not overly bulky nor overly defined like the vein-popping magazine cover men. However, Clay can sprint, hurdle, long and high jump, pole vault and throw such implements as shot, discus and javelin at very respectable levels when each is considered individually.

In the SPARQ (speed, power, agility, reaction and quickness) test commonly used to evaluate NFL prospects, Clay achieved a phenomenal score of 130. In comparison, Reggie Bush, a remarkable physical specimen who won the Heisman Trophy for USC and became a running back for the New Orleans Saints and Miami Dolphins, scored a 93.

Others point to the diverse athletic demands of boxing as fodder for the greatest all-round athlete distinction. Basketball stars such as Kobe Bryant and LeBron James blend an incredible array of skills – speed and endurance, strength and quickness – to perform seemingly superhuman feats. CrossFit.com, a popular exercise web site, idealises the ultimate athlete as a combination gymnast, power lifter and sprinter. For the last word, I'll echo the Primal Blueprint philosophy about dietary habits. The ideal body that you build comes down to personal preference within the broad guidelines of the Primal Blueprint. Do the exercises that turn you on the most – in your mind, your heart and your genes!

Regarding the specific workout plan to reach your Primal Blueprint Fitness goals, it is better to make sure your workout decisions align with your energy and motivation levels than to follow a strict schedule. Sprint once in a while when you are super motivated and energised; take a walk around the block or hike up to the radio tower on Sunday morning if you feel the urge, or stay home and read the newspaper in bed if you're dragging and just don't feel like working out.

'Instead of following a strict schedule, align your workout decisions with your energy and motivation levels.'

This unstructured approach might feel uncomfortable if you are under the influence of flawed conventional wisdom that values consistency, gadgetry and judging your fitness progress by the obsessive tracking of quantifiable data such as miles covered, calories burned, reps completed, time in target heart rate zone, or placing in the race. Grok knew nothing of this superficial silliness. His motivation to exercise was completely pure: to acquire his basic needs of food and shelter or to satisfy the innate human desire for adventure, competition and play and for exploring the boundaries of the human spirit, regardless of what measured results came of it. I urge you to determine the success of your fitness programme by how much fun you are having! Pursue challenges that turn you on instead of worrying about what the magazines say is the best workout or about the marketing hype that glorifies extreme events, such as the marathon or Ironman® triathlon, as the ultimate athletic accomplishments.

ORGAN RESERVE: THE KEY TO LONGEVITY

If you fall somewhere short of fitness freak on the continuum, keep in mind that the benefits of a sensible exercise programme extend far beyond competitive success and looking good. The more lean muscle you maintain throughout life, the better your organs will function as well (up to an obvious point of diminishing returns; e.g. a bodybuilder has heaps of excess muscle that serve little or no functional purpose and requires a lot of caloric energy to sustain). Optimal organ function correlates with maximum longevity and excellent health.

Organs, like muscles, adhere to the 'use it or lose it' natural law: when you hit the deck for 50 push-ups, the conscious decision to engage these muscles in a work effort calls your heart, lungs, liver, adrenals and other organs into action. Blood chemistry changes as you burn glycogen and fat, process oxygen and produce metabolic by-products (e.g. lactic acid) at an accelerated rate. You are asking your organs to keep up with your active lifestyle, in the process strengthening them to better withstand the demands of daily life and the natural ageing process.

In contrast, when your activity diminishes, as in the classic paradigm of ageing, you send signals telling your muscles and organs that can can atrophy. Their function decreases because they are given no reason to remain at 100 per cent efficiency. An unfit person has lower bone-density, less lung capacity (the quantity of air you can exchange on each breath) and stroke volume (the amount of blood your heart pumps with each beat) than a fit person. The ageing process – at least in America – should really be called the 'process of physical decline largely due to inactivity and lifestyle habits that result in mismanaged genes'.

Because all of your organs and body systems work synergistically, you are vulnerable to the often fatal effects of your weakest link. For example, an unfit accident victim or a surgery patient who loses a lot of blood and has a heart operating at only 45 per cent of potential capacity will often fare differently than a fit person with superior heart function suffering the same trauma. Bones break more easily among the unfit. Pneumonia is a common cause of death among the elderly, often due to the inability of their weakened lungs to help clear the germ-laden mucus effectively through coughing.

> *'Walking is the best possible exercise.*
> *Habituate yourself to walk very far.'*
> THOMAS JEFFERSON

PRIMAL BLUEPRINT LAW NUMBER 3: MOVE FREQUENTLY AT A SLOW PACE

While you can benefit from low-intensity aerobic exercise almost indefinitely (e.g. hiking the Pacific Crest Trail or Appalachian Trail all summer is pretty good for your overall health), you can still obtain outstanding health and fitness benefits by engaging in a moderate amount of low-intensity aerobic movement (hike, walk briskly, cycle gently, or jog if you are really fit). You should aim for a bare minimum of two hours and hopefully up to five hours of low-intensity aerobic movement per week, knowing that even five-minute work breaks or 15-minute strolls through the neighbourhood with your dog contribute meaningfully to your genetic requirements for frequent movement. If you can manage a single long hike on the weekend and a few short walks or cardio-machine sessions during the week, you will dramatically reduce your risk of heart disease (in comparison to being sedentary), support optimal metabolism, better control your weight, and, in conjunction with the other two types of workouts, achieve broad athletic competency that characterises Primal Blueprint Fitness.

Remember that these recommendations are averages. I will occasionally go for extended periods of time (thanks to injury or travel) doing no exercise whatsoever. I suffer no ill effects, experience no change in body composition (because I am eating Primally) and invariably pick up right where I left off when I resume normal training. At other times, when the stars align and I have the free time, I'll benefit greatly from doing vastly more than the recommended average (e.g. when going on a backpacking trip or another active vacation).

> *'The ageing process should really be called the "process of physical decline largely due to inactivity"'.*

My definition of *low intensity* movement is sustained exercise at a range of 55 to 75 per cent of maximum heart rate (I will discuss in detail just what this means shortly). With this casual aerobic exercise, your heart and other energy systems work a little harder to handle the extra fuel and oxygen delivery demands, but not so much that you are overstressed. The specific biochemical signals created by this low-level aerobic activity produce numerous health and fitness benefits:

- **Improved Fat Metabolism:** You train your body to efficiently utilise free fatty acids for fuel; a benefit that is realised 24 hours a day, with a higher metabolic rate and a preference for fat over glucose (provided you eat Primally). Low-level aerobic exercise also helps balance blood glucose levels and regulate appetite.

- **Improved Cardiovascular Function:** You increase your capillary network (blood vessels that supply the muscle cells with fuel and oxygen), muscle mitochondria and stroke volume of your heart (more blood pumped with each beat) and also improve oxygen delivery by your lungs.

- **Improved Musculoskeletal System:** You strengthen your bones, joints and connective tissue so you can absorb increasing stress loads without breaking down. This is critical to your ability to perform and recover from your high-intensity Primal sessions.

- **Stronger Immune System:** You enhance the function of your immune system by stimulating beneficial hormone flow and building a more efficient circulatory system.

- **Increased Energy:** You finish workouts feeling energised and refreshed, rather than slightly fatigued and depleted from a schedule of moderate to difficult intensity workouts conducted too frequently.

'I love running cross country …
On a track, I feel like a hamster.'
ROBIN WILLIAMS

ZONING: 'IN' AND 'OUT'

To determine your 55–75 per cent exercise zone numbers, you can perform a strenuous maximum heart rate test (get medical clearance first), or use a formula to estimate your max. You may be familiar with the long-standard '220 minus age' formula, but this is now believed to produce material inaccuracies in some people. I recommend a newer formula from University of Colorado researchers as follows: 208 minus (0.7 times age) = Estimated Maximum Heart Rate. For example, Ken Korg at 40 has an estimated max heart rate of 180 beats per minute [208 – 28 (.7 x 40 = 28)]. Ken's low-level aerobic workouts should thus be conducted in a heart rate range of 99 beats per minute (180 max × 55 percent) to 135 beats per minute (180 max × 75 per cent).

Fifty-five per cent of maximum reflects the bare minimum exertion level to legitimately consider your effort 'exercise'. An unfit person can reach this walking to the mailbox. If you aren't familiar with heart-rate training, you may be surprised to discover just how easy even the upper limit of 75 per cent of maximum heart rate is. At this pace, you break a light to moderate sweat, can easily converse without getting short of breath, and finish feeling refreshed and energised instead of slightly fatigued and hungry, as you might after more strenuous workouts.

You can monitor your heart rate with a wireless heart-rate monitor and chest strap, or just pause during your workout, place your finger against the carotid artery on the side of your neck (the best place to feel a strong pulse) then check your watch and count how many beats occur in exactly ten seconds. Multiply that number by six to determine your heart rate in beats per minute.

Please make an effort to regularly monitor heart rate during workouts when you are warmed up and working at a steady effort. Going by perceived exertion alone can cause you to exceed the recommended zone for long periods of time because a 75 per cent effort feels so comfortable, even for experienced athletes. Disrespecting the importance of regulating intensity can compromise the benefits of individual workouts and your entire training programme, drifting you into the Chronic Cardio category.

The best thing about heart-rate training is that it individualises your experience to ensure you get an optimal workout, particularly when you consider the benefits of staying under 75 per cent versus the drawbacks of exceeding 75 per cent routinely. This critical 'individual' element – one that can make or break your entire exercise programme – has long been ignored by group class instructors, Team in Training coaches, and other social or competitive workout groups working out together. Generally speaking, asking a class or group of workout partners to keep pace together is a recipe for failure, *for all but the fittest members of the group.*

As a final note, please understand that I'm not suggesting that you never exceed 75 per cent of your max heart rate. For extremely fit endurance athletes one or two cardio workouts a week that exceed this will likely be fine, as long as adequate rest and recovery are observed. What I am saying is that maintaining consistently elevated heart rates during long workouts several days per week can be a recipe for failure in the long run (or the long ride).

'Chronic Cardio – a programme followed for nearly 20 years as a marathoner and later as an ironman triathlete – is bad for your health, period.'

A CASE AGAINST CARDIO

In contrast to the comprehensive benefits of a frequent, comfortably paced exercise, getting more serious about working out can really mess you up if you have a flawed approach. Chronic Cardio at heart rates above 75 per cent and up to 95 per cent of maximum places excessive stress on your body, the kind of stress to which you are not genetically adapted. I'd estimate that the vast majority of people you see working out on cardio machines, jogging through the neighbourhood, or keeping pace in the group class are exceeding 75 per cent (often by a wide margin) for the duration of nearly every session.

While an aerobic workout at 75 or even up to 85 per cent of maximum heart rate might not feel terribly difficult at the time, a sustained pattern of Chronic Cardio can lead to numerous problems with metabolism, stress management, immune function and general health. As exercise intensity increases, your preferred fuel choice shifts from primarily fat at intensities below 75 per cent (fat burns well in the presence of oxygen, and fat stores are abundant – even in the skinniest marathoners!) to an ever-increasing percentage of glucose (quicker and easier to burn when oxygen is lacking due to your quickening pace). You'll recall that a major goal of Primal Blueprint eating and exercise is to reprogramme your genes to burn *more* fat – not less.

A routine of Chronic Cardio requires large amounts of dietary carbohydrates each day to support it. While the risks of excess fat storage and hyperinsulinemia (overproduction of insulin) are moderated somewhat by a heavy exercise schedule, they are still significant because of your altered dietary habits throughout the day. When muscles are depleted of glycogen (remember, stored glycogen is converted back into glucose for exercise fuel), your brain sends a powerful signal to replenish with quick-energy carbohydrate foods. Our brains have a tendency to tell us to overcompensate by eating a little too much. This is a genetically programmed survival adaptation against starvation risk, handed down to us from Grok. If you are looking to reduce body fat primarily through vigorous cardiovascular exercise (as conventional wisdom promises), you are quite likely to fail unless you slow down your pace and alter your diet to limit your carbohydrate intake.

Besides the weight-loss issues, Chronic Cardio increases the production of cortisol (in all but the most genetically gifted endurance athletes), which breaks down muscle tissue and suppresses the production of key anabolic hormones, such as testosterone and human growth hormone. This hormonal imbalance caused by over-exercising contributes to fatigue, burnout, immune suppression, loss of bone density and undesirable changes in fat metabolism. Furthermore, the stress of Chronic Cardio increases systemic inflammation (a strong contributing factor to heart disease, cancer and nearly all other health problems) and increases oxidative damage (via free radical production) by a factor of 10 to 20 times normal. This can lead to acceleration of the ageing process. It's ironic that many in their 40s and 50s start engaging in marathon or triathlon training with hopes of improving health and delaying the ageing process when, quite often, it has the exact opposite effect.

BORN TO WALK – AND SPRINT

For those heavily indoctrinated into the conventional wisdom that Chronic Cardio is the path to health, fitness and weight control, consider again the premise of the Primal Blueprint. Because Grok was a lean, strong, extremely active dude, he probably was capable of running long distances at a respectable pace, similar to today's gung-ho endurance athletes, but he most likely very rarely decided to do so. When the concept of organised hunting came along, it appears that Grok relied more on superior tracking ability (using his highly evolved brain) and walking or slow jogging (using his superior fat-burning system), rather than literally chasing down his prey. In fact, squandering valuable energy reserves (and increasing glucose metabolism by a factor of 10) by running hard for long periods of time would have hastened his demise. Imagine Grok chasing some game animal all-out for a few hours and – oops – not succeeding in killing it. He's spent an incredible amount of energy yet now has no food to replace that energy. He has suddenly become some other animal's prey because he is physically exhausted.

A 2007 Taiwanese study published in the *British Journal of Sports Medicine* revealed that an intense *sustained* workout (working at 85 per cent of maximum effort for at least 30 minutes) disrupted immune system function, destroyed some white blood cells and triggered whole body inflammation for up to 72 hours. In contrast, there are literally hundreds of scientific studies confirming the benefits of conducting occasional short-duration, intense workouts (such as interval workouts – spacing work efforts between a particular rest interval). Intervals and sprints quickly and time-efficiently improve key performance factors including VO2 Max (how efficiently you process oxygen during peak exercise effort), competitive performance and body composition.

I cannot emphasise strongly enough the importance of slowing down the pace of your cardio workouts to improve your health and fitness. (Note that I'm speaking to the vast numbers of fitness enthusiasts in the gyms and on the roads who generally take their pace to 'slightly uncomfortable' in the name of pursuing conventional wisdom's definition of 'getting a workout'.) If you already like to take your time and smell the flowers on your walks, hikes and bike rides, congratulations! Just get ready to add a few sprint workouts into the mix. That's where huge benefits will accrue for little investment. As I will detail shortly, slowing down (and adding workouts from Laws 4 and 5) will not only improve health but will lead to outstanding fitness breakthroughs.

> *'You have to stay in shape. My grandmother, she started walking five miles a day when she was 60. She's 97 today and we don't know where the hell she is.'*
> ELLEN DEGENERES

I am fully aware of the many loud and passionate voices extolling the psychological and lifestyle virtues of devoted endurance training and agree that pushing and challenging your body with inspiring competitive goals supports mental, emotional and also physical health (albeit with the significant caveats already discussed). An exercise physiologist friend of mine countered my 'case against cardio' position recently by reminding me that Hawaii Ironman finishers are vastly healthier than the average population. While true, let us not forget, in the words of Jay Leno, the 'average' we are dealing with: 'Today there are more overweight people in America than average-weight people. So overweight people are now average. Which means you've met your New Year's resolution.'

Furthermore, I'll assert that an old has-been like myself (goals: eat Primally, with no processed carbohydrates; nail a couple of brief,

CHRONIC CARDIO DRAWBACKS – POCKET REFERENCE

A consistent schedule of frequent medium-to-high-intensity (75 per cent of maximum or higher) sustained workouts can overstress the body and lead to these negative consequences:

Hormone Imbalance: Chronic Cardio raises cortisol and lowers testosterone and growth hormone. This compromises optimal fat burning, muscle development, energy levels and sex drive. Burnout is a common consequence of pursuing the 'runner's high' too frequently.

Injuries: Recurring muscle fatigue, repetitive impact, restrictive footwear and inflammation from excessive catabolic hormones released in response to Chronic Cardio traumatises joints and connective tissue.

Metabolism: Burning more sugar (at above 75 per cent of maximum heart rate) drives eating more sugar, drives producing more insulin, drives storing more fat.

Stress: Excessive oxidation and triggering of the fight-or-flight response compromise the immune system and accelerate ageing and disease risk.

Use It or Lose It: Chronic Cardio compromises development of power, speed, strength and lean mass and leads to muscle imbalances and inflexibility. Total fitness is sacrificed in favour of narrow, minimally functional aerobic endurance.

intense, strength-training sessions – in the gym or outdoors; conduct one all-out sprint workout; and hang with the young guns for a two-hour Ultimate Frisbee match on weekends) possesses far superior health and comprehensive fitness to the lean, ripped (but often emaciated), physical specimens that strut in their Speedos down the main drag of Kailua-Kona, Hawaii, every October during Ironman week (seriously, they really do strut around shirtless and in Speedos).

Yes, they can all drop me like a shot in a long-distance swim, cycling or running race (it would've have been a different story back in the day, but I digress ...), but their endurance superiority comes at great cost. Collectively, they tend to suffer from recurring fatigue and adrenal burnout, frequent overuse injuries, too-common minor illnesses from suppressed immune function (I get a cold maybe once every five years; a fair number of Ironman triathletes probably get five every year), and, last but certainly not least, high overall life stress-factor scores – something often touted as the number one heart attack risk factor.

Having spent many years immersed in the type A community of driven fitness enthusiasts and competitive endurance athletes, I am aware that many heads will nod in agreement with my message – and then turn around and plug along with their familiar exhausting training regimes. If serious endurance exercise is a centrepiece of your life, I don't wish to deprive you of your passion. That's right, go ahead and hammer that three-hour group ride or that 15-mile trail run with the big boys or big girls but only do these things *once in a while*. This will produce far superior fitness benefits and eliminate the risk factors of repeating highly stressful workouts too frequently.

> 'If you start to feel good during a marathon, don't worry, that will pass.'
> DON KARDONG, US OLYMPIC MARATHONER AND AUTHOR

'BUT THIS FEELS TOO EASY!'

Granted, those with competitive endurance goals may not be satisfied to putter along exclusively at a slow pace and think they can take down the competition with that approach. The most direct performance benefits occur from the intense workouts that approximate the challenge of your competitive goals. However, whether you are a casual fitness enthusiast or a professional athlete, you must establish a strong base of low-level aerobic conditioning before you can introduce more stressful, higher-intensity workouts.

With a strong aerobic conditioning base in place, you then have the ability to absorb and benefit from the *occasional* intense workouts that lead directly to competitive success – if you've chosen such goals. The tertiary benefits of low-level work (better balance, strong postural muscles, increased mitochondria development and capillary profusion, and strengthening of bones, tendons and ligaments to prevent injury) might not be as readily apparent as the direct competitive application of beating your personal record at a time trial, but one cannot happen without the other.

This concept of base first then intensity has been proven successful by the training regimes of the world's greatest endurance athletes of the last 50 years, beginning with the pioneering work of New Zealand running coach Arthur Lydiard. Lydiard's prize students, including 1960 and 1964 Olympic track gold medallist Peter Snell (today one of the world's leading exercise physiologists, based in Dallas, Texas), showed that long-duration, low-intensity training, coupled with intense interval training and adequate rest (rest was another far-out concept for the 1960s), could lead directly to Olympic gold medals and world records at races as short as 800 metres (which lasts less than two minutes).

When I completed my career as an elite marathoner and triathlete and then moved into a career as a personal trainer, my training regime shifted dramatically. I was still out there moving for several hours a day, but I went from banging my brains out with super-fit training partners to dawdling along with a succession of clients on my daily calendar. Unlike many of today's fitness trainers, who stand there and count reps, I got outside with my unfit to moderately fit clients and did their workouts with them. Bike rides that I previously hammered at 20-plus mph for hours were now conducted at 13 mph (it seemed like any slower and we'd tip over!). The long, hard trail runs of my marathon days were replaced with easy jogs where my heart rate barely exceeded 100 beats per minute (only 50 per cent of my max). With a young family and a career filling my days, I rarely had time to do my own specific workouts. I made the most of these opportunities by conducting extremely intense interval sessions once or twice a week – on cardio equipment or with a few quick laps around the track. Usually these sessions lasted around 20 minutes – until my next client came strolling in!

When I jumped into the occasional long or ultra-distance endurance race, the results were shocking to me. My 'by chance' regime of very, very slow workouts coupled with occasional very short, intense workouts was effective beyond my wildest dreams. I was able to be placed among the top competitors in the world in my age group and very close to the standards set by top professionals of that era! Indeed, the Primal Blueprint parameters literally took shape in my mind as I blew by my rivals (who were putting in big Chronic Cardio miles, just like I used to) at races, despite what most experts and prevailing conventional wisdom would deem ridiculously inadequate preparation.

PRIMAL BLUEPRINT LAW NUMBER 4: LIFT HEAVY THINGS

The popular conventional wisdom concept of following a strength-training routine that involves repeating the same workout several days a week is flawed. Your body thrives on intuitive, spontaneous and fluctuating workout habits – not ego-driven regimentation organised around an arbitrary time period of seven days that has no special relevance to your fitness progress. It's the signals created when your muscles are challenged beyond what they are used to that prompt genes to make those muscles stronger. Get creative and integrate the 'lift heavy things' law into daily life, aside from your formal sessions. For example, come the autumn, try raking your leaves vigorously – it's an unsurpassed shoulder, core and abs session, and it will get your garden sorted to boot!

Regarding the particulars of how to balance upper- and lower-body efforts, 'push and pull' workout groupings, lightweight with high reps or heavyweight with low reps: *it doesn't matter that much!* This is not rocket science. The idea is to challenge your body on a regular basis with brief, intense workouts involving full body, functional exercises. The specifics of your workout are based on personal preference. You can do just fine using a park bench and monkey bars, hitting a fancy gym with a high-priced personal trainer, or getting busy in your garage with a few basic weights, stretch cords or creative 'Primal' implements such as kettlebells, slosh tubes and sandbags; or in a hotel room with nothing more than a chair and some floor space. Check out MarksDailyApple.com for hundreds of interesting and challenging resistance workout ideas.

Personally, I'm a devoted gym rat, but my faithful appearance at the local gym a few days a week has a heavy social element. Some days I'll be in there for an hour and 15 minutes, shooting the breeze, preening and talking with my pals – interspersed with some embarrassingly low-effort exercises where I barely sweat. Other days, when I'm feeling fired up, I'll push it hard for 25 minutes of maximum effort sets with short rest. After these workouts, I have trouble slipping my sweatshirt on and sticking my key in the ignition to drive home, but I am exhilarated and recovery is quick. These hard days are few and far between, but they make a big difference. Overall, once you get the Primal Blueprint eating strategy dialled in, you see that it honestly does not require that much time to maintain excellent all-around functional muscle strength and an impressive physique. It's simply a matter of establishing a reasonable baseline commitment of regular workouts, with the occasional super effort that stimulates a fitness breakthrough.

A high-intensity, short-duration workout will stimulate the release of adaptive hormones – particularly testosterone and human growth hormone – so that you become lean, energetic and youthful. Work hard and complete your session in less than an hour, even (or especially) if you are an experienced lifter. That's right, go against the conventional wisdom of long, drawn-out workouts of the same old sets with the same weight and repetitions. A 30- to 45-minute session is actually plenty for most people.

As you improve your fitness, keep your focus on increasing intensity (more resistance, shorter rest periods and tougher exercises) rather than extending the duration of your workouts. Repeated workouts that extend beyond an hour (I've seen some hardcore lifters routinely go for two hours or more!), where you lift moderate weights to failure again and again, can stimulate the excessive release of destructive (also called catabolic) hormones such as cortisol, which lead to fatigue, breakdown and the metabolic problems already discussed at length. Again, think about Grok: he moved some big rocks, which gave his body a shock. But when the quick job was done, he could relax and have fun, basking in the sun.

Always align the difficulty of your sessions with your energy level and don't push yourself beyond what you are motivated and inspired to do. On the other hand, if you feel energised and ready to ramp it up a notch, go for it! You will notice after your first couple of sets whether your reps to failure are worse or better than normal. If you are feeling – and performing – significantly worse than normal, consider skipping or sharply curtailing the workout. If you are feeling significantly better than normal, push yourself beyond your typical routine to achieve a fitness breakthrough.

I should point out that if you are new to strength training you might get too tired to actually complete even 30 minutes of high-intensity effort. Instead, you can work up to it by either compressing your workout time further or taking longer rest intervals between your hard efforts. Even a workout as short as seven minutes can produce outstanding benefits. I know of an ex-collegiate gymnast, still in competitive shape with an amazingly cut physique, who claims only to work out for seven minutes a few times a week, with no resistance equipment, in a tiny floor space in his living room.

'Always align the difficulty of your sessions with your energy level, and don't push yourself beyond what you are motivated and inspired to do. On the other hand, if you feel energised and ready to ramp it up a notch, go for it!'

Impossible? Get a load of his routine: three sets of 20 handstand push-ups, followed by three sets of 20-clap push-ups and 10 one-armed push-ups with each arm, followed by 10 Russian circles, transitioning immediately into 3 sets of 10 leg flairs, then 5 handstand push-ups, followed by, well, you get the picture! His many years of intense daily training have given him a fitness base to accomplish a phenomenal amount of work – and maintain exceptional fitness – with a minimal time commitment. Oh, and he walks a lot and eats right, too!

If you are spent after a 10-minute workout, congratulations! You've pushed yourself to the max and elicited a desirable fitness response in your body. By the way, those seemingly inconsequential hikes and walks will actually contribute substantially to your ability to hit it hard in the gym, thanks to the well-established connection between the cardiorespiratory and musculoskeletal benefits of comfortable aerobic exercise and your ability to perform at peak intensity.

I suggest you try for an average bare minimum of one comprehensive 30-minute session and an abbreviated session of 10–15 minutes per week. If you are a 'more is better' gym rat, I'd argue in favour of increasing the intensity of these three sessions rather than adding in additional workouts.

Feel free to experiment with the types of exercises that are most fun for you and with a routine that fits most conveniently and comfortably into your daily lifestyle. If you like altering your routine per the popular phrase 'muscle confusion', that's fine. If you are a creature of habit and prefer to do the same workout over and over, that's fine too – as long as it adheres to the 'brief, intense, full-body functional movements' description. The *Primal Blueprint 21-Day Total Body Transformation* offers descriptions and photographs of what I call the Primal Essential Movements – four simple, safe, bodyweight resistance exercises (pushups, pull-ups, squats and planks) that can get you super fit in less than an hour a week. We'll also cover these briefly in the Bonus Material at the end of this book.

Realise that this concept of sporadic, intuitive exercise means you have permission to take – and will, in fact, greatly benefit from – holidays. The more extreme your goals and training regime are, the more effort will be required to balance your overall stress levels on both a micro (daily or weekly) and macro (annual) scale. As I discovered for myself (the hard way), trusting the body's need for balance and intermittent stress can lead to results that are superior – in weight loss or peak competitive performance – compared to the die-hard trainaholics who never miss a workout and never get sufficient rest.

To make sure you are adhering to the Primal philosophy, I suggest paying close attention to your energy level and even your emotional state in the hours after a strength workout. After even my toughest sessions, I feel alert, energised and positive – basically I've achieved a natural buzz – for hours afterwards. My muscles, while certainly not eager to repeat the workout in the immediate future, feel pleasantly relaxed, loose and warm. In contrast, if your muscles feel stiff and sore after strength sessions, or you feel like taking a nap, raiding the fridge or snapping at your loved ones, I recommend conducting shorter more intense workouts, perhaps less frequently. If you can only maintain high-intensity effort for seven minutes, then end your workout there and work up to more sets in the future.

In regard to body composition, remember your strength training efforts fall into the fine-tuning 20 per cent category, while 80 per cent of your success is determined by how you eat. This is a sobering statistic if you are working hard at the gym, eating poorly and praying in vain for that six-pack to show up on your midsection. In this scenario, all that hard work in the gym will contribute mostly to a higher shopping bill (okay, and more fleeting pleasure from unrestricted caloric intake), but you'll be wearing the same size clothing when you next head to the shops.

STRENGTH WORKOUT SPECIFICS

Emphasise exercises that engage a variety of muscles with sweeping, real-life movements (squats, pull-ups, push-ups, etc.) instead of a series of isolated body part exercises (this includes those ever-popular, narrow-range-of-motion abs machines!). Remember that you are striving to achieve a high power-to-weight ratio and balanced, functional, total-body strength. Follow an intuitive and fluctuating approach focused on maintaining a proper balance of stress and rest.

This approach is a simpler and safer alternative to those popular routines designed to pack on more muscle than your body is naturally suited to, or to produce disproportionate muscles ('Develop huge guns in six weeks!') in the interest of vanity over functionality. For example, to work my calf muscles in a functional manner, I like to run on an inclined treadmill for a few minutes in socks, without letting my heels touch the ground. This offers a real-life functional test for my calves and works the small muscles, tendons, ligaments and connective tissue in my lower extremities that are otherwise artificially protected and unchallenged in high-tech running shoes. I gradually incline the treadmill to reach from two to five degrees and then steadily increase the speed. I try to make sure my heels don't bear any significant weight or provide propulsion.

Keep in mind that I just made this workout up one day, and you may or may not like it. However, I think it offers an important counter to the time spent working out and walking around in overly cushioned and arch-supported running shoes. Contrast the broad benefits of this exercise with something like donkey calf-raises. This narrow range-of-motion exercise (sit with a weighted bar across your knees and lift your toes off the ground repeatedly) has minimal functional benefit; besides, I'll stack my calves up against any bodybuilder's!

Grok probably never warmed up for his 'workouts' and I'm just not a big fan of doing extensive cardio warm-up periods. (Sorry about that, conventional wisdom.) That said, because you will usually be starting your workout 'cold' (maybe you just left an office where you were sitting all day or you just got out of bed), it does make sense to get a little blood flowing into your muscles before hitting the intense stuff. Therefore, your strength sessions should generally start with a brief three- to five-minute warm-up using light weights or calisthenics specific to the muscle groups you'll be working that day. A few sets of easy push-ups and some jumping jacks might be sufficient.

Because Primal Blueprint Fitness workouts are intended to recruit as many muscle fibres as possible and to build functional strength rather than sheer bulk, I wouldn't worry about following some predetermined and deliberate effort-recovery cycle. Instead, try to be slightly explosive with most of your movements. By that I mean you should apply a controlled dynamic force to each repetition such that you complete it at a speed that allows you to maintain form and a reasonable pace for the number of reps you intend to complete. Do that and, believe me, you'll slow down naturally on that final rep or two! This method will fully load the muscle and trigger the biochemical signal to grow stronger by recruiting new fibres.

While there are disparate schools of thought on the best strength-training techniques, I make this general suggestion here to align with the concept of optimal gene expression and prevention of the all-too-common burnout from chronic workout patterns. If you have specialised fitness goals or an expert personal training support suggesting a different technique, I wouldn't be overly concerned. I'll default here to the big picture and assert that brief, intense workouts are the key to Primal Fitness success.

Much has been written about breathing while lifting weights; some of it is relevant (to protect your back from damage), while some of it is conjecture. When you apply force, you should generally be either exhaling or holding your breath. This will form a sealed air space behind the transverse abdominal muscles of your lower core that protect your lumbar spine. While some camps caution against holding your breath, there is no scientific support to affirm that doing so is harmful. In fact, I find I can bang out two or three reps in a row more effectively when I'm holding my breath and then can catch my breath during a recovery phase.

There are many excellent resources – from certified personal trainers, magazine articles, books, video websites like CrossFit. com, articles on MarksDailyApple.com, and even your imagination (observing certain obvious safety rules, such as spine stability) – to help you create an ideal total-body routine for your needs. The possibilities are nearly limitless if you observe the strategic rules of Primal Blueprint-style training.

STRETCHING: IF YOU DON'T KNOW SQUAT, TRY HANGIN' WITH GROK

'What would Grok do?' It's hard to imagine Grok stretching much beyond a yawning feline-style spine elongation upon awakening, hanging lazily off a branch, or engaging in the timeless, all-purpose stretch of squatting down to the ground. Furthermore, recent research (visit the Primal Blueprint Resources appendix at Marks-DailyApple.com to find relevant materials) seems to refute the benefits of conducting a traditional static stretching routine before exercising. It's now believed the central nervous system may be disturbed by such activity, resulting in what scientists call a neuro-muscular inhibitory response. In plain-speak, your muscles might actually get weaker (by up to 30 per cent) for up to 30 minutes after an inappropriate stretching session (poor technique and/or bad timing – like stretching 'cold' muscles before exercise) and stretching might contribute to more injuries than it prevents.

If you follow a Chronic Cardio or Chronic Strength Training programme that causes recurring muscle fatigue and tightness, you will probably feel an inclination to stretch frequently before and after workouts, even while sitting at your desk. I have a better idea: *slow down!* If you are exercising according to the Primal Blueprint, your muscles should feel supple and strong nearly all of the time. Sure, occasionally you will place extreme challenges on your body (yep, that's a good thing) and become sore and stiff. This is nature's way of saying, 'Back off.' You must also acknowledge the sedentary influences of modern life (such as the loss of hip flexor mobility that comes with sitting in a chair all day) and take corrective action through exercise and some specific dynamic stretches, which I will discuss shortly.

By the way, the old runner's adage that stretching and light exercise the day after a race or tough workout will 'flush the blood' and speed the healing of stiff, sore muscles is questionable. There is strong support for the idea that muscle tissue repair is best accomplished through inactivity, extra rest and sleep, good nutrition and brief, repeated exposure to cold water (particularly immediately after strenuous exercise – read more details about cold-water therapy in the Chapter 2 Endnotes).

As mentioned previously, the best way to prepare your body for any workout is with a few minutes of low-intensity exercise to help shift blood into your extremities from the organs in your working muscles. Even for something like all-out sprints, a few minutes of low-intensity cardio followed by some dynamic stretches, technique drills and then some long, easy strides at 75 per cent effort will prime you for your maximum efforts (as detailed in the Bonus Material's Sprint Workout suggestions).

The best benefits of stretching may be obtained after workouts or to otherwise help move between active and inactive states. My two favourite stretches are (poise your notepad): the *Grok Hang* and the *Grok Squat*. The Grok Hang offers a safe, full-body stretch that leaves you feeling exhilarated every time. It's also an effective strengthening exercise – as Primal as they come. It's as simple as grabbing hold of a bar or tree branch (with overhand grip) and hanging for as long as you can support yourself.

The Grok Squat involves placing your feet approximately shoulder-width apart, feet pointed slightly and comfortably outwards, bending your knees with a straight or slightly arched back and lowering your torso all the way down until your bottom is nearly touching the ground – your torso is between your knees and your arms extended in front of you. This natural movement provides a safe, gentle, efficient stretch for your feet, calves, Achilles, hamstrings, quadriceps, buttocks, lower and upper back and shoulders. For thousands of years people have squatted as a natural 'sitting' position in the absence of chairs (to say nothing of Barcaloungers!). For Grok – and millions of people today in the undeveloped world – squatting is the default position for resting, socialising, eating meals and even eliminating.

Try a Grok Squat for 20 seconds and notice what a comprehensive effect you get from such a basic movement. If it's first thing in the morning or when you're a little stiff from some intense activity or other stressor (e.g. jet or car travel), simply lowering into the position provides a good stretch. When I'm feeling warm and loose, I'll gently rock back and forth and/or extend my arms out further to obtain a deeper stretch. One caution: if you haven't done this for a while, are overweight, or have joint issues, you can begin to ease into this stretch (and keep yourself from going too low or falling over) by holding on to a post or another stationary object.

Beyond the Grok Hang and the Grok Squat, there are certain other dynamic stretches that are very effective, particularly if you have any injuries or joint issues. By dynamic I mean that you are moving your body in a way that achieves a stretch, as opposed to a static stretch where you are putting stress on a muscle while standing still. In the *Primal Blueprint 21-Day Total Body Transformation*, I present a sequence of photos and descriptions of my pre-sprinting routine of dynamic stretches and technique drills.

Enthusiasts of yoga, Pilates and other well-designed workouts that emphasise a balance of strengthening and stretching, can discover effective routines that help improve flexibility, protect against injury and overcome weaknesses and imbalances. What I want you to take away from this discussion is that static stretching may not provide much benefit and could even be counterproductive – especially prior to workouts when your muscles are cold. Even with stretches as simple as the aforementioned, be wary of any discomfort, skip or adapt the movements accordingly, and ease into and out of stretching positions.

> *'My own prescription for health is less paperwork and more running barefoot through the grass.'*
> LESLIE GRIMUTTER

PRIMAL BLUEPRINT LAW NUMBER 5: SPRINT ONCE IN A WHILE

Obviously, Grok's life featured the occasional brief all-out sprint, not for sport but rather to kill or avoid being killed. These bursts of speed were enhanced by the immediate flooding of the bloodstream with fight-or-flight adrenaline-like chemicals. When Grok survived a run to safety from a charging bear unhurt, the resulting biochemical signals prompted a cascade of positive neuroendocrine, hormonal and gene expression events, the net effect of which was to build stronger, more powerful muscles and an ability to go a little faster the next time.

Modern research confirms the Primal Blueprint premise: the occasional series of short, intense bursts can have a more profound impact on overall fitness – and especially weight loss – than a medium-paced jog lasting several times as long. This is because of increases in metabolic rate and appetite suppression (both due to elevated body temperature in the hours after workouts), development of more calorie-burning lean muscle tissue and improved insulin sensitivity (working muscles learn not only to burn glucose efficiently for fuel but also to absorb glucose – transported by insulin – after workouts).

The profound benefits of sprint workouts really hit home for me back in the early 1990s, when I'd take my personal training clients to the Santa Monica College running track. We'd often share this beautiful facility with some of the world's greatest Olympic sprinters. These physical specimens were a sight to behold. Obviously, they were blessed with remarkable genetic gifts, but it was also clear they were training and living in a manner that brought out the best of their genetic potential. In getting to know some of these athletes and their coaches, it became apparent how remarkably different their training methods were to the prevailing templates of the fitness and nutrition industry.

These Olympians were not out there all day circling the track to exhaustion: their workouts consisted of minimal amounts of very slow jogging, casual stretching (between competition-specific drills), unhurried efforts to fuss with their equipment (e.g. starting blocks or resistance tools) and, finally, a brief series of explosive efforts – lasting seconds, not hours. Their banter during these sessions was light; they were always smiling, laughing, joking and clowning around in between the intense focus of their main sprint sets. They also spent some serious time in the gym working very hard with the weights, but these track and gym sessions were interspersed with frequent easy or rest days, including occasionally sleeping in until double figures and taking daily naps. Their training diets were not laden with tofu, frozen yogurt and energy bars; they were more likely to feast on chicken and ribs after a workout. Carl Lewis, considered by many to be the greatest Olympic athlete of all time, with nine sprint and long jump gold medals to his credit, reportedly trained only an hour per day at his peak. And yet sprinters are among the leanest, most well-muscled people on the planet.

Introducing sprinting into your exercise routine is not as easy as lacing up a pair of shoes and heading out the door to go jogging. Sprinting is a physically stressful activity that requires a significant fitness base, muscle strength and flexibility. To reduce injury risk, beginners are advised to choose exercises that are low or no impact. Sprinting up a steep hill (and walking down to commence repeat efforts) offers a lower-impact option than flat running, while stationary cycling presents a no-impact option. I don't recommend outdoor cycle sprints (except for expert riders) due to the danger factor. You can also choose cardio machines (Versa Climber, elliptical, Stair Master, etc.), but I prefer actual running because the weight-bearing nature (and thus the increased degree of difficulty) of the activity offers maximum benefits, such as improved bone density and greater stimulation for muscle gain (or toning, for females) and fat loss. If you are significantly overweight as you start this programme and/or your knees aren't strong enough, cycling or using an elliptical machine might be the best way to start.

For running sprints in particular, you'll want to start the first few sessions gently, gradually increasing the speed and intensity of your sprints over time. You also need significant recovery time after sprint workouts. I recommend conducting a sprint workout approximately once every seven to ten days, and only when you have high energy and motivation levels. That's right, even as little as two to three sprint sessions *per month* can produce outstanding fitness benefits and break you out of Chronic Cardio ruts that may have lasted years. Running is the best but comes with a higher risk of injury if you are out of practice (i.e., you haven't chased down any animals or scored any touchdowns in the last few decades).

Novices can start with three to four sprints, short of full speed, with long rest periods in between efforts. You will likely experience some muscle soreness in the days after these efforts, but your body will quickly adapt to your new workout routine. You can then build up to a workout that includes six to eight all-out sprints – or even a few more as you become stronger. You should never push your body through an intense workout if you have any symptoms of fatigue, soreness, compromised immune system or another malaise. As discussed with strength training, your sprint sessions should be intuitive, intermittent and spontaneous – just as they were in primal life for Grok. The *occasional* sprint workout will elicit the more desirable gene expression effects than performing these workouts come heck or high water just because it's Tuesday.

CLOUSEAU-ROBICS AND DOBERMAN INTERVALS

While I've discussed the fight-or-flight response in the negative context of excessive aerobic exercise or hectic modern life, you should realise that eliciting a stress response is desirable with your sprint workouts. The difference here is that the brief, intense stress is exactly what your genes crave to build fitness and strength and to optimise metabolic function.

Imagine if every so often someone rudely interrupted your jog around the track by turning a vicious Doberman loose! I guess now you'd run as fast as possible, right? Or, like Inspector Clouseau, say you hired a martial arts master as a personal assistant to launch surprise attacks when you least expect it. Preposterous as it sounds, this type of sporadic, intense 'life-or-death' stimulation just might produce far superior fitness benefits than filling in all the blanks in your training log.

One final note: this isn't about speed – it's about effort. It doesn't matter if you aren't covering ground quickly, as long as you exert yourself to the point of going all-out for that brief interval. Age is not an issue here; whether you are 20 or 75, you can find a form of sprint workout that fits your style. For some people, it's simply walking fast up a steeply inclined treadmill for 30 seconds.

SPRINT WORKOUT SPECIFICS

Your sprint efforts should last between eight and 20 seconds, with duration, recovery and number of repetitions determined by your ability level. Sprints of eight seconds or less are fuelled by pure ATP in the muscle cell, sprints of eight to 20 seconds are fuelled by lactic acid, and maximum efforts lasting longer than 20 seconds are fuelled by glucose. While the scientific particulars may only be relevant to athletes trying to hone sport-specific skills and mimic competitive circumstances (track-and-field events of varied distance, football, rugby, etc.), you might like to vary your routine over time to include short, medium and longer sprints.

Longer sprints with short rests develop your anaerobic lactic acid buffering system (a desirable ability for a half-mile or mile race), while the shorter sprints with long rest periods develop your pure speed and explosiveness (such as for a 100-metre race). All types of sprint training will stimulate your fat-burning systems, lean muscle development and beneficial hormone flow, particularly the release of testosterone and human growth hormone (HGH). In this case, even though you will not be burning fat during the actual sprints, your body will become more efficient at burning fats to recover over the long term.

Because the weight-bearing aspect of running makes it significantly more difficult than cycling, running sprints should be shorter than cycling sprints. I prefer going all-out for about 15 seconds (after gradually ramping up my speed) and then taking a full rest period of one minute between efforts. I'll complete six to eight of these efforts, typically on grass, at the beach on hard sand or even in soft sand. Sometimes I'll get lucky and discover a clean path of freshly upturned deeper, soft sand from the beach tractor – begging to be blemished by my footprints! These options stimulate a variety of muscle groups, helping me enjoy a cross-training effect as I have to lift my knees higher to generate maximum turnover.

Ideally, you should sprint on a natural surface with excellent footing, such as a grass athletic field or the beach; use a running track or cement road if you can't find a suitable natural surface. While I like uneven surfaces to develop balance and foot strength for walks and hikes, don't risk it for sprinting. Use a smooth, straight, safe course with excellent footing. I strongly recommend making an effort to minimise your dependency on bulky running shoes and strengthening your feet by going barefoot, if possible, or using specially designed shoes that encourage a fuller range of motion.

On other days, my cycling sprints might consist of six to eight times of one-minute all-out with a two-minute recovery. Regardless of your specific workout choice, the entire sprint session – including brief warm-up and cool-down periods – will require less than 20 minutes. The Sprint Workout Suggestions in the Bonus Material offer several options for novice, intermediate and advanced workouts, including an exciting plyometric workout, a stadium steps workout and a couple of low- or no-impact sprint options, such as sprinting up steep hills or on a stationary bike.

PROPER RUNNING AND CYCLING FORM

While form concerns are relatively minimal in running and cycling compared to other sports, you must respect these important basics:

- **Running:** Torso faces forward at all times, shoulders and pelvis square to your forward direction. Refrain from side-to-side swivelling of the hips or the shoulder girdle. Arms and hands are relaxed as pumping is initiated from the shoulders. Elbows are bent at 90-degree angles. Don't let arms or hands cross the centre line of your body. Focus on fast turnover by striding in a motion similar to pedalling a bicycle. Lift foot quickly off the ground in a dorsiflexed position, drive knees high while keeping the pelvis facing forward. While sprinting, maximum force and drive are generated from the front part, and then initiate the next stride quickly. Your heel should nearly kick your bottom during the recovery phase of the stride. Envision your foot clearing the height of your opposite knee on each stride.

When you experience the inevitable tightening up midway through your sprint, focus on keeping your face, arms and hands loose and relaxed. Notice in videos or photographs of Olympic sprinters how their jaws are slack and their hands are soft and open. Be aware of your breathing rhythm and resist the temptation to hold your breath or pant shallowly. Take deep, powerful breaths by focusing on a forceful exhale.

- **Cycling:** Strive for a rhythmic cadence in a range of 80 to 100 revolutions per minute. Most recreational cyclists pedal at far too low a cadence, putting excessive strain on the muscles instead of balancing the cardiovascular and muscular load with an efficient cadence. Focus on applying circular force to the pedals rather than just stomping down. I highly recommend a clip-in pedalling system to achieve a proper circular stroke. Maintain a level pelvis at all times. Do not rock your pelvis from side to side in an effort to impart more force. Keep your upper body virtually still, with arms, chest, neck and head relaxed and supple, especially when the effort becomes difficult.

Be sure that your seat height is appropriate. A quick test is to place your heel (unclip it from the pedal) on the pedal axle when it's at the very bottom of the pedal stroke. You should be able to extend your leg fully (with pelvis level) and barely touch (or barely miss) the pedal axle. A seat that is too high or too low will stress the knees and also lead to rocking. Resist the temptation to tense your muscles when the effort becomes difficult. Breathe deeply by inflating your diaphragm fully on inhale. Because you are bent over, you should feel your diaphragm pressing against your ribcage when you inhale; then relax and allow a natural exhale.

HAPPY FEET

One of the most annoying non-Primal elements of today's fitness movement is shoes. You heard me, shoes are lame. Sure, typical athletic shoes provide substantial support, cushioning and general protection and are essential for many sports, but they also immobilise your feet inside the shoe – much like being in a cast. Hence, the complex network of 52 bones (a quarter of the total in your entire body) and dozens of tendons, ligaments and small muscles cannot work their magic to provide balance, stability, impact absorption, weight transfer and propulsion.

Constantly wearing shoes during exercise and daily life leads to weakened feet, fallen arches, shortened Achilles tendons and calf muscles, imbalances between the hamstrings and quadriceps, an inefficient gait and, of course, recurring pain and injury (like the old song goes, 'The ankle bone's connected to the knee bone; the knee bone's connected to the hip bone'). The 43 million Americans who experience foot problems daily (we will spend an estimated $900 million annually on foot-care products by 2011) offer another disturbing example of living in conflict with the Primal Blueprint.

Granted, shoes are essential for contact sports or activities involving hard surfaces, such as football, rugby, basketball, volleyball, running on the road and the like. However, for our purposes of conducting basic Primal Blueprint Fitness activities, going shoeless on occasion (and gradually increasing frequency over time) is possible and beneficial. Keep in mind that a lifetime spent in 'casts' – desensitising and weakening your feet for their primary functional purpose – will require that you proceed with extreme caution with your barefoot endeavours.

Here again I'll make a concession for modern life (I don't think Grok had any broken glass to worry about on *his* hikes) by recommending the use of a unique and excellent product called the Vibram FiveFingers shoe. The Vibram 'shoe' consists of a lightweight, form-fitting rubber sole attached to a nylon-like sock and a hook-and-loop closure system. Vibrams slip onto your bare feet like fingers into a glove (with a hole for each toe) and offer excellent grip as well as protection from sharp objects and debris. Duly protected, you can simulate a barefoot experience by giving your feet a complete range of motion during activity. (Search MarksDailyApple.com or VibramFiveFingers.com for details.)

Make an effort to gradually introduce barefoot time into your workouts and everyday life, providing ample time for your feet to adjust and get stronger without undue shock. For example, on my first few long hikes in FiveFingers, I kept my 'normal' shoes in a small pack just in case I needed them. Some mild next-day soreness in your arches is to be expected after your initial barefoot endeavours and is a natural part of the strengthening process (just as with muscle work). However, make sure you don't experience any pain during your efforts to get your feet more Primal. Be particularly careful if you are minimally active or overweight or if you have a history of foot problems or other medical issues. As with most other Primal activities, it is better to ease into a new form of exercise than to overdo it.

You can get some low-risk barefoot time by adopting the Eastern tradition of removing your shoes when you enter your house and otherwise using minimal footwear (flip-flop sandals or the like) whenever you don't need the protection or decorum of more substantial footwear. Try a short stint in socks on the treadmill at your gym and see what you think! Consider complementing your shelf of 'big' shoes with a pair of Vibrams or other choices from the rapidly expanding category of minimalist athletic footwear, using them first for walking around, then for short workouts, and gradually increasing your use as you remain pain-free. Hopefully, one day you'll work up to running some sprints barefoot – it doesn't get any more Primal than that!

'The only exercise some people get is jumping to conclusions, running down their friends, side-stepping responsibility and pushing their luck!'
AUTHOR UNKNOWN

CHAPTER SUMMARY

- **Primal Blueprint Exercise Laws:** Mirroring the active lifestyle of Grok is not a complex endeavour requiring the extensive time, money or specific equipment that conventional wisdom suggests. In particular, you can get extremely fit in as little as a few hours a week, provided you exercise strategically with a balance of extensive low-intensity movement, periodic high-intensity, short-duration strength-training sessions and occasional all-out sprints.

  Best results will come when your exercise routine is unstructured and intuitive, and workout choices are aligned with your energy and motivation levels. Always allow for sufficient recovery and try to pursue goals that are fun and inspiring. Weight-loss goals can succeed by combining Primal eating and frequent low-level exercise (fine-tuning your fat-burning system), with occasional brief, intense strength and sprint sessions (to stimulate an increase in lean muscle and metabolic rate).

- **Primal Blueprint Fitness:** Primal Blueprint Fitness means you have a broad range of skills and attributes (strength, power, speed, endurance – with power-to-weight ratio as a critical benchmark) that allow you to do pretty much whatever you want with a substantial degree of competence and minimal risk of injury. In contrast, narrow, specialised fitness goals are popular today (e.g. for endurance athletes and bodybuilders). These goals often compromise functional fitness and general health. By exercising – and eating – Primal Blueprint style, you will develop the unmistakable physique of a well-balanced athlete and eliminate the drawbacks of narrowly focused, overly stressful exercise programmes.

- **Organ Reserve:** Leading an active lifestyle and maintaining ample lean muscle mass correlates with optimal organ function and longevity, because your organs must keep up with the physical demands you place upon your body. In contrast, inactivity will accelerate the ageing process to the extent that it becomes a greater risk factor than simply getting older.

- **Move Frequently at a Slow Pace:** Two to five hours per week of low-intensity aerobic exercise (heart rate zone of 55 to 75 per cent of max heart rate), such as walking, hiking, easy cycling, cardio machines or (if you are fit) jogging, offer excellent health benefits, including improved cardiovascular, musculoskeletal and immune function and fat metabolism. In contrast, Chronic Cardio (75 per cent of max heart rate and up) workouts can place excessive stress on your system, deplete the body of energy (leading to increased appetite for quick-energy carbohydrates), inhibit fat metabolism, promote overuse injuries and generally result in a burnout condition. Slowing down workout pace and moving around more in daily life lead to improved fitness and health.

- **Lift Heavy Things:** Best results in strength training come from a sporadic routine of brief, intense workouts. These workouts will stimulate the release of adaptive hormones, such as testosterone and human growth hormone, helping improve body composition and delaying the ageing process. Exercises should focus on real human movements (lunges, squats, plyometrics, push-ups, pull-ups, planks and other body weight resistance exercises) instead of isolations on narrow-range-of-motion gym machines. Session difficulty should be aligned with energy and motivation levels: push hard when you feel like it and take it easy or skip workouts when you are tired. With this approach, you will avoid the risk of injury, exhaustion and burnout that comes from trying to follow a consistent schedule of long-duration workouts several times a week. Complete sessions should last around 30 minutes, even for experienced strength trainers. A mini-session of as little as 10 minutes can be extremely beneficial.

- **Sprint Once in a While:** No workout is more Primal than an all-out sprint. Efforts like these fuelled human evolution through survival of the fittest. Today you can enjoy excellent fitness, body composition and health benefits from intense sprinting, modelling the 'use it or lose it' principle. Sprint sessions should be conducted sporadically when energy and motivation levels are high. Intensity is the key – efforts should last between eight and

20 seconds, with complete rest between efforts to ensure maximum performance. Novices can do low-impact options, such as uphill sprints or stationary bicycle sprints.

- **Form and Feet:** Proper form in running and cycling is imperative. For running, the body should always face forward, the centre of gravity should be stable, and wasted motion (i.e., side-to-side movement) should be eliminated. Focus on striding in a circular motion (à la cycling) with centre of gravity always balanced over feet. For cycling, ensure proper seat height and apply circular force while pedalling at a rapid, efficient cadence of 80 to 100 rpm. Make an effort to minimise bulky shoes that restrict natural foot motion and weaken stabilising and propulsion muscles.

CHAPTER 7

THE PRIMAL BLUEPRINT LIFESTYLE LAWS

'IF YOU DON'T SNOOZE, YOU LOSE'

'I am two with nature.'
WOODY ALLEN

IN THIS CHAPTER

So here goes with the five lifestyle laws of the Primal Blueprint: Law Number 6, Get Adequate Sleep; Law Number 7, Play; Law Number 8, Get Adequate Sunlight; Law Number 9, Avoid Stupid Mistakes; and Law Number 10, Use Your Brain. While Grok's diet and exercise patterns were clearly major influences in shaping how his (and our) genes evolved, there were other environmental and behavioural forces that were no less important in perfecting the DNA recipe for a healthy, vibrant human being.

Law Number 6, Get Adequate Sleep, delivers obvious benefits but is widely compromised today. Good sleep entails a basic understanding of the physiology of sleep cycles, establishing consistent habits, taking advantage of the profound benefits of napping (when you need one) and applying effective time-prioritisation skills. Law Number 7, Play is a widely neglected lifestyle law that can deliver widespread benefits and make you quantifiably more productive when balanced effectively with work. Law Number 8, Get Adequate Sunlight, is an area where conventional wisdom has let us down, scaring us into avoiding the outdoors due to the misinterpreted risks of skin cancer. Obtaining optimal levels of vitamin D, synthesised from sun exposure on your skin, is critical to cellular health and cancer prevention.

Law Number 9, Avoid Stupid Mistakes, details how our obsessive desire to control or eliminate all sources of potential danger has made us lazy and inattentive. Cultivating the skills of hypervigilance and risk management is essential to avoid self-inflicted trauma and unnecessary suffering. Law Number 10, Use Your Brain, is about pursuing creative intellectual outlets unrelated to your core daily responsibilities and economic contribution. Finding more stuff to do with your brain may seem counterintuitive to many of us who feel our brain function is maxed out each day. However, the unrelenting pace of modern life and intense pressure to achieve and consume strongly conflict with our genetic make-up and can lead to feelings of restlessness and discontent. Making time for hobbies and personal growth challenges will keep you refreshed and excited about life.

PRIMAL BLUEPRINT LAW NUMBER 6: GET ADEQUATE SLEEP

For billions of years, the evolution of nearly all life forms on earth has been driven by the consistent rising and setting of the Sun. This circadian rhythm (from Latin: *circa*, meaning 'around'; and *dia*, meaning 'day') governs our sleeping and eating patterns as well as the precise timing of important hormone secretions, brain wave patterns and cellular repair and regeneration, based on a 24-hour cycle. When we interfere with our circadian rhythm (through exposure to excessive amounts of artificial light and digital stimulation after sunset, irregular bed and wake times, jet lag, graveyard shift work and alarm clocks, etc.), we disrupt some of the very processes we depend upon to stay healthy, happy, productive and focused.

Admittedly, aligning your sleep habits with the rising and setting of the sun is a challenge in today's world. Depending on where you live and the time of year, your sleep time might increase to the tune of two to six hours a day. I can hear you say, 'Ain't gonna happen anytime soon!' This is not to say you have to turn in at sunset in order to be healthy. For one thing, modernisation has substantially lowered our activity level and the overall degree of difficulty of daily life. (I know commuting is tiring, but imagine *walking* home from the office every day!)

Conventional wisdom usually recommends 7–8 hours per night, while those in the evolutionary health movement call for more. In *Sleep, Sugar, and Survival*, authors T. S. Wiley (anthropologist and medical theorist), and Bent Formby, PhD (biochemist, biophysicist, molecular biologist), urgently call for *nine-and-a-half hours per night* for seven months per year, with less sleep acceptable during the long daylight hours of summer. In addition to obtaining the requisite number of hours, your sleep must be of high quality – not harmed by a disruptive environment, objectionable medications or foods, or behaviours that elevate stress hormone production (vigorous exercise, screen time or other high stimulation) in the hours before bed.

Calm, quiet, dark evenings, and consistent bed and wake times are critical factors for high-quality sleep.

Sleep was long thought to be a passive state; however, we now understand it to be a dynamic process. The brain is active during sleep (but responding to internal stimuli, not external) and it drifts in and out of various sleep stages, or cycles. Our natural sleep pattern is to progress from light sleep (rapid eye movement [REM], when you dream and can be woken easily) into escalating stages of deeper sleep cycles (non-REM sleep, when you are out like a light and experiencing maximum restorative hormone flow, balancing of brain chemicals and cellular repair in muscles and organs). This cycling of REM into non-REM sleep is repeated throughout the night, with each complete cycle believed to last about 90 minutes.

If you divide your night's sleep into three equal time periods, your first third is characterised by the highest percentage of non-REM sleep, while the final third of your sleep time is characterised by a lengthening of the REM cycles and a shortening of the deep sleep cycles (the middle cycle is a balance between the first and the last). Waking up naturally involves letting the cycles play out until finally, after a period of exclusive REM sleep, you wake up effortlessly. (REM sleep is characterised by increases in heart rate, respiration and muscle and brain wave activity, making it easy to rise from this more alert state.)

The sleep hormone melatonin presides over you falling asleep and going through the various sleep cycles. Melatonin is manufactured in the pineal gland near the centre of the brain. As light diminishes, the pineal starts to convert the feel-good hormone serotonin, which has kept your mood elevated all day (and which is why so many of us take SSRI medications – to avoid depleting serotonin), to increasing amounts of melatonin, so that your mind and body will slow down and you'll become sleepy.

With the morning light stimulating your central nervous system, melatonin production is then suppressed and serotonin begins to increase. With melatonin predominating at night, the areas of the brain involved in emotional and social function get the rest they need, helping you face the next day mentally refreshed. A study from Dr Sophie Schwartz and colleagues presented at the 2008 Forum of European Neuroscience suggested that getting a good night's sleep can help the brain 'harden up weak memories which otherwise might fade in time'. Other hormones released during sleep, such as human growth hormone, help your body burn fat and repair muscle tissue.

We hold these truths about quality z-time to be self-evident. However, we are not walking our talk in modern life. A recent study cited by the Harvard School of Public Health found that an increasing percentage of Americans are seriously deficient in sleep (40 per cent of Americans get less than five hours of sleep per night), and an incredible 75 per cent of us suffer from some form of sleep difficulty each night. Chronic sleep deficit may lead to weight gain by affecting how your body processes and stores carbohydrates and by altering hormones that affect your appetite and metabolism. It can negatively affect your mood, concentration and memory retention during the day, making you less productive and more irritable, impatient and moody. Insufficient sleep can also lead to hypertension, elevated stress hormone levels, irregular heartbeat, compromised immune function and drastically increased risk for obesity and heart disease.

Our natural (or actually I should say, 'learnt') inclination to be constantly entertained is difficult to balance with our need for adequate restoration. It's not until we are truly exhausted that sleep moves up the hierarchy of wants and needs. It shouldn't have to be that way. Sure, you can get away with some occasional departures from your routine with no ill effects. Just as with your dietary choices, if you can observe a consistent bedtime 80 per cent of the time (there's that 80 Per Cent Rule again), the 20 per cent of the time where you stay up late, wake up super early, or otherwise skimp on perfect rest will probably be handled by your body more easily. On the other hand, if you have a habit of disrespecting consistent sleep time habits, you create momentum in the wrong direction and will struggle to achieve basic health and fitness goals, especially losing excess body fat.

HOW TO GET AN 'A' IN 'ZS'

Here are some important measures you can take in order to get optimum amounts of high-quality sleep. Visit MarksDailyApple.com for more discussion on this topic, including some helpful tips to beat jet lag.

- **Create an Ideal Sleeping Environment:** It's critical to make your bedroom an area of minimal stimulation and maximum relaxation. Your bedroom should be used only for sleeping (well, okay, that other stuff, too), with absolutely no computer, television or work desk or clutter present. You should have a clear physical and psychological separation between your bedroom and the other areas of the house where you do work or enjoy entertainment. Browse the Internet or flick through design magazines to get a feeling for the beauty of contemporary minimalist bedroom styles.

- **Follow Consistent Bed and Waking Times:** Just as with exercise, think quality over quantity. Establish a consistent, circadian-friendly routine to optimise hormone flows and ensure that you enjoy complete sleep cycles. Remember that melatonin floods your bloodstream on a circadian cue triggered by darkness. For two million years, that meant sunset; today, it means the time that you 'make it dark'. You experience the highest percentage of deep sleep at the outset of your night. Sorry, but if you miss bedtime, sleeping in to reach your typical hourly total will not completely catch you up.

  If you are a night owl, you can probably develop some level of tolerance and effectiveness for a consistent, artificial light-induced, late-night bedtime and an artificially darkened late-morning awakening. If circumstances require that your sleep habits depart from the earth's natural light and dark cycles, make a strong effort to sleep with an eye mask (check mindfold. com for a total darkness sleep mask) in a completely darkened room, since all of your skin cells are sensitive and responsive to light – not just your eyes.

- **Wind Down the Night and Ease into the Day:** Because everything you do after sundown is technically non-Primal, it's important to wind down calmly in the hours preceding your bedtime. Minimise your central nervous system stimulation before going to bed, so you can have a smooth, relaxing transition from your busy day to downtime. Reading is a time-tested popular method to get yourself to wind down, but choose fiction or something light to promote maximum relaxation .

   It may also be helpful to decompress your busy brain by writing down your thoughts before bed. Take five or 10 minutes to write out everything from your day: accomplishments, to-do tasks, stresses and worries. It's easier to arrive at solutions if you don't try consciously to force them. Get them down on paper and then let your sleeping mind do the work for you. You'll wake up feeling clearer and more positive.

   In the morning, awaken gradually and naturally, coming off a complete REM-dominant sleep cycle. Staying in bed for a few minutes to read or talk ('Again, your name was … ?') or starting your day with some light breathing and stretching exercises is preferable to springing up after the fourth snooze alarm and rushing into action. A brief warm shower can help stimulate your central nervous system naturally and get the blood circulating – a particularly good idea if you are going to exercise soon after waking. Hardcore Grok disciples can even try a cold-water plunge on waking up in the summer months – it beats a high-carbohydrate breakfast any day as a morning energiser.

- **Eat and Drink the Right Stuff:** Eat your last meal a couple hours or more before bed so digestion does not interfere with your sleep process. If you are a wine drinker, one fine glass with dinner may help you relax and unwind in the evening hours. The same goes for herbal teas. Camomile in particular is touted for its mild sedative effect. By all means pass on the carbohydrates – all day long and especially before bed. Insulin will interfere with melatonin production.

'No day is so bad it can't be fixed with a nap.'
CARRIE SNOW, STAND-UP COMEDIAN

NAPPING: IT'S NOT JUST FOR CATS ANYMORE

If you are able to obtain all of your requisite sleep at night, there is probably no reason to routinely take naps during the day. On the other hand, if you do have obstacles (job requirements, young children, noisy surroundings, etc.) that prevent you from getting adequate nighttime sleep, napping can help you sustain the focus, energy and productivity you need for an active life.

Many cultures across the world have appreciated nap time throughout their history, especially warm-weather countries in Latin America, Asia, the Mediterranean, North Africa and the Middle East. Furthermore, more than 85 per cent of mammals have polyphasic sleep habits, meaning multiple sleep-wake incidents. Anthropologists believe that Grok likely experienced disruptions to night-time sleep (Primal dangers, caring for young) and took advantage of afternoon down time for napping. Unfortunately, it seems that the fast pace of modern life (combined, perhaps, with some weird puritanical guilt factors) prevents napping being a culturally acceptable lifestyle habit.

'A nap of 20 to 30 minutes will recalibrate your brain's sodium:potassium ratio, a critical factor to recover from nervous system fatigue and wake up feeling refreshed.'

Because the rhythm of sleep cycles is so critical to brain and body restoration, napping can produce remarkable benefits in a relatively short time by helping you catch up on non-REM sleep cycle deficiencies, shortcutting you into the deep sleep cycles characterised by theta brain waves. Many experts recommend a nap period of 20 to 30 minutes. This time frame is believed to be sufficient to recalibrate your brain's sodium:potassium ratio, which is a critical factor in enabling you to recover from nervous system fatigue and wake up feeling refreshed. A nap of this length will not result in the unpleasant grogginess you might experience from a prolonged siesta, nor will it interfere with falling asleep that evening. Notable nappers throughout history include Winston Churchill, John F. Kennedy, Napoleon, Albert Einstein, Thomas Edison and Leonardo da Vinci.

> 'Art is older than production [making things for practical use] for us, and play older than work. Man was shaped less by what he had to do than by what he did in playful moments. It is the child in man that is the source of his uniqueness and creativeness.'
> ERIC HOFFER, AMERICAN SOCIAL WRITER AND PHILOSOPHER (1902–1983)

PRIMAL BLUEPRINT LAW NUMBER 7: PLAY

> 'We don't stop playing because we grow old; we grow old because we stop playing.'
> GEORGE BERNARD SHAW, IRISH PLAYWRIGHT AND POLITICAL ACTIVIST (1856–1950)

Few would argue the importance of play, yet compliance among many health-minded people is low in this area. We have been so heavily socialised into regimented, technological, industrialised life that scheduling time for play (now there's an oxymoron!) is a big challenge. I don't know about you, but I don't think the word *playdate* existed when I was a kid. Oh, we had playdates in my neighbourhood, all right – 365 of them, to be exact. They lasted from the final school bell until the dinner bell, not deterred by mud, rain, sleet or snow (no kidding, I'm from Maine!). We didn't need our mothers making transportation arrangements via email or by phone. We just needed air in our lungs, bike tyres and basketballs.

As the challenges and responsibilities of making a living or managing a family accumulate in our adult years, we collectively adopt the belief that play is only for young people. However, the truth is that play is for everyone, particularly those absorbed in the incredible complexity and breakneck pace of modern life. Regular play – time away from work, home duties, school and other scheduled and unscheduled responsibilities to express the childlike elements of your basic nature – helps quench your thirst for adventure and challenge (physical and mental), improves health, relieves stress, strengthens your connection with friends and community and simply enhances your enjoyment of life.

Learning disability specialist Dr Lorraine Peniston enumerates many research-proven psychological benefits of play, including:

- Perceived sense of freedom, independence and autonomy.
- Enhanced self-competence through improved sense of self-worth, self-reliance and self-confidence.
- Better ability to socialise with others, including greater tolerance and understanding.
- Enriched capabilities for team membership.
- Heightened creative ability.
- Improved expressions of and reflection on personal spiritual ideals.
- Greater adaptability and resiliency.
- Better sense of humour.
- Enhanced perceived quality of life.
- More balanced competitiveness and a more positive outlook on life.

There is plenty of evidence attesting to the fact that we can be more productive when we carve time for play into our busy schedules. A New Zealand study reported that people were 82 per cent more productive following a holiday and enjoyed enhanced quality of sleep – but that 43 per cent of Americans had no plans to get away in 2007 due to work pressures (and that statistic has probably become worse now). A 2006 study published in the *Sunday Times* noted that the percentage of married couples citing lack of quality time due to overwork as the basis for divorce has more than tripled in recent years, while at the same time the leading reasons traditionally cited for divorce, such as violence and infidelity, have dropped sharply. Australian research suggests that frequent breaks from a sedentary work day produce numerous health benefits, including weight control and favourable blood levels of triglycerides and glucose. A study published in the *New York Times* suggests that enjoyable leisure activities boost immune function even more powerfully than stressful events suppress it.

For the majority of us who move far less than we are genetically programmed to, busting loose outdoors, in fresh air and sunlight, for some unstructured physical fun will produce the best physical and psychological benefits. If you are one of the few who have a physically demanding job or daily routine, mellower pursuits (drawing trees in the park, skipping rocks in the pond) might indeed be the ticket.

My favourite activity of the week is a regular Sunday-afternoon pickup Ultimate Frisbee game with my son and several other families at the park. It is a great sport, requiring diverse athletic and strategic skills, and it is fun for players of all ages and ability levels. I'd say it's a 'safe' sport, too, except for my freak accident that resulted in a serious knee injury in 2007 – possibly attributed to a still 17-year-old brain directing a 54-year-old body to get some big air for a circus catch! Most importantly, my enjoyment of playtime has prompted me to reframe my main reason for exercising: I train Primally so I can play hard at whatever I want whenever I choose to, whether it's at Ultimate, snowboarding, soccer, stand-up paddling or golf.

If you can take the spirit of this message to heart, you can make something happen that will change your life. Let's be clear that I'm not advocating selling the shop and becoming a surf rat. All work and no play makes for a dull boy, but all play and no work makes for a foreclosure. Balance is important in all areas of life, and it's up to you to define your level of work–play balance. It might help to keep this popular sentiment in mind: 'No one ever said on their deathbed, "I wish I'd spent more time at work."'

PRIMAL BLUEPRINT LAW NUMBER 8: GET ADEQUATE SUNLIGHT

While the dangers of excessive sun exposure are well recognised and heavily promoted by today's medical community, it's important to challenge conventional wisdom's blanket statement to shun the sun – or lather up with tons of sunscreen as do English Channel swimmers with their lanolin. Adequate exposure to sunlight helps our bodies manufacture vitamin D, which helps regulate growth in virtually every cell of our bodies and prevent a variety of diseases. Vitamin D is essential for healthy teeth, bones and nails; eyesight; the absorption of other key nutrients, such as calcium and vitamins A and C; and immune function. Vitamin D has also been shown to play a role in the prevention of breast, prostate and colorectal cancer; cardiovascular disease; diabetes; autoimmune diseases; and inflammatory conditions, such as arthritis.

Perhaps the most exciting revelation about vitamin D has to do with its critical action on Gene P53 – the 'proofreader' gene. P53 acts as a spell-checker during each of the hundreds of millions of cell replications that occur each day, informing the cell when something has gone awry and instructing it to make any necessary changes. Many scientists believe P53 is an important first line of defence against the kinds of mutations that can develop into cancers. The bottom line is that regular sunlight is essential to excellent health and the *prevention* of skin cancer.

Early humans spent hundreds of thousands of years absorbing powerful equatorial rays over their entire bodies every day. As we migrated farther away from the equator, genetic adaptations occurred (the lightening of skin pigment and hair over many generations) to help us continue to absorb sun optimally even when it was less plentiful. Just as we've suffered devastating health consequences from the relatively recent shift in the human diet away from hunter-gatherer to grain based, the same dynamic holds for our sun exposure – except this lifestyle alteration has been even more severe. Only in the last couple of centuries of industrialisation have millions of people in the civilised world gone for long periods of time with little to no direct sun exposure. Consequently, there has been an alarming increase in health problems related to vitamin D deficiency.

The symptoms of vitamin D deficiency are not as overt as the disturbing image of scurvy-stricken sailors staggering around lacking vitamin C (which was, interestingly, partly a result of their high grain consumption), but the health consequences are devastating nonetheless. The risk increases for those with confined lifestyles (spent in the home, office or car – witness Ken Korg), those with dark skin living distant from the equator, children with vitamin D-deficient mothers, the elderly, or people who are house- or hospital-bound. Recent research suggests that vitamin D levels are also low in those with obesity and Metabolic Syndrome.

Internet and television health advisor and author Dr Joseph Mercola (mercola.com) states:

> *The dangers of sun exposure have been greatly exaggerated and the benefits highly underestimated. Excess sun exposure is not the major reason why people develop skin cancer (many believe poor diet, exposure to environmental toxins such as swimming pool chlorine, and insufficient sun are more significant risk factors). [A study from the Moores Cancer Center at UC San Diego suggested that] 600,000 cases of cancer could be prevented every year by just increasing your levels of vitamin D.*

Granted, the 'fell asleep covered with baby oil at the beach' burn-and-peel ordeals are indeed bad news. Medical experts suggest that even a few severe sunburn episodes in your early years (who hasn't fallen asleep on the beach or chaise lounge as a teenager?!) can generate sufficient ultraviolet radiation damage to potentially lead to the development of carcinoma (less serious growths that are easily removed from skin surface) or melanoma (a more serious form of cancer) in later decades.

However, there is a happy medium between too much sun and too little. Regular exposure of large skin surface areas to sunlight during the months of peak solar intensity at your latitude remains the primary way to obtain an ample amount of the vitamin D. For most people, maintaining a slight tan indicates that you are obtaining adequate vitamin D exposure, while a burn is, of course, unhealthy.

> 'Regular exposure of large skin surface areas to sunlight during the months of peak solar intensity at your latitude (enough for a slight tan) remains the primary way to obtain an ample amount of vitamin D.'

Contrary to conventional wisdom, dietary efforts to obtain vitamin D are almost inconsequential compared with sun exposure. Vitamin D experts recommend you obtain around 4,000 International Units (IU) per day, but the Standard American Diet provides only around 300 IU per day, and the vaunted glass of milk provides only around 100 IU per day. By contrast, 20-40 minutes of direct sunlight can produce around 10,000 IU of vitamin D, which can easily be stored in your cells for future use. In the winter months when the sun's rays are of inadequate intensity to promote vitamin D production, supplements can be useful. For the extremely sun challenged, carefully chosen artificial tanning lights can also boost vitamin D production. Blood tests are available to determine how your vitamin D levels compare to recommended levels. Search MarksDailyApple.com for 'sun exposure' and 'vitamin D' for numerous detailed posts.

The variables of season, climate and skin tone are substantial and should be carefully considered on a daily basis to ensure you obtain adequate sunlight while avoiding risk factors of excessive exposure. Generally, the goal is to expose the large surface areas of your skin (arms, legs, torso, back) to direct sunlight for about *half the amount of time it takes to sustain a slight burn*. This is a pretty low-risk endeavour that allows for plenty of individual flexibility.

Exposing your large surface areas is the key. If you are worried about wrinkling and cancer risk on the skin areas that are at most risk of overexposure and are most visible and sensitive – face, neck and hands – go ahead and cover them with clothing or sunscreen routinely. They represent an extremely minimal amount of your vitamin D potential anyway. Just be sure to bag enough rays during the summer months to manufacture plenty of vitamin D, because in latitudes outside the tropics, there are four to eight months during the year when vitamin D production is impossible. Check the Lifestyle/Medical Care Section in the Bonus Material for sun exposure strategy details.

HOW TO SCREEN YOUR OPPONENT

If you find yourself spending enough time in the sun to encounter a burning risk, you should have a protection plan. Unfortunately, conventional wisdom lets us down again by touting sunscreen as a fail-safe method. Credible research has shown that most sunscreens have historically not blocked the UVA rays that can cause melanoma. And in the case of skin cancer susceptibility, genetics does play a significant role. Those with fair skin, red or blonde hair and light eyes, or those with numerous moles, are six times more likely to develop melanoma than those with darker features. Some researchers even believe that excessive exposure of the skin to swimming pool chlorine is a bigger risk factor for melanoma than ultraviolet sunlight.

Furthermore, many of the popular agents used in sunblock products may have toxic properties, especially when you consider the standard recommendation to reapply these synthetic chemicals frequently to your porous skin. Octyl methoxycinnamate (OMC), a chemical contained in 90 per cent of sunscreen products, could damage living tissue if it penetrates your outer layer of dead skin. Titanium dioxide, another popular sunscreen compound, has been named a 'potential occupational carcinogen' by the US Government due to unclear toxic danger.

If you must be out in the sun for extended periods of time, it is far preferable to use clothing (especially made from fabrics designed to provide extra sun protection), to minimise your exposure to harmful UVA rays and to prevent burning. There are numerous apparel brands touting enhanced SPF (sun protection factor) effectiveness; search the Internet or visit a high-quality speciality sports store to find some. If you are partial to good ol' cotton, realise that it too will offer significant SPF effectiveness. Examining your skin after a day in the sun to make sure it's not burned will reveal just how well your clothing protects you. As a backup to clothing protection, use a premium sunscreen that protects against UVA, UVB and the newly described UVC rays, such as Neutrogena's Helioplex or an opaque zinc-based cream that blocks all rays entirely.

If you are concerned about getting overheated by clothing, it's interesting to note that participants in the Badwater 146-mile footrace across Death Valley in the middle of summer (definitely a non-Primal Blueprint approved event) dress from head to toe in loose-fitting white garments. While it might take a little getting used to, light white clothing has been scientifically proven to keep your skin and core temperature cooler than letting your skin glisten in the sun.

Beyond exposing your skin sensibly and being careful to protect it, a diet high in antioxidants and with a moderated O6:O3 ratio can go a long, long way towards reducing or eliminating any damage caused by sun exposure. In fact, one of the more common testimonials from people who have adopted a Primal Blueprint eating strategy is, 'I can stay out in the sun longer without burning.' On the flip side, a bad diet could be an even more profound risk factor than sun exposure for skin cancer.

Research published by the National Academy of Sciences indicates that dietary O6:O3 ratio is critical to skin cancer prevention. Furthermore, excess consumption of PUFA and chemically altered fats has been known to exacerbate the growth of tumours and other inflammation-related health conditions.

In a future book, I'll address the topic of sun exposure in great detail and help you formulate a customised sun exposure plan. For now, I want you to second-guess conventional wisdom's knee-jerk, fear-based reaction to skin cancer dangers by viewing the sun as evil.

PRIMAL BLUEPRINT LAW NUMBER 9: AVOID STUPID MISTAKES

'I drive way too fast to worry about cholesterol.'
UNKNOWN

Despite common Fred Flintstone-like depictions, early man was far from a numbskull. Grok was almost certainly attuned to his surroundings and was skilful in his ability to avoid making mistakes or getting into situations likely to endanger their health. It is a common faulty assumption that our hunter-gatherer ancestors lived 'solitary, poor, nasty, brutish and short' lives. This was the description advanced by 17-century English philosopher Thomas Hobbes, when he argued for the need to have government structure in civilisation instead of living off the land hunter-gatherer style.

Research suggests that Grok and his family were actually generally healthy (robust is the apropos term), productive and so appreciative of their lives that they felt the need to express themselves through art. There may even have been a selective benefit within tribal units for grandparents – meaning that getting older may have actually had an evolutionary advantage such as babysitting or the transfer of important knowledge and history.

So, if they were so robust and if our genes truly evolved to allow us – and possibly even encourage us – to live long lives, then why was the average life span relatively short? I had always assumed that it was things like deaths during childbirth, infections, accidental poisoning, even tribal warfare that brought the average life span down. But then I got a real-life experience of what might have affected life span more than anything else. Far from nasty and brutish, it was the mundane lapses in judgement, even minor ones, that most likely spelled doom for many primal humans.

My unusually bad dive during an Ultimate Frisbee match in September 2007 resulted in a torn quadriceps muscle, displaced kneecap, ruptured prepatellar bursa and smashed nerve. An X-ray

revealed no other tendon or ligament damage, and my orthopae-
dist said the soft-tissue injury would heal in eight to 12 weeks. He
advised me to use pain as my guide and come back slowly. Because
I had no pain at all (smashed nerve, remember?), I felt like I was
recovering fairly quickly – to the point of resuming my beach
sprints in early December, followed by a snowboarding trip over
the Christmas break. But despite wrapping the knee every day and
taking it fairly easy (wink, wink – and again no pain), I came home
with a very swollen, black-and-blue knee. By the end of the week, I
was unable to bend it more than a few degrees.

An MRI scan revealed a large organised haematoma over the
quadriceps and kneecap that needed to be removed surgically,
otherwise I would carry it with me forever. During surgery, it was
discovered that the original torn quad muscle had never repaired
itself and was leaking blood into the space, causing the haematoma.
So my surgeon removed the haematoma and stitched the quad back
to the patellar tendon.

Here I was, 54 years old, with the body of a 25-year-old and the
mind of a 17-year-old, looking forward to living well past 100, but I
was effectively incapacitated for more than four months by an injury
caused by a random fall. (Truth be told, I had second thoughts as
soon as I jumped.) Of course, I had the luxury of modern surgi-
cal procedures to repair the damage and eventually recovered fully.
Had this happened 10,000 years ago, my inability to run away from
a predator might well have spelled the end for me – all because
of a momentary lapse of judgement. Even today, a small accident
that active younger people barely sneeze at (e.g. a fall from a ladder
while hanging the Christmas lights or turning an ankle on a stair-
case) can mean something entirely different for someone elderly
and sedentary.

THE DARWIN AWARDS – LONG LIVE NATURAL SELECTION

As society continues to modernise exponentially, we are arguably exhibiting less and less common sense in avoiding stupid mistakes. I believe part of the reason is that deep down we know we can afford to make them. Our intricate system of safety nets in modern society has compromised our capacity to take responsibility for our role in the 'accidents' that occur and are chronicled by the news media daily. Look no further than YouTube or the Jackass television shows to confirm that we are actively inviting unnecessary struggle and suffering into our lives. It's all in the name of expressing the youthful sense of adventure that has been stifled by the constraints and predictability of the modern world. The 'Darwin Awards' satirical book and website annually bestow special distinction on those who, with particular brilliance, 'improve the gene pool by removing themselves from it', with particular brilliance. Here are some of my favourite winners from recent years:

- **Hot Rod:** A Texas motorist spilled a petrol can in the back of his car. While searching for the can at night, he flicked on a cigarette lighter to get a better view, igniting the vehicle.
- **Nacho Libre:** A Pennsylvania man was critically injured when he crashed his motorcycle into a telephone pole after being distracted by a plate of nachos on his lap.
- **CSI: Alternative Ending:** A police officer in Illinois was trying to show another patrolman how their fellow officer had accidentally killed himself. While reenacting the shooting incident from the previous week, he forgot to unload his gun and shot himself in the stomach. While driving himself to the hospital to seek treatment, he was killed in an car accident.
- **Up, Up and Away:** A Catholic priest in Brazil attached a garden chair to dozens of helium balloons and launched his homemade craft. Winds picked up and he drifted out to sea. Well prepared for this potential adversity, he fired up his satellite phone to call

for help but could not figure out how to operate his GPS unit to provide an accurate location for rescuers. Rescuers were unable to locate him – ever … although bits of balloon were found later on mountains and beaches.

- **Off the Falls:** A man attempted to pilot a rocket-boosted jet-ski off the side of Niagara Falls. The idea was for the rocket to launch the jet-ski beyond the danger of the falls and then deploy a parachute and float to safety. The damp air caused both the rocket and parachute to fail as he rode off the edge of the falls. Miraculously, he survived the 160-foot drop but drowned because he didn't know how to swim and was not wearing a life jacket.

Each of us must admit that we have brought various levels of misfortune and trauma into our lives from lapses in concentration or critical thinking. As we attempt to reflect on these stupid mistakes, often we default to blaming bad luck instead of reenacting the chain of events with a deep, honest assessment of our accountability. In fact, the concept of taking responsibility seems to have all but disappeared from modern life. If we truly deconstruct the times when we have been the victim of circumstances, it's quite likely we can discover that exact moment when we were distracted, made a poor choice, or ignored the clear warning signal that might have helped us to avoid the entire incident.

HYPERVIGILANCE AND RISK MANAGEMENT

Each of us possesses the genetically hard-wired skills of hypervigilance and risk management. Like any other skill – or muscle – we have to use and develop them or they will atrophy. Unfortunately, the obsessive effort society makes to diffuse all forms of risk and danger suppresses the use of these natural instincts: endless warning signs on roads and in public venues, safety hazard labels on every consumer product and sensationalised news reports about the dangers of toxic playground bark or pyjamas catching fire. Furthermore, continued technological innovations in the name of comfort and convenience collectively push us towards running on autopilot, often to our detriment, through various mundane elements of daily life.

Drive through Europe and you'll notice very few warnings or safety precautions on the roadways – even high in the Alps they don't bother with guardrails. Take a spin through the canyons near my home and you will see miles upon miles of safety barriers, guardrails, runaway truck ramps and diamond-shaped yellow signs with admonitions and icons warning you of assorted dangers that lurk around every corner. Nevertheless, every year tragedy strikes our local community with fatal accidents (typically induced by alcohol and/or speeding) on these obsessively protected roads.

Meanwhile, the historic traffic fatality rates in France, Germany, Great Britain, Switzerland and Scandinavia (per capita and per vehicle miles driven) are significantly lower than those of the United States. Interestingly, some progressive traffic engineers, in the US and elsewhere around the world, are popularising the concept of 'shared space' as a tool to reduce accident rates. The concept relies on human instincts, such as eye contact, in favour of traditional traffic signals and signs. For example, the removal of bike lane striping on a roadway may actually make cycling safer by increasing driver vigilance. This seemingly counterintuitive concept reminds us of the importance of nurturing our natural instincts so that they can help us navigate potentially hazardous situations effectively when we are not pacified by excessive safety measures.

As we strive to succeed in modern life, we must be willing to take personal responsibility for our actions instead of defaulting to speed-dialling a personal injury lawyer whenever we come to misfortune. If you get hit by a motorist running a red light, it is mostly his fault, but you may fare better if you remember to fasten your seat belt and look for oncoming traffic despite the colour of the traffic light. I can't remember if an errant throw or overly aggressive defensive play was involved in my Ultimate accident, as I prefer to focus on the fact that I hurled myself through the air irresponsibly and then tried to come back into action too quickly afterwards. When I take responsibility for my actions, my misfortune becomes a growth experience – an appealing alternative to feeling like a victim or placing any importance on the notion of bad luck.

Similarly, every time I encounter a dicey driving situation, I realise something upon further reflection when things calm down: whenever I mumble 'asshole' to someone who has just cut me up, I should really be saying it to myself, too – for being in a rush, being too aggressive or impatient, or diverting my focus from the road momentarily. Maybe the motorists who incur my wrath truly deserve a little choice feedback, but I can find something I brought to the table almost every time.

This theme also works in a discussion about dietary habits. You can blame lousy food options in airports, your distressing family medical history, or the limitations of your budget, but in each case you may be better served to accept some personal accountability.

Take the extra time to pack healthy snacks for your travel. View your family history as a catalyst to cultivate hypervigilance and risk-management skills instead of as a curse. Take a deeper look at your lifestyle priorities, make some compromises, and stretch your food budget a bit to choose the very best quality ingredients. In this way you can turn negatives into positives and create excellent leverage to be the best you can be, regardless of 'bad luck' or other figments of your imagination that are vying for your attention.

'Everybody gets so much information all day long that they lose their common sense.'
GERTRUDE STEIN, AMERICAN AUTHOR AND FRENCH ART PATRON (1874–1946)

PRIMAL BLUEPRINT LAW NUMBER 10: USE YOUR BRAIN

 While the modern world features plenty of complex thought and a constant and rapid progression in human innovation– technological and otherwise – our over-stimulated lifestyles compromise our ability to use our brains with maximum effectiveness. Even Albert Einstein was reputed to have once said: 'I don't know my phone number because I can look it up easily in the phone book.'

The fact that we are able to outsource brain function is not necessarily bad, but it does reveal that we are having trouble keeping up with today's information overload. In the workplace, the mismanagement of information overload from personal digital assistants (BlackBerry, Droid, iPhone,iPad, etc.), instant chat and the like can stifle creativity and innovation, not to mention our levels of energy, motivation and health. Consequently, many of us operate in a reactive mode, constantly – and often futilely – trying to keep pace with the information with which we are bombarded.

In Mark Bauerlein's book *The Dumbest Generation*, the author blames digital technology for compromising the intellectual development of young people. 'When we were 17 years old, social life stopped at the front door. Now [via MySpace, Facebook, instant chat, texting, Skype, etc.] peer-to-peer contact … has no limitation in space or time,' observes Bauerlein. Hence, time to read, daydream, free-associate, or gain an adequate understanding of current events, history and other mainstays of cultural sophistication goes by the wayside.

If we back up and examine the true definition of *stress* as 'stimulus', it's clear that we require a certain amount of daily stress to thrive, prosper and be happy. 'Evolutionary Fitness' advocate Art De Vany, PhD, author of the *New Evolution Diet,* draws a compelling link between exercising our minds and our genetic nature as free, independent, adventurous human beings. 'Modern life leaves our minds restless and under-utilized because we are confined, inactive and comfortable,' De Vany argues. 'We cannot be satisfied with more and more because we are evolved for another lifeway in which material goods do not matter. The result is that we are deeply unsatisfied with modern life and don't know why.' Our genes simply don't know what to make of all our 'stuff'.

At first glance, few might agree that our minds are restless and underused. Many of us end our days running on fumes, feeling like our minds will explode if we send or receive any more emails. Our minds are indeed overstressed, yet technically under-utilised, because we lack the balance that creative intellectual outlets, play, healthy diet, exercise, sleep and other winning behaviours promote. Eight hours of brainpower is probably a sensible limit to devote to your daily work efforts. However, engaging your mind with things that stimulate your creativity in other ways and that you have a passion for is critical to maintaining good mental health and your overall well-being. Here are few suggestions to model Primal Blueprint Law Number 10: Use Your Brain:

- **Pursue New Endeavours:** Learn a foreign language or musical instrument, take dancing lessons, tackle a jigsaw or crossword puzzle, write a fiction short story – or anything else you can imagine outside of your comfort zone that sounds interesting and challenging.
- **Discipline Your Brain Use:** Pay close attention to balancing your daily intellectual stimulation with rest. Make an effort to avoid (or power down) distracting influences and focus on a single peak performance task at a time.
- **Exercise the Muscle**: Instead of outsourcing as much brain function as possible to technology, make a habit of challenging your brain during your routine daily endeavours. Replay your favourite song on your iPod and try to memorise the lyrics, take down your school yearbook and try to recall the names of your long-lost fellow students, or use your head to add up numbers, instead of always relying on a calculator or notepad. Do a Google search for Sheppard Software's 'Place the States Game' and see how closely you can come to dropping individual states into their correct spot on a blank USA map. There are endless opportunities to keep the brain fresh throughout your day.

CHAPTER SUMMARY

- **Get Adequate Sleep:** Despite being a critical component of good health and stress management, sleep is regularly compromised in modern life due to the pull of technology and hectic schedules. Insufficient sleep can lead to numerous health problems and declines in cognitive function. Try to align your sleep habits as closely as possible with the rising and setting of the sun, with special attention to minimising artificial light and digital stimulation after dark. Create a calm, dark, relaxing sleep environment, observe gradual transitions into and out of sleep, and observe consistent bed and waking times. Occasional brief naps can produce many health benefits, including the reduced risk of disease plus improvements to mood, concentration and physical performance.

- **Play:** The regimented nature of modern life leaves many adults – and even kids – deficient in play. The profound psychological benefits of play are integral to healthy cultures, communities and individuals, including a direct relationship to work productivity. Engage in some unstructured outdoor physical play exertion each day to counter the negative effects of a sedentary, technological existence.

- **Get Adequate Sunlight:** A reasonable amount of daily sun exposure (depending on several variables, including skin pigment and climate) can produce numerous health benefits and alleviate many health risks, because it enables your body to synthesise optimal levels of vitamin D. The dangers of sun exposure are overdramatised and there are many people across the world who in fact suffer from sun deficiency today. Risks of skin cancer are greatly reduced if you avoid getting sunburn and cover or screen the most vulnerable areas of face, neck and hands.

    Pursue a strategy of exposing the large surface areas of your skin (arms, legs, torso, back) to direct sunlight for about *half the amount of time it takes to sustain a slight burn*, during the months of peak solar intensity at your latitude. Dietary sources of vitamin D are vastly inferior to sun exposure for meeting your vitamin D requirements. Vitamin D supplements can be useful in the winter months when sunlight is of insufficient intensity to allow for vitamin D production. Those with particularly severe sun challenges can explore artificial light options. When you've had enough sun, clothing is the best protection, as there are health objections to some suncreams, and certain products may be less effective than advertised.

- **Avoid Stupid Mistakes:** Avoiding stupid mistakes was a critical survival factor for Grok, because the margin for error was much lower in primal times. Today, modern life attempts to shield us from all manner of danger and yet, possibly because we are desensitised by all these protection mechanisms, we still seem to find a way to invite trauma and tragedy into our lives by making stupid mistakes. We must practise our hardwired, evolution-perfected skills of hypervigilance and risk management to navigate successfully through even the mundane elements of daily life to avoid unnecessary suffering and to ensure our own longevity.

- **Use Your Brain:** Human innovation and overstimulation have compromised our ability to use our brains to maximum effectiveness. We must exert great discipline to use technology to our advantage instead of falling victim to it by spacing out, burning out, or otherwise misusing our greatest weapon as human beings: complex thought. Pursue new challenges – such as music, language, hobbies or adventures – which will stimulate your brain and allow you to depart from your daily routine. This will keep your refreshed and energised for your core daily responsibilities and economic contribution.

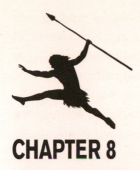

CHAPTER 8

A PRIMAL APPROACH TO WEIGHT LOSS

'A PRIMAL BREAKFAST, A PRIMAL LUNCH AND A SENSIBLE PRIMAL DINNER'

'Desserts is just stressed spelled backwards.'
ANONYMOUS

IN THIS CHAPTER

Here I will give you a detailed step-by-step regime which will enable you to lose an average of one to two pounds (one-half to one kilogram) of body fat per week. You'll learn how to target protein, carbohydrate and fat intake specifically in order to ramp up fat metabolism, maintain high dietary satisfaction levels and avoid the risk of depleting muscle tissue and suffering from the usual rebound-rebellion effect of severe caloric restriction. I will also explain how deregulating food intake and fasting intermittently can be effective calorie-restriction tools and how exercise can accelerate progress towards your body composition goals.

Through the example of two weight-loss case studies (Ken and Kelly Korg, naturally!), and by calculating their average daily caloric expenditure and optimal daily intake of each macronutrient, Primal Blueprint style, to produce targeted and effective fat loss, we'll examine a daily food diary of delicious, nutritious meals that contains a detailed caloric analysis and macronutrient breakdowns for each meal, plus a daily total. The case studies result in a loss of around eight pounds for Ken and 7.75 pounds for Kelly in a single month. Finally, in the following pages there are also some troubleshooting tips which will help you face any possible setbacks and plateaus that arise when trying to lose weight in the real world.

These are the critical elements of the Primal Blueprint weight-loss approach:

- **Minimise carbohydrate intake** to moderate insulin production and enable stored body fat to be burned for energy.
- **Optimise protein intake** to maintain or increase muscle mass.
- **Optimise fat intake** to achieve satiety, provide energy and eliminate hunger.
- **Engage in occasional Intermittent Fasting (IF)** to produce accelerated caloric deficits that lead to greater fat loss.
- **Exercise Primally** to fine-tune fat metabolism and build or tone lean muscle without the drawbacks of Chronic Cardio.

- **Avoid excessive regimentation or obsessing on results** in favour of appreciating the process and viewing body composition goals with a long-term perspective.
- **Remember** that optimal *health* is the underlying goal of living Primally. LGN (looking good naked) is just a pleasant side effect.

By now you've caught my drift that the Primal Blueprint is a way of life as opposed to a regimented, gimmicky crash course diet. I thought carefully about whether to put the presumptuous claim of 'effortless weight loss' on the cover. However, I believe deeply that if you honour the Primal Blueprint principles at least 80 per cent of the time, long-term weight management will happen as a natural by-product of your enjoyable, stress-balanced lifestyle.

Easier said than done, right? While we have literally thousands of success stories compiled at MarksDailyApple.com, we also communicate occasionally with folks whose progress is not always smooth and steady. I'd like to shift gears in this chapter and get a little more precise about macronutrient intake. Following the steps covered in this chapter will enable you to immediately reduce excess body fat without the struggling and suffering inherent in any fat loss programme that's attempted with a carbohydrate-based low-calorie diet.

The idea is to hit the sweet spot where carbohydrates have been reduced just enough so that your body prefers to burn fats and a moderate amount of ketones instead of relying so much on glucose. This carbohydrate sweet spot is between 50 and 100 grams per day for most people. Where you land in this range depends on your size, age, sex and metabolism. Consume more carbohydrates than that (up to 150 grams a day) and you'll maintain body composition quite easily without adding fat, but you'll have to work a little harder to burn it off. On the other hand, it's certainly healthy to take in less than 50 grams per day of carbohydrates once in a while (as we said, you could live on zero carbohydrates for quite a long time), but the idea is to stay just on the fringe of ketosis.

In the sweet spot, you will maintain high energy levels (no more insulin crashes), you can exercise (including regular intense sessions) and recover without getting exhausted, and you won't exhibit any of the unpleasant byproducts of sudden, severely carbohydrate-restrictive diets that put you into ketosis without having prepared you to effectively use those ketones as fuel. These include the annoying 'ketone breath', insufficient vitamin/mineral intake (due to the severe restriction of vegetables and fruits), and poor compliance due to the deprivation and inconvenience involved in trying to bottom out on carbohydrate intake.

As you continue to eat in the sweet spot (or dip into the maintenance zone on certain days, no biggie), your eating habits send signals to your genes to up-regulate fat-burning processes and down-regulate fat-storage processes. You'll become both fat-adapted and keto-adapted, able to derive energy minute-to-minute from your stored body fat. By eating in the sweet spot, you can expect to drop 1-2 pounds (one-half to one kilogram) of excess body fat per week. This may not seem like much in comparison to the headline on the flyer tacked to the telephone pole or the flashing Internet banner ad. However, unless you plan to lose water and muscle tissue (and I know you don't), losing one two pounds of fat per week (your personal maximum rate within this range depends on your existing body weight, metabolic rate and activity level) means an average daily deficit of 500 to 1,00 calories.

You cannot realistically (or safely) lose any more than a pound or two a week of body fat without depleting muscle mass or becoming fatigued.

HOW TO LOSE LIKE A WINNER

The sensible limits on the rate of losing body fat is evident when you consider that one pound of fat contains 3,500 calories and adults only burn between 1,500 to 3,000 total calories per day. What about the 'Biggest Losers' glorified on the television programme, or in before-and-after magazine contests, who alter their body composition dramatically in a short time? These results are achieved with a combination of incredibly intense exercise coupled with severe caloric restriction, an approach that is simply inhumane and impossible to follow long term. Generally, these crash efforts result in a significant reduction in water retention and lean muscle mass, and just a bit of fat.

A crash weight-loss programme (or any other form of extreme stress, such as a family crisis) prompts a fight-or-flight response in your body. Buzzed on adrenalin, you can triumphantly complete your six-, eight-, or twelve-week programme (particularly when the bright lights of television and monetary incentives are there to motivate you). Afterwards, you are likely to collapse in exhaustion when the fight-or-flight response wears off and your body's energy reserves are depleted. In this 'post-traumatic stress' state, many become sedentary (or much less active, in any case) and tend to overeat – a genetically programmed reaction to an ordeal perceived as a starvation threat. Lo and behold, the 'before-and-after' ideal typically becomes a 'before, -and-after and back-to-before … and then some' reality! There is absolutely no reason to have to struggle or suffer to achieve your body composition and health goals. In fact, if you do, I can guarantee that your approach is flawed.

Before the disappointment of hearing 'only a pound or two a week' gets etched onto your face, understand that when you proceed with a embrace the Primal Blueprint lifestyle, a lifelong move out of flawed conventional wisdom's grain-based diet into something aligned with your genetic requirements for health, you'll realise there is no hurry here – you have complete control over your physique the rest of your life. Fine-tune eating habits or workout patterns for a few weeks and you can drop fat and maintaining or add/tone muscle as simply as turning a number on a dial. Stay with the Primal Blueprint and you will always trend towards your ideal body composition.

WEIGHT-LOSS MACRONUTRIENT PLAN

The plan is as follows: obtain a calculable level of protein sufficient to preserve lean muscle mass, strictly limit carbohydrates to an average of 50 to 100 per day, and use fat as the main variable to obtain the satisfaction you need from your diet each day so that you aren't stressed or anxious about your weight-loss journey. To ensure your success and comfort during the fat-reduction period, please make an extra effort to have appropriate snacks available at all times. These include vegetables and certain fruits, and foods high in protein and/ or fat (hard-boiled eggs, macadamia nuts, olives, sardines). If you're feeling deprived during your Primal journey, or have cravings for some of your old grain-based standbys, have a few celery sticks smothered in macadamia nut butter, a hard-boiled egg, then call me!

PROTEIN

As you learned already, you need an average of 0.7 to one gram of protein per pound (.33 to .5 grams per kilo) of lean body weight per day to repair, build, and/or maintain lean muscle mass effectively and to adequately support numerous other metabolic functions dependent upon dietary protein. For an active female with 100 pounds (45 kg) of lean body mass, this is only 400 protein calories per day. For an active male with 150 pounds (67.5 kg) of lean body mass, this amounts to only 600 protein calories per day.

I'm not asking you to undergo an expensive underwater body composition test to pinpoint your lean body mass and then carry around a calculator to nail your exact protein requirements every day. Your appetite will guide you effectively to meet your protein requirements, just as your thirst does for hydration requirements. That said, if you experience low energy or a reduction in muscle mass, you may want to delve further into just what you are eating to be sure the levels are in proper range. Jot down everything you eat for a few days, and then use an online food calculator such as paleotrack.com or Fitday. com to determine how many grams of the various macronutrients you are consuming. I've provided some suggested meals with detailed nutrient breakdowns in this chapter to give you a feel for how healthy and satisfying the Primal Blueprint weight-loss plan can be.

CARBOHYDRATE

Limiting your average carbohydrate intake to 50 to 100 grams per day will effectively moderate your insulin production and optimise

REALLY, IT'S ALL ABOUT THE CARBOHYDRATE CURVE

As you learned when the Carbohydrate Curve was introduced in Chapter 3, your body composition *success* is overwhelmingly dependent on controlling your carbohydrate intake and, hence, your insulin output. Exercising correctly, managing your stress levels, and genetics are minor factors in the equation. Your *failure* to maintain desirable body composition may be related to one of several things – unlucky genetics, an overly stressful exercise programme, insufficient sleep, self-destructive eating and lifestyle behaviours, a sedentary existence and more – but an excess body fat condition *almost always includes excessive carbohydrate intake*.

Limit your carbohydrate intake to 100 to 150 grams per day (depending on size and gender) and you will not store more fat (unless you have an extremely severe overeating problem – but even then it will be hard!). That's the maintenance zone. Limit your carbohydrate intake to 50 to 100 grams or less per day and you will begin to lose stored body fat. Your rate of fat loss will also be affected by your exercise efforts, sensible eating of healthy fats and protein and, lastly, genetic factors. Here again is the Carbohydrate Curve and the general effects that various levels of average daily carbohydrate intake have on your body.

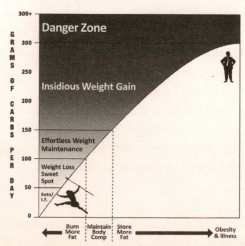

your fat-burning process. At this level of carbohydrate intake, your body will be stimulated to burn more stored fats and manufacture a little extra glucose in the liver through gluconeogenesis. In this case, however, dietary protein will provide the substrate for gluconeogenesis instead of your precious muscle tissue. I've discussed the gluconeogenesis process as a bad thing in the context of the fight-or-flight response triggered by Chronic Cardio or a protein-deficient extreme diet, but it can just as easily be a wonderful energy balancing mechanism when you eat Primally.

As an added benefit of this process, your liver will generate a moderate level of ketones which will help spare muscle tissue and provide added fuel for cells that might otherwise require glucose. Hence, limiting your carbohydrates to well under 100 grams per day will put you in a very mild (and desirable, because you'll be burning fat like crazy) state of ketosis. You probably won't even notice it, but for the appreciable increase in steady-state energy now available. If your batting average drifts above 100, your increasing blood glucose levels will start to redirect energy pathways more towards glucose burning.

I'm not asking you to split your carrot sticks down the middle or to skimp on salad portions to stay under 100 grams. As you can see from this chapter's examples, you can still enjoy abundant servings of vegetables and ample servings of well-chosen fruit (nutrient-dense foods that are particularly important to consume when you are restricting calories and exercising diligently) and land in the optimum range for insulin control and weight loss. The key to meeting this seemingly strict guideline effortlessly is to virtually eliminate processed carbohydrates from your diet – then it's truly a breeze. If all you do is get rid of sugars, desserts, soft drinks, pasta, bread, cereals and beans (and starchy tubers such as potatoes – especially if you eat them and their derivatives frequently – for the time being) you won't even have to track the remaining carbohydrates.

FAT

Coupling your protein requirements with your strict limitations on carbohydrates (at 50 to 100 grams per day during the fat-loss phase), it's easy to see how you can reduce body fat at an accelerated rate. Even an active male will be under 1,000 calories per day before considering fat intake. Hence, the variable for your energy needs and total calorie consumption ends up being fat. If you are committed to success, you will make a concerted effort to eat only what you need (in fat, and in total calories) to feel satisfied and energised. Because fat has such a high satiety factor, a little will go a long way. Even something like a small handful of nuts can sustain you for hours when you skip meals or need a quick snack to keep you going. With the right meal choices and healthy snacks around, your intensive weight-loss experience will not involve the typical struggling and suffering of a 'diet'. After you reduce the amount of body fat you desire, you can consume even more liberal amounts of fat without worrying about gaining weight.

While the 'eating fat is okay for weight loss' idea might seem contradictory at first glance, it is valid; without insulin, eating fat will not make you fat! If you don't produce insulin, your body has no way to store the excess calories as body fat. Note, however, that if I give you an inch and you take a mile (pounding high-fat foods all day 'as directed by Mark Sisson'), you will not succeed in losing fat either. As you build up momentum with more and more weeks of eating low insulin-producing meals, notice how your genes become reprogrammed to not require regular high-carbohydrate feeding sessions to stay awake and functional. Your appetite will 'self-regulate' to a point at which you eat when you are hungry and become comfortable eating only as much as you need to feel satisfied. As your old, ravenous 'eat-every-three-hours' sugar-burner hunger gives way to the new 'energy-all-the-time' fat-burning furnace you have created, capitalise on your progress now and then by skipping meals – noticing that you can actually crank away all morning without eating an all-American breakfast. In fact, your new breakfast might now be the 500 calories of fat you are currently sitting on or that's hanging over your belt (no offence) ready to be burned off as energy. Proceed with your dietary transition at a pace most comfortable to you, and realise that this is the essence of Primal living: rejecting a dependence on dietary carbohydrates as facilitated by the standard American diet and reclaiming your *Homo sapiens* genetic factory setting as a fat-burning beast!

KEN KORG: SUGGESTED EATING FOR PRIMAL WEIGHT LOSS

Let's look at a case study of our old friend Ken Korg, a 40-year-old, five-foot-eleven (177.5 cm), 197-pound (89 kg), moderately active male with 25 per cent body fat (metric equivalent: 25 per cent; sorry, still too much!) who wants to lose weight aggressively (near the maximum suggested rate of two pounds per week) following the Primal Blueprint. We'll calculate Ken's estimated daily caloric expenditure and suggested macronutrient intake based on Primal Blueprint guidelines. Then, I'll present a list of suggested meals and snacks with accompanying macronutrient analysis. The day's example will show how Ken can enjoy sensible, satisfying meals and snacks and still achieve a dramatic improvement in body composition by meeting the average macronutrient guidelines for a single month.

Throughout these examples, remember to focus on the concept of *averages*. While it's instructive to examine a detailed daily example of both expenditure and intake to understand how we can properly achieve caloric deficits, in reality you will have days where you exceed your carbohydrate limit, fall short of your protein limit, and exercise more or less than the averages in our calculations. Ultimately, this isn't about counting and tracking, but about developing an intuitive sense of what works best for you.

CALORIC EXPENDITURE

The basal metabolic rate (BMR) estimates were derived using a BMR calculator (many are available on the Internet, such as one at bmi-calculator.net). BMR factors your age and weight to estimate the number of calories your body burns if you simply stay in bed all day. An Activity Factor adding additional calories to the daily estimate is derived using the Harris Benedict Formula (also available at bmi-calculator.net), which takes into account various typical levels of activity. You can input your personal variables and generate similar estimates for total daily caloric expenditure.

CALORIC EXPENDITURE

- **Basal Metabolic Rate:** Number of daily calories Ken burns to support basal metabolic functions (at his age and body composition) = 1,923.
- **Activity Factor:** Harris Benedict Formula for additional calories burned when 'moderately active': BMR × 0.55 = 1,057.
- **Total Average Daily Calorie Expenditure:** BMR (1,923) + Activity Factor (1,057) = 2,980.

MACRONUTRIENT CALCULATIONS

- 197 pounds (89 kg) at 25 per cent body fat = 148 pounds (67 kg) of lean body mass
- Moderately active = 0.7 grams per pound (.33 grams per kg) factor for protein intake per pound of lean body mass
- 148 pounds (67 kg) × 0.7 = 104 grams of average daily protein intake
- Goal of losing 8 pounds (3.6 kg) per month = 932 calories per day average caloric deficit
- Desired average caloric intake per day = 2,048 (2,980 average caloric expenditure less 932 deficit)
- Desired protein grams = 104 (416 calories) – per previous calculations
- Desired carbohydrate grams = 75 (300 calories) – to get into in the Sweet Spot on the Carbohydrate Curve
- Desired fat grams = 148 (1,332 calories) – to back into the 2,048 daily total

You can see right away that the suggestions will not be difficult for Ken to follow. That amount of fat calories will provide ample energy and satiety at each meal, while the number of protein grams will ensure that his body recovers from exercise stress and continues to burn at his average daily rate of 2,980 calories – or higher. In his past dieting efforts, Ken tried to cut back on calories in general, slightly reducing normal intake of fat, protein and carbohydrates. More likely, he probably made a little extra effort to cut back on fatty foods but was not nearly diligent enough with carbohydrates and possibly compromised some lean body mass (depending on how devoted his efforts were) by falling short of protein requirements.

Each time he tried to lose this way in the past, Ken's energy and exercise level declined slightly but insulin was still prevalent to drive consumed calories into fat cells. Hence, his body fat percentage has stayed pegged at 25 per cent for years despite repeated efforts to reduce it. Let's see how the results can differ when eating Primal Blueprint style.

FOOD DIARY

Breakfast: Primal Omelette

Eggs (three medium) with cream (1 ounce/25 grams) and shredded Cheddar cheese (1 tablespoon)

Chopped mushrooms, red onions and red peppers (¾ cup total)

Topped with sliced avocado (2 ounces/50 grams) and fresh salsa (2 tablespoons)

Fresh blueberries (¼ cup)

Cup of black coffee

Breakfast FitDay.com Analysis

Total Calories: 463

Protein: 23 grams, 89 calories (19 per cent)

Carbohydrates: 22 grams, 82 calories (18 per cent)

Fat: 33 grams, 292 calories (63 per cent)

Lunch: Primal Salad

Mixed salad greens (2 cups)

Chopped onions, carrots, red peppers and cherry tomatoes (2 ounces/ 50 grams each)

Chopped or shredded chicken (3 ounces/75 grams)

Sesame seeds (⅓ ounce)

Chopped walnuts (½ ounce/15 grams or 7 halves)
Oil-based dressing (2 tablespoons)
Lunch FitDay.com Analysis
Total Calories: 585
Protein: 31 grams, 124 calories (21 per cent)
Carbohydrates: 30 grams, 120 calories (21 per cent)
Fat: 38 grams, 341 calories (56 per cent)

Dinner: Salmon and Vegetables

Grilled wild salmon (6 ounces/175 grams)
Steamed asparagus and courgette (6 ounces/175 grams each) with
  butter (1 tablespoon)
Red wine (5-ounce/140 ml glass)
Dinner FitDay.com Analysis
Total Calories: 560
Protein: 39 grams, 157 calories (28 per cent)
Carbohydrates: 16 grams, 63 calories (11 per cent)
Fat: 26 grams, 232 calories (41 per cent)
Alcohol: 16 grams, 108 calories (21 per cent)

Snacks

Hard-boiled egg
Macadamia nuts (1½ ounces or 17 nuts)
Venison jerky (one 4-inch strip)
Snacks FitDay.com Analysis
Total Calories: 437
Protein: 14 grams, 58 calories (16 per cent)
Carbohydrates: 8 grams, 32 calories (7 per cent)
Fat: 41 grams, 347 calories (79 per cent)

Daily Totals

Calories: 2,045
Protein: 107 grams, 428 calories (21 per cent)
Carbohydrates: 78 grams, 297 calories (15 per cent)
Fat: 139 grams, 1,212 calories (59 per cent)
Alcohol: 16 grams, 108 calories (5 per cent)

- Caloric deficit from average daily expenditure (2,980) = 935
- Projected net fat loss over 30-day period: 8 pounds (3.6 kg)

YOU WON'T BELIEVE WHAT'S PRIMAL!

The diary entries for Ken and Kelly illustrate the concept that Primal Blueprint weight loss does not have to be a Spartan exercise of weighing and measuring bland food, choking down powdered 'replacements' for real food, or otherwise engaging in repetitive, restrictive eating habits. While the rules of Primal Blueprint macronutrient intake are clear cut, there is tremendous opportunity for flexibility within these guidelines.

At MarksDailyApple.com, we have hundreds of recipes, shopping tips and detailed meal-planning strategies that will help you actually enjoy the process of eating healthily, perhaps to an even greater extent than you did your pre-Primal dietary habits. You may also enjoy *The Primal Blueprint Cookbook* and *The Primal Blueprint Quick and Easy Meals*. Take a glance at this list of recipes that are posted on the website – yep, they're all Primal-approved!

- Arugula Endive Salad with White Wine Vinaigrette

- Spicy Thai Coconut Soup

- Broiled Halibut with Garlic Aioli and Steamed Broccoli

- Crustless Quiche with Spinach and Scallions

- Baked Mahimahi with Pesto and Tomatoes

- Grilled Flank Steak with Sautéed Beet Greens and Creamy Horseradish Beets

- Smoked Salmon with Asparagus and Poached Egg

- Spicy Korean Seaweed Salad with Shrimp

- Sautéed Broccoli Rabe with Sundried Tomatoes and Pine Nuts

To make up for the caloric intake deficit, Ken will derive his additional 935 daily calories from stored body fat – what is now his primary energy mechanism to fuel a busy day. Quite an improvement from his previous roller coaster of carbohydrates, caffeine, insulin, fatigue and insufficient exercise.

> 'Ken is now using stored body fat as his primary energy mechanism to fuel a busy day, instead of his previous roller coaster of carbohydrates, caffeine, insulin, fatigue and insufficient exercise.'

KELLY KORG: SUGGESTED EATING FOR PRIMAL WEIGHT LOSS

Now let's evaluate Kelly Korg, our 40-year-old, five-foot-four (162 cm), 148-pound (67 kg), very active female with 27 per cent body fat. While her goal of losing nearly eight pounds of body fat (3.6 kg) in a single month is ambitious for a female, she is fit enough to tolerate intense exercise and create substantial caloric deficits with sensible Primal Blueprint meals. She will actually reduce her total weekly exercise hours and corresponding calories burned in favour of a more sensible programme with slower-paced cardio, more rest and shorter, more intense workouts.

CALORIC EXPENDITURE
- **Basal Metabolic Rate:** 1,411
- **Activity Factor:** Harris Benedict Formula for additional calories burned when 'very active': BMR × 0.725 = 1,023
- **Total Average Daily Calorie Expenditure:** BMR (1,411) + Activity Factor (1,023) = 2,433

MACRONUTRIENT CALCULATIONS
- 148 pounds at 27 per cent body fat = 102 pounds of lean body mass (46 kg)

- 1.0 grams per pound (.5 grams per kg) factor for protein intake per pound lean body mass (due to high stress levels and history of heavy exercise requiring more protein than a moderately active person like her husband)
- 102 pounds lean mass = 102 grams of average daily protein intake
- Goal of losing 7.66 pounds of body fat per month = 894 per day average caloric deficit
- Desired average caloric intake per day = 1,539 (2,433 average caloric expenditure less 894 deficit)
- Desired protein grams = 110 (408 calories) – per previous calculations
- Desired carbohydrate grams = 79 (316 calories) – to get into the Sweet Spot on the Carbohydrate Curve
- Desired fat grams = 91 (816 calories) – to back into the 1,539 daily total

You can see right away that the diet will be much more pleasant for Kelly to follow than were her previous efforts, by which she severely restricted calories and interspersed this approach with inevitable carbohydrate binges. The fat calories will provide satiety at each meal (missing from her last diet, which featured heavily processed liquid shakes). The protein calories will ensure that her body recovers from exercise stress and also maintains and even builds some attractive lean muscle tissue, and that her metabolic rate stabilises at 2,433 calories daily.

FOOD JOURNAL
Breakfast: Steak and Fruit
Flank steak (4 ounces/100 grams)
Blueberries (½ cup)
Peach (½ of whole)
Green tea (1 cup)
Breakfast FitDay.com Analysis
Total Calories: 238
Protein: 25.0 grams, 106 calories (44 per cent)

Carbohydrates: 15.7 grams, 56 calories (24 per cent)
Fat: 8.5 grams, 76 calories (32 per cent)

Lunch: Chicken Club Lettuce Wrap

Lettuce (3 large leaves)
Diced cooked chicken (4 ounces/100 grams)
Sliced red pepper (½ cup)
Plum tomato (1 medium)
Avocado (½ of whole)
Mayonnaise (1 teaspoon)

Lunch FitDay.com Analysis

Total Calories: 397
Protein: 38.5 grams, 159 calories (40 per cent)
Carbohydrates: 17.2 grams, 62 calories (14 per cent)
Fat: 20.5 grams, 176 calories (44 per cent)

Dinner: Beef Stir-Fry

Sliced beef steak (4 ounces/100 grams)
Olive oil (2 tablespoons)
Sliced zucchini (1 medium)
Sliced mushrooms (1 cup)
Spinach (1 cup)
Sliced bamboo shoots (½ cup)
Sesame seeds (¼ ounce)

Dinner FitDay.com Analysis

Total Calories: 611
Protein: 37.6 grams, 150 calories (25 per cent)
Carbohydrates: 9.5 grams, 35 calories (6 per cent)
Fat: 48.1 grams, 426 calories (70 per cent)

Snacks

Hard-boiled egg (1 large)
Apple (1 large)
Almond butter (1 tablespoon; spread on apple)

Snacks FitDay.com Analysis
Total Calories: 283
Protein: 9.3 grams, 35 calories (13 per cent)
Carbohydrates: 33.1 grams, 121 calories, (43 per cent)
Fat: 14.8 grams, 127 calories (45 per cent)

Daily Totals
Calories: 1,529
Protein: 110.4 grams, 450 calories (29 per cent)
Carbohydrates: 75.5 grams, 274 calories (18 per cent)
Fat: 91.9 grams, 805 calories (53 per cent)

It's essential to reject the ridiculous prevailing mentality that weight loss can be achieved quickly with extremely severe measures. You want to lose 10 pounds in just a few hours? I've done it – at the 1973 Boston Marathon. The intensity of the competition at the world's most prestigious marathon coupled with an unseasonably humid day left me totally depleted and dangerously dehydrated at the finish. I'll never forget roaming around in a daze in the finishers' area (an underground parking garage) and passing by a full-length mirror. I paused, locking eyes with the gaunt image in the mirror (he seemed to recognise me as well …), and asked, 'Hey, how did you do?'

- Caloric deficit from average daily expenditure (2,433) = 904
- Projected net fat loss over 30-day period: 7.75 pounds (3.5 kg)

WEIGHT-LOSS EXERCISE PLAN

While my view that 80 per cent of your body composition success is determined by how you eat is difficult to prove scientifically, the anecdotal evidence is overwhelming. Go to the starting line of a major marathon or ironman triathlon and take note of the surprising level of excess body fat sported by many of these very highly trained athletes. The same goes for the droves of gym rats and aerobics queens with flawed diets and physiques that belie their tremendous devotion to fitness. There's no better proof that regardless of how many calories you burn, consuming excessive processed carbohydrates ultimately inhibits your ability to access and burn stored body fat efficiently around the clock. Instead, all that arduous training results in an increased appetite, again thanks to insulin-driven sugar cravings from poor food choices combined with, or as a consequence of, overly stressful workouts. Unless you are a genetically gifted, extremely devoted endurance athlete (i.e. racing at the front of a pack with a motorcycle escort), it's a vicious cycle that you cannot escape no matter how hard you exercise.

While it's true that exercise moderates the insulin response (i.e., a sugary energy gel consumed during a tough workout will be burned quickly and will not prompt an insulin release like it would if you sucked it down at your desk), burning lots of calories (particularly with Chronic Cardio) and eating lots of carbohydrates throughout the day will simply make you carbohydrate-dependent for energy. Invariably, left to its own devices, your body will want to overcompensate by tempting you to eat slightly more than you need to refill the tank, as if it's actually thinking, 'What if this clown decides to do this again tomorrow? I'd better be ready!' This is how so many people have programmed their genes over the years, protecting them against depletion by stimulating an appetite increase in response to hard exercise.

Beyond the appetite increase, chronic exercise patterns have been scientifically shown to make you lazier throughout the day. Seriously, it's known as the *compensation theory*! Perhaps some of this compensatory behaviour is conscious ('Sure, why not take the elevator? I already ran five miles this morning'), but there is also a subconscious component. The compensation theory asserts that you move generally less energetically throughout the day and are more liberal with your 'appetite' and caloric intake. Buoyed by a deep-down sense of accomplishment from your chronic workouts, you essentially grant yourself free licence to pig out!

The bottom line is that you will not lose fat effectively with exercise-driven weight-loss efforts unless you moderate insulin production.

Of course, a sensible exercise programme will improve your health, sense of well-being and muscle tone and somewhat minimise the negative effects of the high-carbohydrate diet by making you more insulin-sensitive, but it won't get rid of that spare tyre. On the flip side, I have been able to maintain my ideal body composition effortlessly, even working out only one-tenth as much as I used to, since I evolved to eating very low-carbohydrate Primal Blueprint foods (getting increasingly observant over the past 10 years and eventually reaching what you might call 'very strict' Primal, beginning in 2002). During my recovery from knee surgery in 2007, I was able to maintain my exact weight and 8 per cent body fat on zero exercise for a month and very limited exercise for a few more months after that.

> '*The bottom line is that you will not lose fat effectively with exercise-driven weight-loss efforts unless you moderate insulin production.*'

Of course, we all have genetic differences that create the reality of 'results may vary'. Regardless, you must focus on the concept of triggering the ideal expression of your own genetic potential through the combination of Primal Blueprint diet and exercise behaviours. Consider an age when you were pleased with your fitness level and physique. It *is* possible to approximate your appearance and energy levels at age 18 or 21, reversing years or even decades of suboptimal diet and exercise practices, in a relatively short time.

Be content with uninterrupted gradual improvement in your body composition and a wholehearted enjoyment of the process. This improvement may not be a linear 'pound or two a week' experience; instead you may have some months, or seasons, when you will really lean out, while at other times you will experience inevitable plateaus (I'll discuss how to handle these shortly). With this mind-set – that you are taking care of your health and constantly progressing towards your goals (at a speed you determine, mainly by dialing in your carbohydrate intake) – your motivation and compliance levels will be strong even years down the line.

By the way, you are welcome to pursue the programme with more enthusiasm and discipline to produce accelerated results, but you must align your efforts with your fitness level. Serious athletes who have added a few pounds in the off-season can ramp up training easily and return to their ideal weight relatively quickly.

An old-time pro triathlete I coached was once asked how long it took to drop the typical seven pounds gained over the off-season after resuming training: 'couple of long rides,' he deadpanned. On the other hand, a novice unaccustomed to regular exercise must follow a more patient approach to avoid burning out. So here are some Primal exercise recommendations which will help you to turbo-charge your weight-loss efforts.

> *'Be not afraid of growing slowly, be afraid only of standing still.'*
> CHINESE PROVERB

RAMP UP LOW-LEVEL ACTIVITY

As discussed previously, when you exercise at moderate heart rates you run little risk of fatigue or burnout. Increase your daily activity level in every possible way – walking or cycling instead of driving to do local errands, taking the stairs, parking at the furthest edge of the car park, strolling the neighbourhood after dinner and enjoying leisurely hikes on the weekends. One friend of mine makes business calls while walking briskly on a treadmill (a great icebreaker, by the way: 'Hey, what's that hum in the background?'). Considering that the average American watches 28 hours a week of television, we could possibly cure obesity if we all casually pedalled stationary bikes during our viewing time (and of course regulated our insulin production by eating Primally)!

MAKE YOUR HARD WORKOUTS HARDER

Focus on intense strength training and sprint sessions, ensuring that you are well rested and fully recovered between efforts. Remember, it's not the frequency of your intense workouts that matters as much as their quality. When you exercise a muscle to short-term exhaustion at 12 reps or deliver a maximum effort for 10 pull-ups, you'd be surprised what your body can do two minutes later if you repeat the effort. If you think you've pushed it to the limit at your typical 25-minute intense workout, take a five-minute water break and then go back out there for another 15 minutes of high intensity. If you pat yourself on the back after your typical eight sprints, rest for five minutes then go back and do a couple more!

CHILL OUT AND BREAK THROUGH

I cannot emphasise strongly enough how important it is for you to reject the conventional wisdom mindset towards weight loss that obsesses on daily calories burned, strictly controlled portion sizes and other dictatorial nonsense. If you are hungry, eat (the right stuff); if you are motivated, exercise (the right way); and if you are tired, rest! When you are dragging, your energy is going towards rebuilding broken-down muscles and energy systems. Pushing a fatigued body through exercise will only lead to depletion, burnout and undesirable sugar cravings.

The key to the exercise component of weight loss is in expertly balancing stress and rest to allow for peak efforts to be reached in conjunction with adequate recovery and rebuilding. With the athletes I advise, I call these peak efforts *Breakthrough Workouts* – sessions that are difficult and challenging enough to help you 'break through' to a higher fitness level (or, in our context here, stimulate a reduction in body fat). Whether you want to reduce your 10k time or drop 10 pounds, it comes down to directing optimal gene expression: primarily through diet and secondarily through an effective workout plan with occasional Breakthrough sessions. From our understanding of the selection pressures of evolution, it's clear that taking fat off is more difficult than packing it on. Only by harnessing your energy with careful attention to stress management and the occasional bouts of brief, very intense, good old-fashioned hard work can you expect something different from the 'same ol' same ol'": scale numbers, clothing sizes, race times and so forth.

SHHH! SISSON'S SIX-PACK SECRETS

'How to have washboard abs on a high-fat diet, no cardio and no ab exercises' was the title of one of my most popular MarksDailyApple.com posts. In the weeks after the post, my shirtless photo accompanying the article was 'tagged' and spread all over Facebook, necessitating a crash course on the amazing technology of cyber social networking in order to protect my name and likeness. While a 'six-pack' is the universal hallmark of a lean, fit, well-toned man or woman, getting there following conventional wisdom protocol (gruelling crunches and sit-ups to the point of nausea, burning endless calories on a treadmill and then obsessively limiting what you take in – especially those high-fat foods so reviled by diet and fitness personalities) is too daunting to be a realistic goal for all but the most devoted (and least employed) gym rats.

The truth is, we all have washboard abs – underneath whatever fat might currently be obscuring them. Remember, 80 per cent of your body composition success comes from how compliant you are with Primal Blueprint eating. A possible genetic predisposition to storing extra belly fat might indeed limit your ultimate potential to land on a magazine cover, but I'm willing to bet many times the price of this book that you can bring to the surface impressive ripples you never knew existed (or at least haven't seen since your college days) by hitting the sweet spot with your carbohydrate intake and naturally engaging your abs throughout daily life. In fact, washboard abs can be considered an effortless side-effect of living Primally.

Grok had to have a great set of abs in order to be an effective thrower, climber, runner, jumper, crawler and lifter. Not that abs themselves lift, throw, catch or push, but the whole complex of abdominals (rectus and transverse abdominis, internal and external obliques and pyrimidalis) provides the foundation for nearly every athletic and everyday movement you do. Thus, they are part of today's popular 'core' training – the ultimate functional muscle group. But rather than isolating them on some fancy $4,000 gym machine or getting carpet burns on your bottom from doing a bazillion crunches in your living room (you know who you are), the best way to work your abs is to **involve them in almost every other movement you do** – every time you do it.

When you do push-ups, you should make a concerted effort to tighten your abs (pressing the navel towards the spine); the same is recommended during pull-ups, squats, lunges, curls and other complete body exercises. Raking leaves, carrying your toddler, reloading the bottom drawer of the copy machine, lugging shopping out of the car and onto the kitchen counter and infinite other daily activities (including simply sitting at your desk or in your car) can all be considered opportunities for a mini abs workout. I bet I did more than a thousand of these efforts sitting at my desk writing this book!

When you are engaged in basic movement, sitting or walking, you should tighten your belly as if you are going to be punched in the gut while blowing out the candles on your birthday cake. Hold it for 10, 20 or more seconds a few times every hour. Now do it while slightly tilted to one side. Repeat for the other side. For even better results and a stronger core, you can also simultaneously contract your buttock muscles. Do these short exercise bursts while you are driving to pick up the kids or when stuck in traffic. After a while, it will become second nature to squeeze your abs spontaneously. I do some of my best abs work while bent over doing sprints on the stationary bike. It's really all about squeezing, tightening and trying to isometrically shorten the distance between your sternum and your pubic bone. Engage your abs, eat right and in no time you'll be sporting that six-pack! Furthermore, a strong, functional set of abs will help you avoid back problems as well as perform all outdoor activities safely and with less risk of injury.

SUGGESTED EXERCISE WEEK SCHEDULE

Walk, walk, walk. Hike, hike, hike. Move, move, move. This might seem like strange advice to help you get lean and ripped like our primal friend Grok. However, by now you should have a clear understanding of why ill-advised, frequent, moderate- to high-intensity workouts simply burn glucose and increase appetite and that your exercise programme on the whole is only dealing with the 20 per cent slice of the weight-loss pie. After all, walking around the block or hiking up to the water tower doesn't burn enough calories to contribute noticeably to weight loss. However, increasing your daily movement will build you from the inside out: toning muscles, joints and connective tissue to enable you to thrive on the high-intensity workouts that strongly influence body composition.

Coupled with Primal Blueprint eating habits, your active lifestyle will refine your fat-burning skills so that you become an efficient fat-burning machine around the clock and easily reach your ideal weight in a matter of weeks or months, as seen with the Korgs' case studies. Best of all, as you scan the suggested daily meal plan (earlier in this chapter) and the weekly exercise plan (next), you'll see that it's easy to eat and exercise in a Primal manner for the rest of your life. Here's a sample of what Kelly and Ken can do to 'go Primal' with their workouts:

- **Sunday:** Two-hour hike at low intensity. (The Korgs can do this together and get quality time as well.)
- **Monday:** Easy 45-minute spin on a stationary bike and a 15-minute walk after dinner.
- **Tuesday:** 30-minute intense strength-training session. Go for an 8 to 10 effort on a 10 scale. Try the, simple, functional, body-weight resistance exercises I call the Primal Essential Movements (pullups, pushups, squats and planks). These are described in the Bonus Material at the end of this book. Further details are available at MarksDailyApple.com in the free download eBook, *Primal Blueprint Fitness*, as well as the *Primal Blueprint 21-Day Total Body Transformation*. Add in a 15-minute walk after dinner.
- **Wednesday:** Rest.
- **Thursday:** Easy 45-minute stationary bike ride or hike.
- **Friday:** Sprint session at grass field, school track or even the beach. You can also sprint indoors on a treadmill, elliptical or stationary bicycle. Duration, including warm-up and cool-down, is about 30 minutes. Choose from the recommended sessions based on ability level in the Bonus Material at the end of this book.

- **Saturday:** 10-minute intense strength-training session. Go for a 6 to 7 effort on a 10 scale.

MARK'S EXERCISE WEEK ANALYSIS

- **Total Duration:** Around five hours – most of it comfortable cardio.
- **Total Calories Burned:** Who cares? Enough to accelerate fat reduction and get in shape without suffering.
- **Muscle Groups Exercised:** Arms, legs, core and everything in between or attached.
- **Total Scenery Enjoyed:** A ton more than someone on a treadmill or in a spinning class.
- **Total Fun Had:** Lots!

What a far cry from Kelly Korg's exhausting regime of pre-dawn high-intensity workouts, mundane malnutrition shakes replacing real meals, and the resulting fatigue, energy-level swings and sugar cravings.

On the Primal Blueprint plan Kelly could wake up leisurely with the rest of the family and enjoy comfortable exercise sessions (possibly including some of her less-than-optimally-active family members?). Instead of suffering several mornings a week, she could pick a few key opportunities with high-intensity Breakthrough Workouts that leave her exhilarated and accelerate her fat reduction. In six months' time, she'll have shed some 24 pounds of body fat and will likely have added a few pounds of well-placed, lean, toned muscle tissue. She'll be happier and more energetic and she'll look better than she has in decades, through less effort and less struggle than before.

Meanwhile, Kelly's neighbour Wendy (remember her, the peppy network marketing enthusiast who dropped eight pounds in two weeks?) will almost assuredly weigh the same or more than she did when she started her cleansing diet six months previously. Further-more, because 99 per cent of network marketing participants lose money (from a survey of the largest and most reputed network marketing operations – after considering all expenses and inventory purchased from the company for resale), she'll probably have a lot of cleansing diet kits gathering dust on the garage shelves.

IF YOU WANT TO LOSE EVEN MORE FAT, TRY IT!

As we reflect on the tidy examples of Ken and Kelly Korg nailing their daily caloric deficits with delicious, fulfilling meals, I must stress once again the concept of averages and expanding your timeline for measured progress out from a day or week to at least a month-by-month view. The meal diaries for Ken and Kelly obviously represent a good – make that perfect – day. In real life, your ability to optimise your meal choices and caloric intake will be more difficult than the examples (based on some of my own favourite meals!) printed here.

I realise there will be days, and even longer periods, when you slip away from ideal. However, you can get back on track and even make up ground easily because of the metabolic leverage you create with Primal Blueprint eating habits. When your insulin production is moderated and your fat metabolism is optimised, you have a greatly reduced need to snack or even eat regular meals. As you'll see from my 72-hour personal journal panel in the next chapter, my own day-to-day caloric intake frequently varies by 250 per cent or more! I didn't even realise this until I completed the journals and evaluations for this book.

When your body has reprogrammed gene expression to be able to get energy from fat whenever it wants, hunger tends to subside and blood sugar and energy levels stabilise. Why not tap into this new 'skill' and take full advantage? You can not only easily make up lost ground when you slip a little, but you also accelerate the process of fat reduction to virtually whatever speed you want (up to the maximum mentioned previously) by engaging in a classic Primal strategy called *Intermittent Fasting* (IF).

Your choices of just when and how to practise IF should fit with your personality, lifestyle schedule and unique habits and preferences. Both meticulous planners and spontaneous types can succeed with these varying styles. I suggest trying a mixture of unplanned meal skipping combined with structured fasts of 12 to 24 hours, or even longer for devoted and experienced fasters. There are few rules or strict guidelines to follow with IF. Most readers will be well-served to simply break free of their habituation (does that sound nicer than 'addiction'?) to regimented mealtimes and other cultural traditions, such as always having dessert after dinner, eating until you are stuffed, or freaking out if you skip a meal.

Numerous studies show that IF offers a multitude of benefits, including lowered blood pressure, improved insulin sensitivity and glucose uptake, loss of body fat (obviously), a decrease in oxidative damage and even a kick start for tissue repair. I personally fast when I feel a disturbance in immune function, such as a sore throat or stuffy head, and feel that my recovery is quicker due to this practice. These benefits are achieved when certain genes are 'turned on' to repair specific tissues that would not otherwise be repaired in times of surplus. One could surmise that this genetic adaptation allows certain cells to live longer (as repaired cells) during famine because it's energetically less expensive to repair a cell than to divide and create a new one. That might help explain some of the phenomenal longevity results produced by studies on animals eating restricted-calorie diets. With mice, longevity continues to improve as calories are restricted by 10 per cent, 20 per cent, and even 50 per cent of normal.

IF has also been shown in animal studies to reduce spontaneous cancers in animal studies, which could be due to a decrease in oxidative damage or an increase in immune response. Pockets of research around the globe strongly suggest that deregulated meal timing and generally moderated caloric intake produce many health benefits (particularly for those who are overweight) and promote longevity with virtually no negative side-effects. How about that for an alternative to the zillion-dollar pharmaceutical and agricultural industries?

Whatever method of caloric restriction you engage in, the net effect is to send signals to your genes to up-regulate fat burning and down-regulate glucose burning, as well as to turbo-charge your body's calorie processing system. It's a similar dynamic to that invigorating feeling you get from a splash in cold water, an afternoon nap, or an intense workout. Your body likes to be stimulated and challenged with these brief, *natural, positive* stressors that fine-tune gene expression and numerous other functions and evolutionary skills. In contrast, your body rebels and weakens from chronic *artificial* stressors such as jet travel, working long hours indoors, pushing through a long, uncomfortable cardio workout, or eating until you are full three times a day for your entire life. Here is a quick overview of some ways you can achieve IF:

- **Skipping Meals:** Listen to your body carefully and you may discover that you're not always hungry when your regular mealtimes come around. Take advantage of this occasionally and skip or significantly delay a meal or two. You will learn to appreciate food even more when you use it to truly nourish and energise yourself, instead of habitually shoving stuff down the pipe just because it's six o'clock or because everyone else is partaking.
- **Condensed Eating Window:** Condense your daily food intake into a set period of four to seven hours, based on your preferences. This allows for a sustained fasting period until the next day, when you factor in sleep time.
- **Early and Late:** Enjoy an early-morning meal and a late-afternoon/early-evening meal. This is a good option for people who have stressful jobs or otherwise have difficulty carving out a relaxed time period for lunch in the middle of the day.
- **Planned Fast:** Enjoy dinner and then fast until the following evening (24 hours), or continue to fast until the next morning (about 36 hours). Many have success doing this once a week. You may want to start by trying it once a month and then work up to doing it more frequently. For a deeper cleansing effect, you can try an occasional alternating day fast that lasts for a week. You can

drink water, tea or small amounts of juice on your fasting days and eat normally – or almost normally – on your alternate days.

Regardless of what approach you use, be sure that you don't over-eat when you do sit down to meals. After a skipped meal or fasting period, you will be especially attuned to your body's hunger signals and satisfaction levels when you resume eating. Overeating is a largely psychological response to the anxiety of altering a familiar routine. Expert fasters typically ease out of their fast with several sparse meals to gently reengage the digestive system.

By seamlessly integrating IF into your Primal Blueprint eating routine, you will prove to your conscious brain that you can survive quite nicely without constantly needing food. This is easy to handle when you control insulin production with Primal Blueprint foods and really, really hard when you are entrenched in a typical American diet with lots of carbohydrates and insulin highs and lows. If you have tried fasting or skipping meals in the past but (as with Kelly Korg) concurrently ate a diet moderate to high in carbohydrates, you can likely relate to becoming irritable and exhausted when you miss even a single meal.

In my days as an endurance athlete I burned so many calories (and relied so heavily on carbohydrate to repeatedly refill the glycogen stores I drained on a daily basis), I'd feel like I was on the verge of a hypoglycaemic coma if I did so much as skip breakfast or otherwise failed to stuff my face several times a day. Now I marvel at how often I forget to eat – and the fact that doing so has no impact on my energy levels. That's the true power of shifting from being a sugarburner to becoming an efficient fat-burner.

I cannot emphasise enough the magic of this transformation. Freeing yourself from an addition to regular doses of energy from ingested calories is the essence of 'going Primal'. Experiencing these Primal 'symptoms' yourself ('Hey, I'm actually not hungry!') will recalibrate your entire belief system about food and meals. Or, as one friend of mine commented about his dropping excess body fat by eating Primally and being more sporadic with his meals, 'Hey, food is overrated!'

If you take a moment to reflect on the principles of evolution and homeostasis, it's clear how messed up our modern eating culture is. It should not be this hard for humans to sustain daily energy levels and optimal body composition, we just make it hard by constantly pumping our bodies with foods that we have not adapted to eat. Eat Primally for 21 days to allow your genes to up-regulate fat burning mechanisms and get used to moderated insulin levels, then start playing around with Intermittent Fasting. I promise that you will experience this epiphany: that you are eating in the way evolution designed you to (perhaps for the first time since you were an infant) and that it is easy and fun and leads to incredible breakthroughs in the frustrating challenge of fat loss and long-term weight management.

WEIGHT-LOSS TROUBLESHOOTING

If you are making a sincere effort to drop body fat with the Primal Blueprint and are not satisfied with your results, here are some suggestions as to how you can alter your routine and which issues you should investigate further to find out what might be tripping you up.

GET INTO THE SWEET SPOT AND STAY THERE!

When you limit your carbohydrates to 100 to 150 grams per day, you can pretty much maintain your weight and body composition indefinitely. You will probably even experience a gradual and sustained reduction of body fat if you come from eating a typical Western diet of double or triple that many carbohydrates and carry a bit, or a lot, of excess fat. However, if the fat is not coming off quickly enough after a month or two of Primal Blueprint efforts, the best remedy is to tighten the reins even further over your carbohydrate intake and stay in the sweet spot for several weeks.

While you may experience difficulty adjusting to the severe reduction of dietary 'staples' (e.g. grains and pleasure foods, including sweetened beverages and snacks), your body will quickly adapt to an eating style that is aligned with your genes. Yes, I know, getting your carbohydrates down to 50 to 100 grams a day is easier said than done. It is on this issue that many people get stuck in the mode of 'trying' to cut back instead of making a firm commitment to modify their habitual intake of certain foods and replace them with ample servings of foods that are more nutritious and technically more satisfying to your body than your favourite carbohydrate treats. For what it's worth, some investigators believe Grok's average daily intake of carbohydrates was as low as 80 grams per day for months on end – and he thrived on that!

Keep in mind that there are days when your carbohydrate intake will go well above 100 or even 150 grams, thanks to the reality of prevalent carbohydrate choices and cultural traditions that can entice you away from a strict Primal Blueprint eating style. It will require great discipline to maintain an average of 50 to 100 grams (remember, most of us are accustomed to throwing down 300 grams per day or even more), but you only have to do it for a short time, say a month or two, depending on your starting point and how ambitious your goals are. By 'great discipline' I'm not talking about suffering with a cloud of anguish and guilt hanging over your head; it's more like, 'Eat reasonably generous amounts of eggs, meat, chicken, fish, nuts and seeds, plus all the vegetables you want and fruits (with a little bit of restraint and selectivity), and stay away from all grains and processed foods.'

If you find yourself struggling to meet your weight-loss goals, I strongly recommend using an online food calculator so that you know exactly where you stand instead of 'guessing'. I find the mere act of having to write down everything I eat for two days increases my awareness of dietary habits and provides an effective check and balance against idle grazing or overeating when awareness is low. Chart everything you eat for a few days and then enter the results on a site such as paleotrack.com or FitDay.com to get a truly accurate indication of where your carbohydrate intake is. Even today, with what I consider a pretty decent knowledge of the macronutrient content of many foods, I continue to be surprised at some of the results that the online calculators spit out when I input my data.

MODERATE STRESS LEVELS

Body fat reduction simply doesn't work well when you are skimping on sleep, working too hard, or experiencing high levels of emotional and psychological stress. Scientific research is validating the connection between things like lack of sleep and hormone levels that hamper fat metabolism or increase appetite. To succeed long term with changing your body composition, you must have the time, energy and patience to devote great attention and care to the topic. Rushing through meals or reaching for sweet foods when you are stressed is not aligned with the simple lifestyle of the Primal Blueprint.

While the insulin control and intense sprint sessions might be the more exciting elements of the Primal Blueprint weight-loss plan, you should not discount the importance of the supporting lifestyle elements that can make or break your success. Getting enough sleep (including naps, which trigger positive hormone flow, balanced appetite, more energy for and faster recovery from exercise) and sunshine (vitamin D enhances all cellular function, including fat metabolism), playing, relaxing and using your brain will assist your weight-loss goals on many levels. It's time to start walking your talk, stop burning the candle at both ends and make the right choices to allow your genes to express themselves optimally. When you follow the laws of the Primal Blueprint, the weight you want to lose will come off naturally.

ADOPT A POSITIVE MINDSET

I believe there is a bigger picture to observe that involves optimism, positive thoughts and enjoyment of the process when you pursue body composition changes.

The subject of body composition is laden with failure, deprivation, restriction, self-limiting beliefs ('I have the fat gene') and superficial judgement from society. Here's a sampling of *Shape* magazine article teasers: 'Cellulite Solution', 'Firm Your Trouble Spots', 'Get Flat Abs By 1 August; Firmer, Sexier Buns in One Move'). It's critical to approach the subject with a positive attitude and an appreciation for the process. Your primary motivation must be to enjoy a higher quality of life and better health. The by-product of a change in body composition is not something to obsess about, measure and judge as success or failure each day or each week, but instead to experience effortlessly as a consequence of lifestyle change driven by higher ideals than wanting to look good in a bikini for your summer holiday (although there is nothing wrong with that goal).

ACCEPT YOUR PLATEAUS, THEN CARRY ON – PRIMALLY

After a few months of progress, you often arrive at a frustrating point where the weight stops coming off, the sustained run of high energy levels fizzles a bit or you stop building extra muscle. That makes sense from an evolutionary perspective, because the body is so well tuned to adapt to any situation. Even with carefully restricted carbohydrate intake, your body may react to a sustained period of fat loss by taking subtle actions to drift closer towards homeostasis. For example, genes could 'down-regulate' insulin receptors and other metabolic systems in the interest of preserving fat – a crucial survival mechanism that has been in place for millions of years. In many cases, this plateau is just an example of the body saying, 'I like this new weight. It's easy to maintain, I have more energy all the time and I never get sick.'

Accept that your genetically ideal weight might be a bit higher percentage of body fat than a magazine cover model, and that there is nothing wrong with that. You might decide that it's not really worth the additional effort and focus to go beyond your 'healthy, energetic, comfortable weight' to your ultimate ripped weight. Accept that plateaus are going to happen and exercise a little patience when you reach them. Weight loss does not happen in a linear manner; there are simply too many variables and homeostatic forces at work. When I say you can 'average a pound or two a week' of fat loss, I'd like you to consider this statement with a four- or six-month timeline attached. I know we are conditioned to a 'what have you done for me lately' mentality, but we are dealing with lifestyle change here, not journal entries of happy faces or frowns each day based on your scale numbers or food calculator graphs and charts.

I guarantee you that making some elementary Primal changes (e.g., eliminating grains from your diet to regulate your carbohydrate intake at below 100 grams per day average; adjusting your exercise programme to refrain from Chronic Cardio and adding some brief, intense sessions to the mix) will result in a certain amount of effortless weight loss. However, there is a range of outcomes based upon individual factors (e.g. compliance rate as discussed in Troubleshooting, life stress levels and how long and how severely you have diverted from Primal Blueprint laws before embarking on this journey). A female might effortlessly go from 185 pounds to 152 in six months, at which point she might long to drop into the 140s but find the process a bit more difficult.

One of my favourite sayings – whether it has to do with business, fitness or balancing the varied demands and responsibilities of daily life – is: 'If it were easy, everyone would be doing it.' There is a reason why you don't see 80 per cent of American adults sporting single-digit body fat or dozens of joggers flying by in the park at a pace of six minutes per mile. If you are unsatisfied with your results after months of devoted effort, refer to the Troubleshooting tips and consider making an increased commitment to achieve superior results. Rest assured that there are no mysteries involved here, or even much of the genetic 'good luck' that we are so conditioned to believe is important. It's all up to you, and how you can direct your genes to do the right thing.

AVOIDING THE THREE BIGGEST REASONS FOR WEIGHT LOSS FAILURE

1. Lack of awareness and/or lack of commitment to actually moderate your carbohydrate intake to 'sweet spot' levels. If it turns out from your online pie graph results that you have been a little loosey-goosey here and there, I promise you that even a few days of Primal-style low-carbohydrate eating will cause noticeable changes in your appetite and an increase in your energy level – and lead you on the path to the promised land. Start your day tomorrow with a Primal Omelette and notice how your inclination to snack in the hours afterwards is eliminated. Keep the momentum going with a Primal Salad for lunch, followed by a meat and vegetable dinner, and you'll see how these (and many other) Primal Blueprint-approved meals leverage one another to get you off the carbohydrate/insulin/stress-response/sugar-craving cycle and into round-the-clock fat burning.

2. Failure to stock up on Pimal Blueprint-approved foods. Dropping from several hundred grams of carbohydrates down to a range of 80 essentially means you can eliminate the foods that once served as major energy sources (albeit very poor, quick-burning sources) throughout your day. If you have no logs around (filling, nutritious, long-burning food) and your flame is petering out, your reaction might naturally be to fan the flames with wads of newspaper (cheap carbohydrates). Make absolutely sure that you stock your home, car, office and backpack with Primal Blueprint-approved snacks. (Including my favourites mentioned in the Chapter 4 panel. The Primal Approved – At a Glance panel at the end of the book summarises healthy eating choices and also what foods to avoid.) Reach for these any time you need an energy boost or feel a sugar craving coming on.

3. Lack of awareness/commitment to Primal Blueprint-style exercise programme. Many exercisers are unaware of their working heart rates and the effect they have on metabolic rate and stress levels. Because the perceived exertion of aerobic exercise (75 per cent or less of maximum heart rate) is extremely moderate, most exercisers (again, misguided by conventional wisdom) equate significant exertion – suffering – with getting in shape. Walk through the room of a typical Spinning or Step class or along the window line-up of cardio machines at an urban health club and note the suffering etched on the faces of the participants. Even America's devoted exercisers – a culturally elite anomaly in the world's fattest, most sedentary nation – are quite often burning sugar and tiring themselves out through their well-meaning efforts. Remember: exercise is about the movement, not the calories burned.

CHAPTER SUMMARY

- **Primal Weight Loss:** You can lose one to two pounds of body fat per week (one-half to one kilogram) by targeting optimal intake levels of each daily macronutrient, fasting intermittently, doing Primal Blueprint-style workouts and approaching the challenge with a positive, process-oriented, big picture attitude.

- **Macronutrients:** Adequate protein intake – 0.7 to one gram per pound (.33 to .5 grams per kg) of lean body mass, depending on activity level – will preserve muscle tissue (and metabolism) during calorie-restriction efforts, avoiding the 'crash and burn' effect of most diets. Maintaining the 'sweet spot' of 50 to 100 grams of carbohydrates per day will moderate insulin production and allow stored body fat to be your primary energy source. Fat intake will be the main variable to ensure you are satisfied and nourished at each meal, making your weight-loss efforts effective, realistic and even enjoyable.

- **Korgs' Weight Loss:** Ken and Kelly Korg can achieve their ambitious fat-reduction goals eating delicious, nutritious Primal Blueprint-style meals. When the carbohydrate intake sweet spot is observed and protein requirements are met, ample amounts of fat will provide a high satiety factor at meals but will not result in excess fat storage, thanks to low insulin levels.

- **Exercise:** Exercise can complement the main variable of optimal macronutrient intake to support and accelerate weight-loss success. Increase low-level activity, make hard workouts harder (and maybe even shorter, if you've been in a chronic pattern), and understand that the commitment to changing your body requires focus and dedication.

- **Intermittent Fasting:** IF, whether deliberate or as a natural course of fluctuating mealtimes (now that stored body fat instead of ingested carbohydrates is your preferred energy source), will create natural caloric deficits that lead to fat reduction and effortless long-term maintenance of ideal body composition. You can engage in IF by skipping meals, eating in a condensed window of time, eating morning and night but not in between, or engaging in planned fasts lasting for 24 hours or more.

- **Troubleshooting:** If your progress slows, try being more diligent in hitting the carbohydrate intake sweet spot (use an online nutrient calculator to know exactly where you stand), moderating your life stress levels (put into practice the Primal Blueprint lifestyle laws), adopting a positive mindset, and realising that plateaus in your progress rate are natural and acceptable, thanks to your body's innate desire for homeostasis.

CHAPTER 9

CONCLUSION

TIME TO PARTY LIKE A GROK STAR

'A person will sometimes devote all his life to the development of one part of his body; the wishbone.'
ROBERT FROST

As we near the end of the book, I want to call attention to the special place in my heart that Chapter 2, 'Grok and Korg', occupies. I've been fascinated by the Primal concept for nearly two decades. (I self-published my *Training and Racing Duathlons* book using the name Primal Urge Press in 1988!) As an athlete and a coach, I've reflected on the Primal theme constantly, inspiring athletes to balance the unnatural act of endurance training with proper recovery and life-style support and to temper our competitive human instincts with common sense to avoid burnout.

My work in the fields of nutrition and personal training and my immersion into the health community on the Internet have enlightened me about the realities of everyday modern life for the masses. While society is making progress in some ways, I am increasingly disturbed by the seemingly inexorable drift further and further away from natural, healthy, evolutionary behaviour in the techno-logical world.

As my staff and I worked through the stages of Chapter 2 – conceptual, research, first draft, editing, soliciting external feedback and revisions – I finally had the chance to print a fresh copy of the text, sit on a lounge chair in my yard and truly 'read' the material for the first time. I have to admit I was downright horrified. I questioned whether people would think the commentary was sensational or unrealistic and be turned off accordingly. So I returned to my computer, reviewed all the references, connected more research and generally made darn sure this was an accurate and realistic picture of modern life.

Unfortunately, the draft withstood my own devil's advocate scrutiny as well as that of numerous health, medical, nutrition, psychology and sociology experts. Family and career men in their 40s and 50s take prescriptions left and right, families frequently feel that life is too hectic and stressful to align with the broad definition of *health*, and teenagers often feel overpressured and disconnected from parents. Today's kids have too much body fat and too little physical fitness. We eat too much beige stuff and not enough green stuff. We avoid exercise and sit at desks all day staring at a screen in the name of increased productivity. We go home at night and stare at a bigger screen in the name of relaxation. We stay up too late and then awake to the stressful screech of an alarm clock. We are stressed by bills, traffic, air, noise, digital pollution, the past, the future and all kinds of anxiety that we manufacture in our restless minds. Our first line of defence when our genes react as they are programmed to by these lifestyle habits is to reach for prescription drugs, which treat symptoms quickly but, over time, weaken our natural ability to achieve homeostasis.

As we bombard our genes with these lifestyle risk factors, they respond the only way they know how to, in an often futile attempt to maintain homeostasis and a desperate effort to keep us alive in the short term: with inflammation, early cell death, insulin resistance, atrophy and so on. If you consider the dietary habits, activity level and body composition of your family 'above average' for Americans, you can congratulate yourself while remembering that 'average' is actually borderline obese (64 per cent of American adults are classified as overweight, of which one-third are classified as obese).

In California, 40 per cent of 10-year-old schoolchildren fail to attain a bare minimum aerobic conditioning performance stand-ard known as the Healthy Fitness Zone (established by the Cooper Aerobics Institute), meaning that hundreds of thousands of 'average' kids in California (what I consider to be a progressive, fair-weather state with a population arguably fitter than that found in the United States as a whole) are technically classified as 'at risk' of develop-ing serious health problems related to inactivity because they can't complete a mile run at a slow jog. *40 per cent!* Take a big fat zero off that figure and I think you'd approximate the relevant statistic during the time of my youth.

As we reflect on how far we have drifted from Grok's simple life-style and ponder how we can better honour and reprogramme our genes by following the Primal Blueprint, it is critical to proceed with a clean slate and a deep conviction that you are doing the right thing. This is not an easy task; numerous elements of the Primal Blueprint flat out oppose the mainstream dogma that the Western governments espouse, or that big pharmaceutical companies promote at the expense of billions of advertising and marketing dollars.

One must also wonder how society has strayed so egregiously far from the healthy living that Grok devolved to the carbohydrate-overdosed, pill-popping, overfed, overweight, overstressed Ken Korg. How can the conventional wisdom that you have believed for years and decades, have read about in respected publications, or have heard because it has been handed down from trusted elders be wrong and even dangerous? The truth is, human nature is to blame. Just like Grok, we have programmed into our genes a desire to manipulate and rule our environment for our benefit; to pursue a more advanced, more comfortable life. Our indomitable human spirit has accomplished many great things but it has also created tremendous fallout from our constant quest for 'progress'.

Man has conquered the world; as a species, he is the fat cat, he is on top of the heap. Yet now, peak physical and intellectual performance and self-discipline are no longer requirements for survival. Man has become self-indulgent and has reverted to behaviours that provide short-term gratification. Like the miners who stripped and poisoned the land and water during the gold rush, we have committed a similar crime with regards to our bodies in the name of making life easier, more convenient and more productive.

In Eric Schlosser's *Fast Food Nation*, he reveals how the fast-food phenomenon exploded in popularity because this sort of food made life easier. No more cooking or lengthy waits for expensive meals, now everyone can live the good life by dining out on delicious food! Unfortunately, the fare served up was disastrous not only to the human body but also to the human spirit, destroying a centrepiece of family fabric that was the shared, home-cooked meal.

When there is interest and demand to make life easier, profit seekers often swarm in and exploit this element of the human spirit. Nowhere is this more evident than in my own field of health. While I am all in favour of capitalism and making a profit, it seems that where health is concerned we have allowed forces to run amok to the extent that today we must question the approach, motives and trustworthiness of many of the traditional pillars of health, human compassion and expert medical knowledge.

We must admit that doctors, despite their extensive knowledge, training and loyalty to the Hippocratic Oath, are focused on treatment rather than prevention. As with drugs, it's wonderful to have extensively trained and prepared doctors standing ready when we need them. The sad reality is that most of them are so busy dealing with illness there's little time for prevention. This means their business comes from dealing with the symptoms, not the causes, of easily preventable conditions (as evidenced by the remarkable comment from a solo family practice doctor I know, who lamented that his 'business was down' due to America's 2008 economic recession!). The fact that doctors receive so little training in nutrition is nothing short of abysmal. Our government's nutrition policies and diet education efforts (grain-heavy Department of Health Eatwell plate, anyone?) are seemingly driven by poorly informed scientists who misinterpret research, and I am suspicious of the impact lobbyists for the meat, grain and dairy industries have on this. In the media, the historical checks and balances provided by the impartial investigative journalist have been deemphasised and devalued by giant profit-driven corporations. Salacious stories that elicit fear, anger or other strong emotions are what sell, regardless of their legitimacy. Even our educational community experiences free market influences that potentially bias the objectivity and even the premise of many studies.

THE KORG KOMEBACK

Let me reiterate my distaste for a perfectionist mentality towards diet, physical appearance, lifestyle change and even school, career and competitive athletics. Respecting the broad definition of health and the legacy of the simple lifestyle that our ancestors lived, we need to reject the measuring and judging forces of society and pursue fun and peace of mind in conjunction with health and fitness goals.

Admittedly, the comprehensive and emphatic nature of the Primal Blueprint might seem intimidating, and your efforts to go Primal will possibly require some serious departures from and adjustments to your comfortable modern existence. If you feel overwhelmed or take occasional exception to my strong positions (e.g. 'Everything in moderation, including moderation'), keep in mind my 80 Per Cent Rule as well as the suggestion to take one step at a time.

While the Korgs seem quite far down a disastrous road, they can also easily turn things around, step by step. No, they are not going to be perfect anytime soon, but they will be happier, healthier and fitter with minimal pain, suffering, negativity or disruption of the things they love to do in life. If Ken modifies his late-night activities by snacking on macadamia nuts instead of cheesecake, watching less television in favour of reading or a quick stroll around the block with the dog; and turning the lights out at 10:30pm instead of midnight, he'll fall asleep more easily and wake up refreshed the next morning, without having to rely on Ambien. This means more quality time with the kids, including walking young Cindy to school.

If Ken brings the macadamias, some carrot sticks for snacks at work and chooses lunch wisely at the supermarket deli (one-third pound of sliced beef stuffed inside a red bell pepper costs less than Chinese buffet), he'll maintain stable energy levels all day long, increase his productivity and be better able to handle workplace stress. Ken could then leave the office at 6pm feeling ready to enjoy and appreciate the leisure and family time options that await him.

If Kelly reduces the stress of her exercise programme and eats delicious, satisfying Primal Blueprint meals, she will get her blood sugar and energy levels under control and tap into her stored body fat for a steady, reliable source of energy. And as for the younger Korgs, with a few sensible and consistently enforced limits on digital entertainment and bedtimes, Kenny can reconnect with the family, focus better in school and consider the option to stop taking his medication.

Talk about little things making a big difference! There is no better example to illustrate this maxim than the momentum (particularly the unbridled increase in physical energy) created by healthy lifestyle changes begetting further healthy lifestyle changes. If all you do after reading this book is cut way back on grains, you will still dramatically improve your health. With more stable energy levels and better immune function, your dietary alteration could trigger an increased interest in exercise. Equally, if all you do after reading this book is simply back off your taxing jogs and step classes in favour of long hikes, brief neighbourhood strolls and the occasional sprint workout, you'll have more energy and less cravings for carbohydrates, which will likely lead to improved dietary habits and general health. Forget diet and exercise for a moment; if you took only four letters of the entire book to heart and added more *play* to your busy life, this could still stand as one of the most important, life-changing things you ever do.

ON YOUR OWN

Opening our eyes to the direction in which the bullet train carrying modern society is heading is sobering to say the least. In my opinion, the heaviest realisation of all is that *you are on your own*. The imagined safety net of government, modern medicine or the food or pharmaceutical industries looking after your health is a façade. Oh sure, you'll be cared for very, very well if something catastrophic happens – whether it's a high-risk childbirth, serious injuries from a car accident, or one of the small fraction of cancers that are not lifestyle related – but when it comes to eating healthily, getting in shape, avoiding stupid mistakes and even building a career and a nest egg – the world can lead you astray and separate you from your cash (and other assets, such as health, sanity, etc.) in the blink of an eye.

A discernible pattern emerges when I relate the story of Grok to friends and casual acquaintances. After first expressing disbelief that Grok was leaner, stronger and healthier than modern humans, most are captivated by the story of his uncomplicated life and the 10 surprisingly simple behavioural laws that dictated his (our) evolution. After a few moments of silence to absorb the information, people then commonly call attention to the most unpleasant aspects of Grok's life – a surreptitious way of asserting their superiority over some vulnerable, primitive caveman.

It seems we are scared of what's beyond our comfort zone of comfort foods, conventional wisdom, typical exercise routines, the prospect of wasting time with unstructured play, and the rest. We have a tendency to get in our own way, manufacturing self-limiting beliefs and knee-jerk defence mechanisms when confronted with our frailties or the prospects of lifestyle change.

THE ELITIST RACE

Recently, I read with amusement the occasional critiques of the Primal Blueprint eating style, as being 'elitist' – too expensive [eschewing inexpensive grains and switching from commercial animals and plants to the pasture-raised or organic variety] and impractical for the average person to follow. Furthermore, astute observers point out that there are not enough local, pasture-raised animal products or organic produce 'to sustain our society at its current population.' My gut reaction is, 'You're damn straight it's an elitist diet!' Expensive? Depends on your perspective. Eating Primal Blueprint style for the rest of your life is much cheaper than long-term prescription drug regimes or extensive doctor visits or hospital stays for cardiac bypass surgery or cancer treatments.

The evolutionary theme pops into mind here. Our increasingly sedate modern life disguises the fact that the concept of survival of the fittest still permeates our being. Competition is everywhere in the world, with human nature programmed for '*Citius, Altius, Fortius*' – the Olympic Games motto (in Latin) meaning 'faster, higher, stronger'. Make no mistake, we are in a competition with a massive number of entrants worldwide to achieve good health and prosperity. Economically, you need only glance through Fareed Zakaria's *The Post American World* to see the writing on the wall for the world's leading superpower. America is heading steadily down the pop charts while larger, hungrier, more strategically minded societies, such as China and India, will soon catch up and surpass our economy. (Poor investment in education and technology in favour of billions spent on the military are some key reasons for our impending downfall, according to Zakaria.) Imagine if all the money recently spent on bank bailouts had been channelled into diet, fitness and health education!

Over the past century of rapid technological progress, we've figured out how to manufacture and package food and mass produce animals, producing huge profits without regard to the health, humane or environmental consequences. Stepping back for a moment to grab a wide-angle view of the wide angles in the buffet line at a Vegas casino, it's evident how ridiculously out of control this situation has become. No offence, but America looks like one giant yard of fattened cattle ready for slaughter, complete with a significant percentage of 'downers' (a term for sick cattle that can't stand up; they are dragged with giant hooks to slaughter).

In comparison, being 'elitist' doesn't seem bad at all. Theoretically, if everyone wanted wild salmon and organic strawberries we would indeed run out in the short term (however, demand would also stimulate increased production, thereby changing the world one person at a time through the power of our wallets). Right now, the race is on and you are welcome to participate. So suck it up and pay for the pasture-raised animal products at the farmers' market, and organic leafy greens, especially if you are pregnant or have a two-year-old in his most crucial brain-development stage. Come to think of it, make that especially if you are *not* pregnant; are age 20, 30, 40 or 50 and have an interest in enjoying a long, healthy, happy life.

'When it comes to eating right and exercising, there is no "I'll start tomorrow." Tomorrow is disease.'
V. L. ALLINEARE

'I put a dollar in one of those change machines. Nothing changed.'
GEORGE CARLIN, AMERICAN COMEDIAN/WRITER

AROUND THE WORLD (OR AT LEAST TO DALLAS AND BACK) IN 72 HOURS

I'm often asked by interested readers at my MarksDailyApple.com posts to reveal my life-style 'secrets'. The truth is, I'm short on secrets but big on guidelines and practical tips that will help you successfully navigate the particulars of your daily life, including the innumerable challenges to being Primal that we face in the modern world. Because the Primal Blueprint is a blueprint and not a regime, what I do has less relevance to your success than *what you like to do*. That said, I hope my real-life experiences give you some perspective that I'm a regular guy trying to raise a family, make a living, achieve peak health and fitness levels, forage Primal foods in a modern world and, most of all, enjoy the heck out of my life.

The exercise of keeping an accurate journal for 72 hours to produce this panel helped me realise that even the times when I slip from ideal are no big deal. When 'stuff happens' to take you off track, it's a great opportunity to develop your 'go with the flow' skills, staying positive and relaxed instead of stressed. Consider the following example from my Tuesday journal where my teenage son Kyle called me, begging for a ride to the valley to see friends while I was en route to the gym for a precious final workout before a business trip. My 30 minutes of captive teen audience time in the car was a far more precious experience than yet another workout.

Furthermore, when I was driving home alone after dropping Kyle off, ruminating about my missed workout, I realised that the concept of *hormone manipulation* supersedes the need to nail all of your food choices and workout goals every single day. When you direct insulin, glucagon, cortisol, testosterone, growth hormone and other agents in the correct pathways by following the Primal Blueprint, you can easily handle the unexpected because you have built a healthy, efficient foundation. A little sugar here, a few missed workouts there, or an occasional sleep-deficient sleep can be effortlessly righted with, respectively, low-carbohydrate follow-up meals, a maximum-intensity workout and a power nap! Likely you can attest to the phenomenon of returning from an extended exercise absence (due to illness, vacation or whatever) and picking up right where you left off – or performing even better, thanks to the rest.

The Primal Blueprint message that you can achieve robust health and ideal body composition without obsessive calorie restriction or exhausting exercise is the best takeaway lesson I can offer from sharing my routine. I regulate my carbohydrate intake naturally by simply avoiding sugars, grains and other processed foods. It's no trouble, because by all measures I enjoy a satisfying – you could even say indulgent – diet. I engage in an average of a few brief, intense exercise sessions per week that deliver the precise signals my body needs to stay strong and lean, with minimal time commitment. I also have occasional extended stretches where I do embarrassingly little – and nothing bad happens! And then there are weeks when my body and mind are geared up to exercise many consecutive days in a row; when I am enjoying every minute of being in the gym, sprinting on the beach or hiking the trails — and so I'll go a week or so without a single day of rest.

I follow the Primal Blueprint lifestyle laws naturally, thanks to family, friends, a lifelong appreciation of the outdoors, a stimulating career and a positive attitude – one that I've worked hard to cultivate over the years. I've seen the alternatives and travelled a long, long way down that marathon road to nowhere, the vicious cycle of a carbohydrate-based, sugar-burning, fat-storage diet, the struggle-and-suffer approach to fitness goals and the inevitable anxiety and disappointment that come from such a tenuous approach. Here then are my journal entries for a three-day stretch from January 2009, featuring a business trip to Dallas bookended by typical weekdays at home in Malibu.

TUESDAY: TRAVEL DAY

6.30am: Wake up and drink a large cup of strong coffee with heavy cream. Read the paper (almost finish *LA Times* crossword puzzle; Law Number 10, natch!). Move to desk and answer emails, blog and pack for afternoon flight to Dallas.

10.15am: Down protein shake (30 grams protein powder and 17 grams net carbohydrates). Head to the gym for quick workout.

10.30am: En route to gym, Kyle calls me begging for a ride to the valley (gotta love winter break!). Return home, pick up Kyle.

11.30am: Return from valley trip with no time for workout or lunch. Depart for LAX and 3:00 pm flight to Dallas. Can you say, 'Been there, done that'? I've flown this route 150-plus times in the last 10 years. Destination: a suburban television studio (I've never once been to downtown Dallas; I hear it's nice) to tape regular appearances on my friend Doug Kaufmann's show – *Know the Cause* – a nationally distributed daily cable talk show on health and nutrition.

8.00pm: (6:00pm PST): Check into hotel, enjoy leisurely dinner at Outback Steakhouse (flank steak with asparagus and red wine, hold the potato). Time change contributes to late bedtime of 11:30pm.

Elapsed time stuck in metal boxes today = about six hours (counting drive to and from valley and to airport – featuring traffic jam on Pacific Coast Hwy – shuttle bus rides and a three-hour flight).

Tuesday Micronutrient Calculations:

- Coffee, heavy cream
- Protein shake (1.5 servings of Primal Fuel protein powder)
- Apple
- Flank steak (175g/6oz), asparagus, red wine
- FitDay.com Analysis
- Total calories: 774
- Protein: 88g, 352 calories (41 per cent)
- Carbohydrates: 56g, 224 calories (24 per cent)
- Fat: 22g, 198 calories (22 per cent)

WEDNESDAY: DALLAS DAY

7.00am: Wake-up call comes after not sleeping well (hate it when that happens). Turn on early news and conduct short, intense Primal routine (one-minute rest between exercises):

3 × 60 pushups, 3 × 35 squats, 3 × 25 abbreviated dips between armchair and coffee table, 3 × 60-second abs planks. Elapsed time from first effort to stepping in the shower: 17 minutes.

8.00am: Breakfast of four-egg chile-chicken omelette at IHOP. Extra sour cream and Cholula hot sauce. Try as they might (and they try hard), they still can't get me to take the pancakes (or toast or English muffin) that come free with the order. Coffee with cream and packet of sugar.

9.00am: Arrive at studio for four to five hours of taping. Drink a couple bottles of water (the most water I drink all week!) just to keep my vocal chords lubed.

2.30pm: Late lunch with the production team. All the ribs you can eat (which isn't all that much) and iced tea at a local rib joint. I'd prefer a salad bar, but this is where the crew wants to eat and we are in Texas, so who am I to say no? Skip the mashed potatoes, potato salad, corn, cornbread, apple-sauce and bug juice, thus relieving my system of well over 200 grams of carbohydrates in one fell swoop.

4.00pm–5.00pm: Walk the Irving Mall (low-level aerobic activity) and make phone calls the whole time. Head to airport.

6.00pm: Dinner at TGI Friday's (in the terminal) – pecan-crusted chicken salad and a glass of cabernet. One of my favourite travel meals. Board plane, fly home.

Wednesday Micronutrient Calculations:

- Coffee with cream and packet of sugar
- Four-egg chilli-chicken omelette, extra sour cream and Cholula hot sauce
- Ribs (6 ounces/175 grams) and iced tea
- Pecan-crusted chicken salad and glass of cabernet

- FitDay.com Analysis

- Total calories: 2,087

- Protein: 153g, 612 calories (29 per cent)

- Carbohydrates: 92g, 368 calories (17 per cent)

- Fat: 123g, 1,107 calories (50 per cent)

Note: this was a long day of hard work, but even with the three sit-down meals, I ate fewer calories than I normally do. I often use travelling as a great opportunity to engage in Intermittent Fasting. Because the food options on the road are generally inferior or difficult to find, I hone my foraging skills and look for nothing but protein and vegetables.

THURSDAY: MALIBU DAY

7.30am: Wake up and shake off the effects of jet lag with a quick plunge in the pool (I'd estimate low-60s temp) and a coffee with cream. Head to desk to catch up.

10.00am: Down four-egg omelette, sprinkled mozzarella cheese, sliced mushrooms and green peppers, topped with sliced avocado and a scoop of fresh salsa. Back to desk.

11.00am: Head to gym for a 'pull and sprint day':

4 sets of cable rows, starting at 20 reps at 100 pounds and adding 10 pounds per set.

10 × 10–15 reps of wide -grip pull-ups, with as little rest as possible (maybe a minute between).

4 × 15 inverted rows, (sort of an inverted pull-up).

3 sets of two-arm cable curls) while in squat.

Jog to car, drive to beach to catch low tide. Three-minute dynamic stretching warm-up drills, followed by 10 barefoot sprint sets (each consisting of jog 10 complete strides, transition to run 12 complete strides, transition to sprint 15 strides all-out), one-minute rest between. Easy jog to cool down, followed by brief 'Grok Squat' stretch. Gym and beach total time: 50 minutes. Head home and shower.

1.00pm: Make my world-famous Primal Big Ass Salad (check video at MarksDailyApple.com) with 12 veggies and a scoop of canned salmon, drenched in olive oil-based dressing. Nothing to drink. Granny Smith apple for dessert. Back to work in the office.

4.00pm: Handful of macadamia nuts and break from desk to throw tennis ball to a very old, very slow yellow lab named Buddha. En route back to desk, a challenge is issued by my son, Kyle. Challenge accepted. Detour from office to garage for a battle royale championship match on Wii Rock Band. Obtain perfect score of 100 on Rock Band vocals to reign supreme in Sisson family (PB Law Number 7, Play ... and kinda Law Number 9, Avoid Stupid Mistakes!).

7.30pm: Grass-fed steak, three cups of steamed broccoli dripping in real butter, glass of merlot. Okay, one more. Doesn't get any better than that!

8.30pm: Watch TiVo replay of our favourite 30-minute sitcom, followed by 60-minute ESPN Sports Center broadcast. Watch both broadcasts in only 52 minutes total.

10.00pm: Five-minute outdoor walk with Buddha, retire to bed for some pleasure reading. Lights out, and out like a light, at 10.30pm.

Thursday Micronutrient Calculations:

- Coffee with cream
- Four-egg omelette with sprinkled mozzarella cheese, sliced mushrooms and green peppers, topped with sliced avocado and a scoop of fresh salsa
- Primal Big Ass Salad
- Granny Smith apple
- Handful of macadamias
- Grass-fed steak (10 ounces/300 grams), three cups of steamed broccoli dripping in real butter
- Two glasses of merlot

- FitDay.com Analysis
- Total calories: 2,676
- Protein: 168g, 672 calories (25 per cent)
- Carbohydrates: 108g, 432 calories (15 per cent)
- Fat: 170g, 1,530 calories (57 per cent)

AVERAGE OVER THREE DAYS
(Allows for rounding margin of error)

Calories: 1,842

Protein: 136g, 544 calories (38 per cent)

Carbohydrates: 86g, 344 calories (18.5 per cent)

Fat: 106g, 954 calories (51 per cent)

RETHINKING YOUR GOALS

You may have noticed in the tips throughout the book that I empha-sise the long-term approach and the enjoyment of the *process* of healthy lifestyle change. In discussing weight loss, I take great pains to position this eventuality as a *byproduct* of healthy eating, exer-cise and lifestyle habits. We must reflect on the importance of this distinction because we are so conditioned to approaching lifestyle goals with a short-term, results-oriented approach.

We wear heart-rate monitors and use GPS technology to provide objective data about whether we are reaching our goals – or failing. We use fancy training logs to record every possible bit of information about our workouts (such as time, distance, strength-training reps, calories burned – even 'shoe mileage!' [to determine when to buy a new pair]. We strain, struggle and suffer to obtain predetermined times, paces and distances of our workouts, thinking that our bodies and spirits will actually appreciate a robotic approach to fitness.

Consider for a moment the possibility that setting and pursuing goals is screwing us up more than it's helping. We live in a superficial world where everything we do is measured and judged, and success (and often happiness) is thus defined by what we accomplish and accumulate, rather than what kind of character we have. For athletes, the world hits us with, 'How far did you run?' 'What was your time?' 'What place did you take in the race?' 'Did you beat your previous time or your opponent?' All these interrogations typically come before the more relevant questions we should ask ourselves about a workout or race: how about, 'Did you have fun?' or, when my son and his volleyball team lose a competition and thereby admit it wasn't much fun, I might ask, 'Was it a positive experience? Did you learn and grow as a team, as an athlete and as a person through a hard-fought battle – even though it ended in defeat?'

My fervent desire to achieve my athletic goals – to run in the Olympic trials, average 100-mile weeks and beat my training partners – ruined my physical health and my running career. When I returned to competition as a triathlete, I had a more relaxed attitude. I enjoyed the challenge of a new sport and pushing the limits of human endurance, just for the heck of it. Gun-shy from my injury history, I adopted a more relaxed approach. I listened to the signals from my body and backed off when energy levels declined or aches and pains crept up. I enjoyed longer, slower bike rides into the mountains, connecting with nature and enjoying a sense of adventure in exploring new routes. I built my fitness in a comfortable manner and felt refreshed, energised and inspired about my training – a far cry from the out-and-out suffering I endured from recurring intense running sessions with a fit pack of training partners. Lo and behold, with my casual approach I became the fourth fastest Hawaii Ironman triathlete in the world one year, avoided injuries, and had a great time.

After retiring from professional racing and pursuing a 'real' career, I continued competing just for kicks on the amateur level, well into my late 30s. I had no goals, structured training programme or logbook. I was just having fun, inspiring my personal training clients, and mixing with the professional athletes that I coached at the time, but I was ranked among the top racers in the world in my age group. Often I would see the 'game faces' worn by others (amateurs as I now was, mind you) on race morning: tense, anxious, snapping at their loved ones, looking like they weren't having much fun.

It's simply no fun to predicate your happiness on whether you reach your goals. Failing to reach your goals will lead to disappointment and dwindling motivation levels – and even reaching your goals can lead to a dead end and a flawed mentality. Many 'winners', in sports and other competitive arenas, such as business, develop a distorted sense of self-worth, leaving them vulnerable to up-and-coming opponents or negligent in behaving themselves in ordinary society because of our twisted hero-worshipping of winners and the wealthy.

There is a phenomenon in endurance sports known as the post-marathon blues (or post-ironman blues for triathletes), which is so common that it's been discussed in psychological journals. It seems that on the occasion of the glorious achievement for which they've trained diligently for months, or even years, many athletes get that 'now what?' feeling that leads to a profound sense of letdown. Ideally, we would use our physical accomplishments as catalysts for continued growth (including perhaps moving on to less extreme fitness pursuits), exploration and challenge, not an excuse to get depressed and pig out on jelly beans in the weeks after the big event.

We must take a close look at the goal-setting process to avoid these common pitfalls and bring a relaxed, fun-first approach to our diet, fitness, body composition, career and other lifestyle pursuits. The primary reason for switching to a Primal Blueprint eating style should be enjoyment – eating foods that taste great, stabilise your energy levels, optimise the function of all the systems in your body, provide long-lasting satisfaction and alleviate the psychological stress of regimentation and deprivation that accompany many diets. Yes, you will look better, become stronger, have more energy, avoid illness, disease and obesity and enjoy other quantifiable results, but these motivators pale in comparison to the instant gratification you get at every single meal from eating the foods that your body was meant to eat.

If you have any psychological stress about your diet, reject it flat out and start eating foods and meals that make you happy, drawing upon the long list of foods and minimal logistical restrictions of the Primal Blueprint eating style. Do whatever you need to do to enjoy your life, including indulging once in a while with a clear conscience and a big smile. If you are not having fun with your current workout regime, junk it and figure out other endeavours that will turn you on. Instead of struggling and suffering to keep pace (with your peppy group exercise instructor or your training partners), adopt the Primal Blueprint suggestions to make your sustained workouts comfortable and energising so they become fun again. Throw in some fun fast stuff occasionally to get you excited about pushing your physical limits and enjoying tangible breakthroughs, including weight loss, more energy and peak performance. Play once in a while. Forget the notion of consistency in this context and align your exercise programme comfortably with your energy level, mood and life responsibilities. Push yourself when you are rested and motivated and rest when you are tired.

When you discard unnecessary goals that are mentally and emotionally stressful, you can focus your attention on process-oriented goals. Goals such as having fun, aligning workout choices with energy levels and tackling new endeavours should define your exercise mentality. That said, great champions have an esteemed ability to blend a process-oriented approach with a strong competitive drive to achieve measurable results. It's certainly okay to aspire to specific results (e.g. losing 10 pounds or completing a 10k, marathon or triathlon), but you must never lose sight of the concept that the rewards come from the chase, not from reaching the finish line.

You can lose 10 pounds very quickly via any number of ill-advised methods (remember that skeletal guy at the Boston Marathon?). The true joy from changing your physique comes not from a surgeon's knife, a brutal calorie-restriction diet coupled with an exhaustive workout routine, nor even accolades from the cocktail party crowd. The most lasting rewards come from the positive, fun lifestyle changes you implemented to make it happen.

It is time for you to accept the grand purpose of the Primal Blueprint and reject other motivators that are confusing, petty or contradictory to your health and well-being. To get more connected with the ideal represented by Grok, we have to pare down, not accumulate. The power and the magic are in the simplicity; a refreshing break from the complexity of modern life, the sordid influence of the ego on your endeavours and emotional state, and the dizzying admonitions on the bookstore shelves that can easily make you feel like a loser if you aren't as tight as the beautiful person on the cover.

Grok did not traffic in any of this nonsense. Granted, he was preoccupied with survival, and we surely don't need to regress to that point to adjust our mentalities. What we *can* do is use the Primal Blueprint laws in our daily lives to become healthier, fitter, happier and more connected with our basic nature as human beings. Make it your goal to honour your genes and your destiny to make the most of your life on earth, without attachment to any outcome.

What are you waiting for? Let's get Primal!

BONUS
MATERIAL

PRIMAL APPROVED – AT A GLANCE

DIET

Beverages: Water (in moderation according to thirst), unsweetened tea.

Coffee/Caffeine: Enjoy in moderation (cream and minimal sweetener okay); don't use as an energy crutch.

Dairy: Enjoy in moderation (only if able to digest comfortably). Raw, fermented, high-fat and organic products (including cheese) are preferred.

Eggs: Organic preferred for high omega 3 content. Yolks especially!

Fats and Oils: Coconut, dark-roasted sesame, first-press extra virgin locally grown olive, hi-oleic sunflower/safflower, marine (supplements), palm, high omega 3 oils (borage, cod-liver, krill, salmon, sunflower seed, hemp seed). Refrigerate and use quickly. Animal fats (chicken fat, lard, tallow), butter and coconut oil are best for cooking.

Fish: Wild-caught from remote, pollution-free waters. Small, oily, cold-water fish are best (anchovies, herring, mackerel, salmon, sardines).

Fruits: Locally grown, organic (or wild) in-season preferred. Berries are premier choice. Go strictly organic with soft, edible skins. Moderate intake of dried fruit and those with higher glycaemic/lower antioxidant values. Wash thoroughly.

Fruit/Vegetable Juice: Fresh-squeezed only, in moderation. Home-juiced with organic produce preferred.

Herbs and Spices: High-antioxidant, anti-inflammatory, immune-supporting, flavour-enhancing.

Indulgences: Dark chocolate (high cocoa content), alcohol sensibly (red wine best choice). If forced under duress to have dessert, select premium-quality, high-fat (low-sugar) options and enjoy guilt-free.

Meat and Poultry: Organic, free-range, grass-fed/grass-finished, hormone-free designation is critical. If you must eat conventional meat, choose the leanest possible cuts and trim excess fat to minimise toxin exposure.

Nuts, Seeds and Their Derivative Butters: High omega 3, nutritious, filling snack. Refrigerate and use butters quickly (cold-processed, organic if available.)

Snacks: Celery with cream cheese or almond butter, cottage cheese with nut or fruit topping, canned tuna or sardines, berries, hard-boiled eggs, nuts, seeds, olives, trail mix and other high-fat and/or high-protein, low-carbohydrate Primal foods.

Starchy Tuber Vegetables: Enjoy yams and sweet potatoes (instead of white or brown potatoes) in moderation. Good choice for athletes needing extra carbohydrates.

Supplements: Multivitamin/mineral/antioxidant formula, omega 3 fish oil capsules, probiotics, protein powder. Choose premium quality to supplement healthy diet.

Vegetables: Locally grown, organic, in-season preferred. Go strictly organic for large surface area (leafy greens) and soft, edible skins (peppers). Wash thoroughly.

Wild Rice: Enjoy in moderation (instead of white or brown rice).

EXERCISE

Low-Level Cardio: Two to five hours (or more) per week of walking, hiking or other exercise at 55 to 75 per cent of maximum heart rate.

Schedule: Vary workout type, frequency, intensity and duration, always aligned with energy levels. Make it fun!

Shoes: Gradually introduce some barefoot time (in low-risk activities) to strengthen feet and simulate natural range of motion. Choose shoes with minimalist design (Vibram, Nike Free) to prevent cuts and other injuries. Ease into it!

Sprinting: All-out efforts lasting 8 to 60 seconds. Total workout duration under 20 minutes. Conduct every 7 to 10 days when fully energised.

Strength Training: Brief, intense sessions, always under an hour, and often just 7 to 30 minutes. Full-body, functional exercises that promote balanced 'Primal Fitness.'

Stretching: Full-body, functional stretches to transition from active to inactive: *Grok Hang* and *Grok Squat*.

LIFESTYLE/MEDICAL CARE

Medical: Medication and invasive care for serious or acute conditions. If you are on prescription medication, combine with aggressive lifestyle modification in pursuit of drug-free health. Request additional blood tests for CRP, Lp2A, A1C, fasting blood insulin levels and vitamin D.

Play: Change attitude – it's not just for kids! Enjoy daily, outdoor physical fun to enhance work productivity and manage stress.

Sleep: Consistent bed and wake times, calm evening transition, 'empty room' environment, and sensible evening eating. Strive to awaken naturally without alarm. Take 20-minute power naps when necessary.

Stupid Mistakes: Cultivate hyper-vigilance and risk-management skills (e.g. 'green light = look around, confirm it's clear *and only then proceed*' mentality).

Sunlight: After adequate exposure (for vitamin-D), use clothing (or approved sunblock) to protect from burning.

Use Your Brain: Engage in fun, creative intellectual pursuits to stay sharp and enthusiastic for all of life's challenges.

PRIMAL AVOID – AT A GLANCE

DIET

Beverages: Avoid sweetened 'energy drinks' (Red Bull, etc.) and 'teas' (Snapple, Arizona, etc.), soft drinks, powdered drinks and performance drinks used outside of workouts (Gatorade, etc.).

Coffee/Caffeine: Avoid excessive use or use as energy crutch in place of adequate sleep and healthy lifestyle habits.

Dairy: Limit or avoid GMO or conventional products due to hormone, pesticide, antibiotic, allergenic and immune-suppressing agents.

Eggs: Limit eggs from chickens commercially raised in cages and fed with grains, hormone, pesticides and antibiotics. Go organic first!

Fats and Oils: Avoid all trans and partially hydrogenated, canola, cottonseed, corn, soybean, all other high polyunsaturated (safflower, sunflower, etc.) oils, margarine, vegetable shortening and deep-fried foods.

Fast Food: Avoid chemically treated, deep-fried, insulin-stimulating fare that is devoid of nutritional value: French fries, onion rings, burgers, hot dogs, chimichangas, chalupas and all the rest.

Fish: Avoid fish from farms, polluted waters or from the top of the marine food chain (shark, sword and others that might have more concentrated levels of contaminants).

Fruits: Limit or avoid GMO, remote grown, or conventionally grown with soft, edible skins. Find local or organic alternatives.

Fruit/Vegetable Juice: Avoid juices with added sugar or that are heat processed, or come from pesticide-laden produce. Limit total consumption, even for good juice.

Grains: Avoid wheat, rice, corn, oats, cereals, breads, pasta, muffins, rolls, waffles, pancakes, croissants, baguettes, crackers, doughnuts, swirls, Danishes, tortillas, pizza, other grains (barley, millet, rye, quinoa, amaranth, etc.), and other baked or processed high-carbohydrate foods. Even avoid whole grains due to higher levels of objectionable phytates, lectins and gluten. Everyone is allergic to grains at some level!

Indulgences: Avoid high-carbohydrate (sugar or flour based), heavily processed treats: biscuits, cakes, pies, brownies, sweets, ice cream, doughnuts, iced lollies and other frozen desserts.

Legumes: Limit or avoid alfalfa, beans, peanuts, peas, lentils and soybeans due to high insulin response and lectin content.

Meat and Poultry: Limit or avoid commercially grown, grain-fed ranch animals (with concentrated hormones, pesticides and antibiotics). Limit or avoid smoked, cured or nitrate-treated meats (hot dogs, salami, etc.).

Processed Foods: If it comes in a box or a wrapper, think twice!

Snacks: 'Energy' bars, granola bars, pretzels, crisps, puffed snacks (Cheetos, Goldfish, popcorn, rice cakes, etc.) and all other grain-based snacks.

Sugar, Soda, and Grains: The less you consume, the less you'll want! Get off the 'high-low, high-low' carbohydrate-insulin-stress response cycle to regulate your energy and improve your health.

Supplements: Avoid cheap, bulk-produced vitamins and supplements with additives, fillers, binders, lubricants, extruding agents and other synthetic chemicals.

Vegetables: Limit or avoid GMO, remote grown or conventionally grown with large surface areas or edible skins (leafy greens, peppers).

EXERCISE

Chronic Cardio: Avoid a consistent schedule of sustained cardio workouts at medium to high intensity (above 75 per cent of maximum heart rate). Occasional sustained hard efforts are okay; allow for sufficient recovery.

Chronic Strength Training: Avoid prolonged, repetitive workouts conducted too frequently (e.g. hour-plus sessions featuring exhausting, non-functional, isolation exercise sets).

Schedule: Avoid consistent workout type, frequency, intensity and duration (compromises health, energy and motivation levels).

Stretching: Avoid stretching 'cold' muscles, prolonged sessions (either before or after exercise), or isolated muscle group stretches, except by professional recommendation for injuries/imbalances.

LIFESTYLE/MEDICAL CARE

Medical: Limit or avoid prescription medication for minor health problems easily corrected by lifestyle changes. Reframe 'fix it' mentality into a 'prevention' mentality.

Sleep: Don't burn the candle at both ends. Avoid excessive evening digital stimulation, morning alarms after insufficient sleep, or fighting off a much-needed nap with caffeine.

Stupid Mistakes: Avoid multi-tasking, zoning out or trusting that the world will keep you safe (e.g. *'Green light = Go!'* mentality). Don't blame others for your stupid mistakes.

I've taken advantage of the infinite capacity of the Internet to augment the Primal Blueprint with continually updated supporting material to make this not just a book but a starting point for a complete life-style movement. I encourage you to visit MarksDailyApple.com and explore our conveniently organised appendices, featuring Primal Blueprint text references and suggested reading, extensive Q&A with deeper insights about book content, and detailed strength and sprinting workout suggestions, not to mention daily diet and fitness insights, recipes, videos and more, 'with a side of irreverence' at MarksDailyApple.com. Following are *The Primal Blueprint*-related categories published at MarksDailyApple.com when this book went to print.

INTERNET APPENDICES

Primal Blueprint Text References, Resources and Suggested Reading
Primal Blueprint Q&A: Everything You Always Wanted to Ask ... but Were Afraid to Know

All About Grok
Dispute About Recent Human Evolution
Details About Genes Directing Cellular Function
Reconciling Evolutionary Rationale with Religious Beliefs
Grok and Korg Nicknames
Diet
Differing Scientific Conclusions
Insulin-Balanced Meals
Fibre
Diet Sodas
Exercise
Compliance for Low Body-Fat Athletes
Cortisol
Natural vs. Synthetic Human Growth Hormone and Testosterone
Lifestyle

ENDNOTES

INTRODUCTION ENDNOTES

1   *Physiology of Sport and Exercise*, by Dr David Costill and Jack Wilmore.
2   The Central Intelligence Agency's World Factbook reports that the 2008 US overall life expectancy at birth is 78 (75 for males; 81 for females).
3   The 2008 American Heart Association 'Heart Disease and Stroke Statistics', available for download at americanheart.org, reported that, in 2004, 869,000 deaths were attributed to heart disease and 550,000 to cancer. 2005 CDC stats indicate the percentage references, but recent headlines suggest cancer has surpassed heart disease as the number one killer. (cdc.gov/nchs/data/nvsr/nvsr56/nvsr56_10.pdf)

CHAPTER 1 ENDNOTES

1   **Origin of Man**: The 'out of Africa' theory is also known as the Recent Single-Origin Hypothesis (RSOH), Replacement Hypothesis, or Recent African Origin (RAO) model. The theory, originally proposed by Charles Darwin in his *Descent of Man*, modernised by Christopher Stringer and Peter Andrews and strongly supported by recent studies of mitochondrial DNA, says that anatomically modern humans evolved solely in Africa between 200,000 (first appearance of anatomically modern humans) and 100,000 years ago, with members leaving Africa 60,000 years ago and replacing all earlier human populations, including *Homo neanderthalensis* and *Homo erectus*.

2   **Origin of Agriculture**: Dr Jared Diamond, evolutionary biologist, physiologist and Pulitzer Prize-winning professor of geography at UCLA, is the author of *Guns, Germs and Steel: The Fates of Human Societies*, which discusses the advent of agriculture and its effects on civilisation and human health. Chapter 5 of *Guns, Germs and Steel* details agriculture's origin (including which crops were cultivated) in several locations around the globe.

   The Emergence of Agriculture by Bruce Smith details the great transition of humanity from a hunter-gatherer lifestyle to agriculture and thus to civilisation. *Guns, Germs and Steel* and Richard Manning's *Against the Grain* detail the negative aspects of humankind's shift to agriculture, blaming it for large-scale disease, imperialism, colonialism, slavery and an inexorable progression to global warfare. All this thanks to the abuse of 'free time' resulting from the specialisation of labour and the pursuit of power – over resources, humans and geography – goals that were previously irrelevant in the largely egalitarian hunter-gatherer societies.

3   **Primal Human Life Span:** The estimate of 'maximum lifespan potential' from *Homo sapiens* 15,000 years ago of 94 is actually higher than the corresponding figure attached to modern humans of 91! This material comes from the work of Dr Richard G. Cutler, molecular gerontologist and longevity expert, who has produced more than 100 papers on the subject. Dr Cutler was a research chemist at the Gerontology Research Center at the National Institute on Aging, National Institutes of Health for 19 years. Dr Cutler's estimate is derived from laboratory analysis of skeletal material, with particular emphasis on the ratio of body weight to brain size. Other factors involved in making accurate life span calculations are age of sexual maturation to life span ratio (a 5:1 ratio is common among humans) and rates of caloric intake and expenditure.

4   **Grok:** In Chapter 2 we talk about Grok as the patriarch of a primal family. However, in the interest of political correctness and ease of reading, you can view Grok as a not-necessarily gender-specific euphemism for primal ancestor(s) whom we aspire to emulate in lifestyle behaviours. For example, 'Grok never ate sugar, and neither should you.'

CHAPTER 2 ENDNOTES
Grok Family References

1   **Life Expectancy:** According to Wikipedia, life expectancy during the Paleolithic era (2.5 million years ago to 10,000 BC) was around 33 years, factoring in the high rates of infant mortality. If Grok reached puberty, life expectancy increased up to age 39 and if he reached 39, he could expect to live until 54. And this was a ripped, energetic 54, not a guy struggling to hang on. The fatal hazards that befell Grok during his lifetime were entirely primitive: infections, accidents and predators – not heart disease, diabetes or obesity.

The advent of agriculture and civilisation caused life expectancy to drop significantly, reaching a low of 18 years during the Bronze Age of 3,300 BC to 1,200 BC . Life expectancy remained low (between 20 and 30) through AD1500 and then climbed only gradually, reaching 30 in 1800 and 40–50 in 1900 in the USA and Europe. The past century has seen a dramatic increase in lifespan in civilised countries, thanks mainly to medical advances that limit infant mortality and protect against disease plagues.

A 2004 study published by Rachel Caspari at the University of Michigan and Sang-Hee Lee at the University of California at Riverside revealed that a dramatic increase in human longevity that took place during the early Upper Paleolithic Period, around 30,000 years ago. The scientists studied dental information derived from molar wear patterns of *Australopithecines*, *Homo erectus* and *Neanderthals* and discovered a five-fold increase in the number of individuals surviving to an older age (defined by doubling reproductive age – so humans could become grandparents) around that time period.

The scientists speculated that 'this trend contributed importantly to population expansions and cultural innovations that are associated with modernity.' Elders could pass on critical life knowledge to younger generations, social networks and family bonds were strengthened and Grok could generally become a better parent by living longer.

'There has been a lot of speculation about what gave modern humans their evolutionary advantage,' Caspari said. 'This research provides a simple explanation for which there is now concrete evidence: modern humans were older and wiser.'

2   **Cold Water Benefits:** The healing properties of water have been recognised for thousands of years. Public baths were a common feature in ancient civilisations. The Romans, Greeks, Egyptians, Turkish, Japanese and Chinese all believed water was helpful for muscle recovery, sleep and immune protection. In the early 1800s Vincent Priessnitz, an Austrian farmer, pioneered the use of hydrotherapy as a medical tool. During the mid to late 1800s, a Bavarian monk named Father Sebastian Kneipp gained wide recognition for his water therapy work. He cured himself of pulmonary tuberculosis (a common and typically fatal condition referred to then as 'consumption') by regularly plunging into the icy Danube River to stimulate his immune system. Kneipp wrote extensively on the subject of hydrotherapy and other natural healing topics, gaining such notoriety that he attracted people from across the world to visit his clinic.

Several studies support the historical anecdotes that cold water offers health benefits. One study conducted by the Thrombosis Research Institute at London's Brompton Hospital found that exposure to cold baths boosted sex hormone production, and improved fertility, chronic fatigue conditions, immune function and blood circulation – reducing cardiovascular disease risk. Numerous studies indicate that the invigorating effect of cold water stimulates the release of endorphins by the autonomic nervous system. Anyone who has taken a plunge and emerged energised can attest to the powerful effects of cold water on the body.

3   **Napping:** Data from the National Sleep Foundation suggests that 'a well-timed afternoon nap may be the best way to combat sleepiness.'

Gregory Belenky, MD, Research Professor and Director of the Sleep and Performance Research Center at Washington State University, says naps can help make up for insufficient sleep and that 'it's even possible that divided sleep is more recuperative than sleep taken in a single block,' noting how popular the afternoon siesta is in countries across the world. Dr Mark Rosekind's studies with NASA pilots indicated that napping pilots had a 34 per cent increase in performance and 54 per cent boost in alertness that lasted for 2–3 hours. Harvard University studies show that 60–90 minute naps help the brain integrate new knowledge similar to night-time sleep. A study published in the research journal *Sleep* suggests that naps ranging from 10 to 30 minutes are optimal for improved cognitive performance and alertness. The Center for Applied Cognitive Studies says that 'the length of sleep is not what causes us to be refreshed upon waking. The key factor is the number of complete sleep cycles we enjoy. Each sleep cycle contains five distinct phases, which exhibit different brainwave patterns.' Leading sleep researcher Dr Claudio Stampi found that naps taken in the afternoon (a common low-energy period in our circadian rhythms) were comparatively higher in the most restorative slow-wave sleep. During a 10–20 minute afternoon nap, your brain cells reset their sodium and potassium ratios, which are thrown out of balance after long periods of intense brain arousal, as in a typical busy day. 'This is the main cause of what is known as "mental fatigue,"' the Center says about this nutrient imbalance. 'A brief period in Theta (slow-wave sleep) can restore the ratio to normal, resulting in mental refreshment.'

4 **Quality Time:** The Office of National Statistics 'Time Use Survey' study indicates that today's average working parent spends 19 minutes of digital distraction-free quality time per week.

Korg Family References

5 **Commuting:** The Public Policy Institute of California reports that 18 per cent of Californians commute over 45 minutes each way, while 3.4 million Americans commute 90 minutes or more each way. The US Census reports that the average commute time nationwide is 25.5 minutes each way, with Californians commuting 10 per cent longer than the national average. Tracy, CA, near the Korg's home of Stockton, had one of the longest average commute times in the state in 2000: 42 minutes each way.

In a United Kingdom survey of over 400 people, performed by the International Stress Management Association, 44 per cent said that rush-hour traffic was the most stressful part of their lives. A Hewlett Packard study of UK commuters found that blood pressure and heart rate were 'higher than those experienced by fighter pilots going into combat and police officers facing rioting mobs'.

A study by researchers at the New York University Sleep Disorder Center found that 'long commuters' (those who travel one hour and 15 minutes or longer) have more sleep disorders and other health problems than the general population. There is also a significant danger of multi-tasking while commuting. The Harvard Center for Risk Analysis found drivers using cell phones are responsible for 2,600 traffic deaths per year and 330,000 traffic injuries (motorists on the road make 40 per cent of all cellular telephone calls).

6 **Digital Media Disturbing Sleep:** Daniel Reid's *The Tao of Health, Sex and Longevity* details how television disturbs the ocular-endocrine system.

A US study showed that rats exposed to invisible television rays (screen was blackened) for six hours per day became hyperactive and extremely aggressive for about a week, then suddenly become totally lethargic and stopped breeding entirely. A Columbia University Study conducted in New York suggests that 'watching late-night television may put people in a state of heightened alertness and physiological arousal, preventing them from falling asleep with ease. In addition, being exposed to many hours of the bright light of the television screen may throw people off their sleep-wake cycle, while too little physical activity may cause people to become restless and struggle with sleep.' A Rhode Island study published in the *Journal of American Academy of Pediatrics* suggests children's sleep is disturbed by watching TV before bedtime – causing them to become 'over-stimulated, disturbed or frightened by the content of programmes … particularly those containing violence.'

7 **Sleep Medication:** Thirty million people in the USA take sleep medications (*American Academy of SleepMedicine*), an estimated 50 per cent jump since 2000. With an ode to the 'over x billion served' signs adorning McDonald's franchises, Sanofi-Aventis, maker of Ambien, boasts an aggregate total of 12 billion nights of patient use worldwide – $2 billion was spent on the drug worldwide in 2004. According to *Live Science*, global sales for sleeping pills are estimated at $5 billion annually.

Daniel Kripke, UC San Diego psychiatry professor and author of *The Dark Side of Sleeping Pills*, conducted a revealing six-year sleep study with over one million adults. Kripke reported that the health risk of taking sleeping pills daily was not much different from the risk of smoking a pack of cigarettes a day! A study by researchers at Beth Israel Deaconess Medical Center and Harvard Medical School found that treating insomnia with habit and attitude modification was more effective – both immediately and over the long term – than using Ambien. The sleep success techniques Kripke recommends include: don't go to bed until you're sleepy, get up at the same time each morning, avoid excessive stimulation or worry before bed, avoid caffeine for six hours before bed, avoid alcohol before bed and spend adequate time outdoors.

8   **Teenage Sleep**: A 2007 Mayo Clinic article suggests that teenagers require about nine hours of sleep to maintain optimal daytime alertness, but few actually get that much sleep due to jobs, homework, friends, digital media and other distractions (the National Sleep Foundation reports that 25 per cent of teens report sleeping 6.5 hours per night or less). 'Puberty changes a teen's internal clock, delaying the time he or she starts feeling sleepy until 11pm or later (before adolescence, circadian rhythms direct most children to naturally fall asleep around 8 or 9pm).' Staying up late to study or socialise can disrupt a teen's internal clock even more.

The article also notes that sleeping in or forcing an early bedtime are not adequate solutions, since they are not aligned with the teen's unique circadian rhythm. The Mayo Clinic staff suggests that you darken rooms at desired bedtime and expose teens to bright light in the morning, discourage naps longer than 30 minutes, discourage caffeine use and establish a consistent, quiet relaxing routine before bed – free of digital media.

9   **Artificial sweeteners:** An online review mentioned by Dr John Briffa indicates that '100 per cent of industry-funded studies proclaim aspartame to be benign; more than 90 per cent of independent studies and reports in the scientific literature say otherwise.' Numerous studies suggest that intense artificial sweeteners increase appetite for sweet foods, promote overeating and may even lead to weight gain. One study with rats from Purdue University concluded that 'consuming a food sweetened with no-calorie saccharin can lead to greater body-weight gain and adiposity than would consuming the same food sweetened with higher calorie sugar.' However, there are some other studies that refute the concept entirely. Perhaps the most relevant evidence is how obesity rates continue to climb even with the advent and increased used of artificial sweeteners in the modern diet.

10 **Cardiovascular exercise heart rates**: My position that Chronic Cardio is harmful and that low-level aerobic work is beneficial is based on personal experience over three decades as an elite athlete, personal trainer to clients of all ability levels and coach to elite professional triathletes. The extensive work of legendary coach Arthur Lydiard is a major influence as well. Lydiard, who pioneered the concept of overdistance endurance training for track and field athletes, developed numerous Olympic gold medallists and world record holders in his home country of New Zealand and for various other national teams. Elite athlete/authors including former professional triathletes Mark Allen (*Total Triathlete*) and Brad Kearns (*Breakthrough Triathlon Training*), former Olympic marathon runner and

popular author and speaker Jeff Galloway, and Joe Friel's popular series of 'Training Bibles' for various endurance sports all echo these fundamental principles of endurance training:

Building a base of comfortable aerobic activity is critical for success.

High-intensity exercise should be strictly limited as a small percentage of total exercise volume and conducted only when a sufficient aerobic base is present. Conversely, the American College of Sports Medicine recommends exercise intensities of 55–90 per cent of maximum heart rate, a ridiculously disparate range that stimulates vastly different metabolic responses in the body. Sadly, this information is widely circulated by health clubs, personal trainers, group exercise programmes, books and magazines to the detriment of the average fitness enthusiasts. Exceeding 75 per cent of maximum heart rate regularly (particularly for a non-elite athlete) will greatly inhibit the development of a strong aerobic base and invite increased risk of injury and burnout. Your cardio exercise range should be 55–75 per cent of maximum heart rate, with occasional high-intensity sessions where heart rate approaches maximum during short sprints.

11 **Statin Side Effects**: A Columbia University Study published in *The Archives of Neurology* suggests that even short-term statin use depletes CoQ10 levels, a possible explanation for common statin side effects of exercise intolerance, muscle pain, and other indicators of muscle dysfunction.

The conventional wisdom connection between cholesterol levels and disease risk (and thus the popularity of cholesterol-reducing statins) is increasingly being called into question. Seventeen studies on lowering dietary cholesterol were assessed in a 2005 *Annals of Internal Medicine* article. Overall, the studies led to an average 10 per cent decrease in cholesterol levels, but there was no decrease in overall risk of death. A long-term study published in the *New England Journal of Medicine* (in 1986, 1987 and 1991) showed that people who are taking multiple cardiac medications have a 40 per cent higher risk of mortality after four years than those who take nothing. Several other large studies (10,000 men in Europe, published in the *European Heart Journal*, 1986; 61,000 men in Europe, conducted by the World Health Organization and published in the *Lancet*; 12,000 men in America, published in the *Journal of the American Medical Association*; and a study in Finland published in *the Journal of the American Medical Association*, 1991) reported the same conclusion – medication either increased mortality or didn't increase survival time.

12 **Walking To School**: CDC indicates that the percentage of children who live within a mile of school and who walk or cycle to school as their primary means of transportation has declined almost 25 per cent over the past 30 years (from 87 per cent to 63 per cent) and that children who walk

or cycle from any distance has declined 26 per cent (from 42 per cent to 16 per cent).

13 **Poor compliance** with doctor-prescribed exercise programmes is a major reason for the widespread condition of lower back pain, poor recovery from surgery and prolonged elevated risk factors for heart disease and cancer.

A 1998 *Journal of the American Medical Association* article noted that even when it comes to taking medication, the average compliance rate is only 50 per cent. An article from *AlignMap – Beyond Patient Compliance*, further suggests that 'noncompliance is underreported, typically hidden, and rarely detected by clinicians', and 'research studies consistently reveal high levels of inadequate adherence to treatment recommendations throughout the healthcare spectrum, including cases of life-threatening illnesses. The indisputable conclusions are that medical noncompliance is, by any measure and from any perspective, pervasive, and that health-care's failure to successfully address such a problem comes at the cost of diminished outcomes, unnecessary expense, and avoidable patient morbidity and mortality.'

One Canadian study of heart attack victims published in the *Canadian Medical Association Journal* indicated a 43 per cent noncompliance rate with rehabilitation and treatment recommendations. A Texas study of bariatric surgery patients revealed a noncompliance rate of 41 per cent (female) and 37 per cent (male).

14 **Caffeine**: The average American uses about 230 milligrams of caffeine per day according to the Mayo Clinic. Side effects of consuming too much caffeine vary by individual (based on body weight, levels of physical and psychological stress and other drug use – according to MayoClinic.com), but can include 'increased heart rate and urination, anxiety, headaches, nausea and insomnia', according to the online medical encyclopedia provided by the US National Library of Medicine and the National Institutes of Health. The Mayo Clinic calls caffeine the 'most popular behaviour-altering drug', with nine of out ten Americans consuming some type of caffeine regularly.

15 **Family Finances**: A 2003 book by Elizabeth Warren and Amelia Warren Tyagi called *The Two Income Trap: Why Middle Class Mothers and Fathers Are Going Broke*, details the financial challenges faced even by working families who enjoy income levels far higher (even adjusting for today's dollars) than previous generations. While many point to the '*Affluenza*' mentality (the widespread cultural ill of excessive consumption habits detailed in John De Graaf's book of the same name) for the middle class's financial challenges, the authors make the convincing case that the larger,

less optional expenses are the biggest culprit. Expenses for childcare, car payments, college tuition and particularly surburban homes result in millions living in financial distress. Homes sold to families with children skyrocketed 79 per cent in inflation-adjusted dollars from 1983 to 1998. The two-income couple (comprising some three-quarters of all married couples) is a key component of the skyrocketing inflation of suburban home prices over the past 25 years. Hence a vicious circle emerges: home prices rise because many two-income couples can afford them … because they have two incomes! This sounds like 'keeping up with the Joneses' times fifty million.

The *New York Times*, in 2003, revealed that a 'typical household' (two income earners and one or two children – a demographic responsible for half the nation's personal consumption expenditures) making $60,000–80,000 per year spends 70 to 75 per cent of their take-home pay on essentials such as home costs, food shopping, vehicles and fuel, education and health care. The authors of *The Two Income Trap* point out that the figure for these expenses was only 54 per cent in the early 1970s. Furthermore, the remaining 25 per cent of disposable income, typically categorised as 'discretionary', is further eaten up by expenses that might be better defined as 'essential' due to social pressures and norms: cell phones, cable or satellite TV, Internet service, high-definition TV sets, digital entertainment such as iPods. Arguably the category could extend to fashion, cosmetics and popular diversions such as movies and vacations.

16 **Childhood Obesity:** The CDC reports that nine million kids ages 6–19 are overweight or obese, and that 33 per cent eat fast food every day (American Academy of Pediatrics). The prevalence of children (ages 6–11) who are overweight has increased from about 4 per cent in the 1960s to almost 19 per cent in 2004 (Dr Richard Troiano and Dr Cynthia Ogden.)

17 **Children Recreation:** Dr Sandra Hofferth and colleagues report that the way children spend their discretionary time has changed – less time is spent in unstructured activities (e.g. free play) and more time is spent in structured activities (e.g. sports and youth programmes). Other changes of interest include a doubling of computer use.

18 **Massive Multiplayer Online Role-Playing Games:** The popularity has skyrocketed from zero in 1998 (due to poor graphics quality, slow Internet connections, and a consequent lack of interest) to an estimated 30–60 million active users in 2007, according to a Giga Omni Media article. Some consider this a vast underestimate, due to millions of Chinese playing in Internet cafés for four cents per hour but not registering as paid monthly subscribers. *World of Warcraft* (8.5 million users), *Hobbo*

Hotel (7.5 million) and *Runescape* (5 million) are the leading games. Pre-teen games *Club Penguin* (4 million) and *Webkinz* (3.8 million) are also extremely popular. A survey published on Adpoll.com indicated that 45 per cent of kids play for 10 or more hours per week.

19 **ADHD Prescriptions**: Diagnosis rates of Attention Deficit Hyperactivity Disorder (ADHD) have skyrocketed 500 per cent since 1991, according to the Drug Enforcement Administration. An estimated seven million schoolchildren are being treated with stimulants for ADHD, including 10 per cent of all 10-year-old American boys, according to an article published in the *Journal of the American Medical Association*.

A 1998 study by researchers Adrian Angold and E. Jane Costello found that the majority of children and adolescents who receive stimulants for ADHD do not fully meet the criteria for ADHD. The efforts of neurologist Dr Fred Baughman, ADHD diagnosis critic, led to admissions from the FDA, DEA, Novartis (manufacturers of Ritalin) and top ADHD researchers around the country that '*no objective validation of the diagnosis of ADHD exists.*' A Maryland Department of Education study found that white, suburban elementary school children are using medication for ADHD at more than twice the rate of African American students.

20 **Life Expectancy of Today's Child:** A 2005 report published in the *New England Journal of Medicine* suggests that the prevalence of obesity is shortening average lifespan by a greater rate than accidents, homicides and suicides combined. Children today will lose some two to five years of life expectancy due to the prevalence, and earlier onset, of obesity-related diseases such as type 2 diabetes, heart disease, kidney failure and cancer.

Dr David S. Ludwig, director of the obesity programme at the Children's Hospital in Boston, said in the report, 'Obesity is such that this generation of children could be the first basically in the history of the United States to live less healthful and shorter lives than their parents. There is an unprecedented increase in prevalence of obesity at younger and younger ages without much obvious public health impact. But when they start developing heart attack, stroke, kidney failures, amputations, blindness and ultimately death at younger ages, then that could be a huge effect on life expectancy.'

21 **American Television:** A. C. Neilsen reports that the average American watches 28 hours of TV per week and that 66 per cent of households have three or more televisions at home (A. C. Nielsen Co.). Dr Donald Roberts and colleagues and Victoria Rideout and colleagues with the Kaiser Family Foundation report that children between the ages of eight and 18 years spend an average of nearly 6.5 hours a day with electronic media.

INDEX